For Dummies
BESTSELLING BOOK SERIES

Mind-Body Fitness
For Dummies®

Cheat Sheet

W9-CMI-748

Basic Mind-Body Movements for Everyday

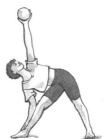

Triangle (Chi Ball)

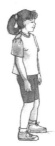

Standing Makes Perfect (Qigong)

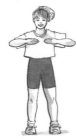

Standing Like a Tree (Qigong)

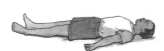

Corpse Posture (Yoga)

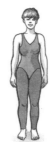

Mountain Posture (Yoga)

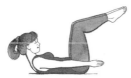

Hundreds (Pilates)

Centering Step (Tai Chi)

Hold Balloon (Tai Chi)

Three Keys to Successful Mind-Body Fitness

1. **Be mindful:** Use your mind in a meditative and inwardly focused manner during postures, movements, and exercises.
2. **Breathe:** Exhale and inhale fully as you do the movements. Breathe while holding positions, too.
3. **Move:** Use your muscles in some way, even lightly.

For Dummies™: Bestselling Book Series for Beginners

Mind-Body Fitness For Dummies®

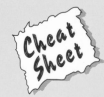
Cheat Sheet

Seven Basic Principles

1. **Turn off your gray matter:** Mind-body workouts are about the process not the goal. So don't analyze, time, judge, or critique yourself. Just feel the way your body moves.

2. **Breathe:** Keep the oxygen moving in and out of your body. Breathing helps you stay focused, keeps your muscles relaxed, and generally rejuvenates your mind and body.

3. **Relax:** Avoid tensing and clenching muscles, hands, toes, jaws, eyes — you name it. Remind yourself to release and let your body move.

4. **Warm up and cool down:** Use a couple of minutes not only to get your muscles ready, but also to get your mind ready for the challenges ahead. Same after you're done: Ease both your body and mind back into your daily life.

5. **Perfect your posture:** Stand tall with your chest open, neck long, and spine straight without tucking your pelvis under or letting it sway backward. Some methods advocate letting your belly be loose and relaxed, and not pulled-in tight, others want you to use the belly more. Either way, a relaxed belly doesn't mean sagging shoulders and a swayback.

6. **Find your power center:** Your center, somewhere around your belly button, is your power core. Use your core for strong movements, strong breathing, and strong meditation.

7. **Let your energy flow:** Try to breathe and release any blocks. Imagine a freely flowing stream circulating through your body. Let that energy move you.

Breathing Basics

A full inhalation moves all the way down your abdomen and inflates your belly a little without causing your chest to move much at all. Points to remember about breathing as you do your mind-body workouts:

✔ **Breathe consciously:** Breathing may be involuntary, but you can block it, stop it, and make it jerky, choppy, or uneven. Try to keep your breathing relaxed and flowing.

✔ **Breathe fully:** Let the breath move the full length of your torso, not just to your chest.

✔ **Breathe with the movement:** The hardest part is keeping your breath moving fully and freely *while* you're moving. Be conscious about applying this basic to get all the mind-body benefits.

Be Neutral, O Spine o' Mine

To keep your posture perfect and your breath moving freely, keep your spine neutral. That means practicing keeping your pelvis aligned — not tipped too far forward or backward. To find your neutral spine:

1. Place your palms on your belly with your fingers pointing down and the base of your palms on your hip bones. Your hands should be perpendicular to the floor.

2. Tip your pelvis forward or back to bring your hands perpendicular to the ground if you need to. You are now neutral.

3. Remember how the neutral position feels and practice it all day long.

Copyright © 2001 IDG Books Worldwide, Inc. All rights reserved.

Cheat Sheet $2.95 value. Item 5304-6.

For more information about IDG Books, call 1-800-762-2974.

For Dummies™: Bestselling Book Series for Beginners

Praise for Mind-Body Fitness For Dummies

"Record numbers of Americans are turning to mind-body workouts such as Yoga, Tai Chi, and Pilates. This comprehensive guide offers the tools and information you need to recap the numerous benefits of these timeless techniques."

— Ken Germano, American Council on Exercise (ACE)

"At a time when IDEA surveys show rising popularity for Yoga, Pilates-based exercises, and other mind-body activities, this book is a clear guide on how to take advantage of these programs. *Mind-Body Fitness For Dummies* is an important contribution in making these exercises more accessible to everyone."

— Kathie Davis, Executive Director of IDEA,
The Health & Fitness Source

"It's challenging to present a complex topic like mind-body fitness with the clarity so helpful to the novice and the sophistication which informs the initiated. Therese Iknoian does so with wit and knowledge."

— Judith Hanson Lasater, Ph.D., physical therapist, and author of *Relax and Renew: Restful Yoga for Stressful Times* and *Living Your Yoga: Finding the Spiritual in Everyday Life*

"*Mind-Body Fitness For Dummies* is terrific. Finally we have a book on mind-body exercise which puts it all together in one neat package. This book gives you the definitions and background information on a whole gamut of mind-body techniques along with plenty of user-friendly exercises — all described in down-to-earth language which is filled with humor and inspiration. A must-have book for all fitness professionals and for those looking for real meaning to their movements."

— Mara Carrico, owner of Yoga Lady®, INK, and author of *Yoga Journal's Yoga Basics*

"To all my friends who have wondered what was the difference between Yoga, T'ai Chi, Pilates, and the rest; and to all my students who have begged for more information about how their T'ai Chi practice could be good exercise ("when it just felt like gentle fun") — at last I have a good book to recommend! Therese has just the right touch, the right balance between the east and the west, between traditional wisdom and the modern science. I think this is a book both beginners and Mind/Body purists can get their fingers around."

— David-Dorian Ross, a.k.a. Dr. T'ai Chi, well-known and respected instructor

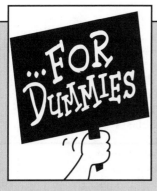
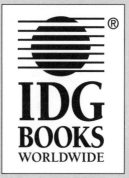

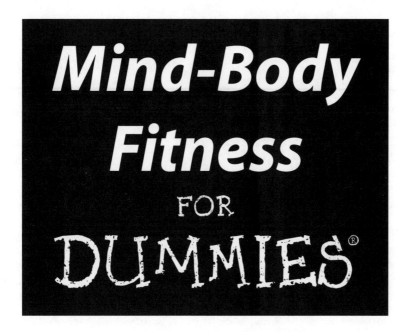

Mind-Body Fitness FOR DUMMIES®

by Therese Iknoian

Foreword by Ralph La Forge

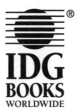

IDG BOOKS WORLDWIDE

IDG Books Worldwide, Inc.
An International Data Group Company

Foster City, CA ◆ Chicago, IL ◆ Indianapolis, IN ◆ New York, NY

Mind-Body Fitness For Dummies®

Published by
IDG Books Worldwide, Inc.
An International Data Group Company
919 E. Hillsdale Blvd.
Suite 400
Foster City, CA 94404
www.idgbooks.com (IDG Books Worldwide Web Site)
www.dummies.com (Dummies Press Web Site)

Library of Congress Control Number: 00-109399

ISBN: 0-7645-5304-6

Printed in the United States of America

10 9 8 7 6 5 4 3 2 1

1O/QR/RR/QQ/IN

Distributed in the United States by IDG Books Worldwide, Inc.

Distributed by CDG Books Canada Inc. for Canada; by Transworld Publishers Limited in the United Kingdom; by IDG Norge Books for Norway; by IDG Sweden Books for Sweden; by IDG Books Australia Publishing Corporation Pty. Ltd. for Australia and New Zealand; by TransQuest Publishers Pte Ltd. for Singapore, Malaysia, Thailand, Indonesia, and Hong Kong; by Gotop Information Inc. for Taiwan; by ICG Muse, Inc. for Japan; by Intersoft for South Africa; by Eyrolles for France; by International Thomson Publishing for Germany, Austria and Switzerland; by Distribuidora Cuspide for Argentina; by LR International for Brazil; by Galileo Libros for Chile; by Ediciones ZETA S.C.R. Ltda. for Peru; by WS Computer Publishing Corporation, Inc., for the Philippines; by Contemporanea de Ediciones for Venezuela; by Express Computer Distributors for the Caribbean and West Indies; by Micronesia Media Distributor, Inc. for Micronesia; by Chips Computadoras S.A. de C.V. for Mexico; by Editorial Norma de Panama S.A. for Panama; by American Bookshops for Finland.

For general information on IDG Books Worldwide's books in the U.S., please call our Consumer Customer Service department at 800-762-2974. For reseller information, including discounts and premium sales, please call our Reseller Customer Service department at 800-434-3422.

For information on where to purchase IDG Books Worldwide's books outside the U.S., please contact our International Sales department at 317-572-3993 or fax 317-572-4002.

For consumer information on foreign language translations, please contact our Customer Service department at 1-800-434-3422, fax 317-572-4002, or e-mail rights@idgbooks.com.

For information on licensing foreign or domestic rights, please phone +1-650-653-7098.

For sales inquiries and special prices for bulk quantities, please contact our Order Services department at 800-434-4322 or write to the address above.

For information on using IDG Books Worldwide's books in the classroom or for ordering examination copies, please contact our Educational Sales department at 800-434-2086 or fax 317-572-4005.

For press review copies, author interviews, or other publicity information, please contact our Public Relations department at 650-653-7000 or fax 650-653-7500.

For authorization to photocopy items for corporate, personal, or educational use, please contact Copyright Clearance Center, 222 Rosewood Drive, Danvers, MA 01923, or fax 978-750-4470.

is a registered trademark under exclusive license to IDG Books Worldwide, Inc., from International Data Group, Inc.

About the Author

With degrees in journalism and exercise physiology, and a long reputation as a fitness author and instructor, **Therese Iknoian** used every tool of her trade to research and write *Mind-Body Fitness For Dummies.* She spent a decade as a newspaper reporter before launching a freelance career specializing in sports and fitness writing and instruction and earning her master's degree in exercise physiology. She has been a nationally ranked race walker, and is an internationally published freelance health & fitness writer whose work has appeared in *Men's Health, Fitness, Backpacker, Shape, Women's Day, Walking,* and *Parenting,* among others. Aside from magazine and book writing, she is also a partner in GearTrends LLC — www.GearTrends.com — the premier information Web site for products and trends in the fitness, outdoor, paddle, snow, and bike markets. Her other Web site, Total Fitness Network — www.TotalFitnessNetwork.com — is filled with her stories about all areas of fitness and training and was recognized as a 1999 Golden Web award winner.

Long known as "The Walking Woman" because of her two walking books and personal competitive race walk history, Therese Iknoian breaks out of that stereotype with *Mind-Body Fitness For Dummies.* Though proud of the walking label and her advocacy for that activity, she continually takes on other fitness or sports challenges and has never met one she didn't want to experience . . . if she hasn't already. From rock climbing to running to rafting, Therese is the first one to say "Let's go!" — sometimes much to the chagrin of her husband, parents, and friends. As someone who has also tried assorted mind-body techniques over the last two decades, she was eager to research — and dabble in — them all even more. Her family likes it better when she stands still and moves slowly.

Therese has authored two books on walking, two instruction/music audiotapes for walkers, and has developed fitness and walking programs for several inter-national companies. She is an American College of Sports Medicine-certified Health/Fitness Instructor and holds enhanced credentials in nutrition, is a gold-certified ACE instructor, and a USA Track & Field Level II-certified coach who focuses on working with kids. As a race walker, she was ranked 24th overall woman in the country in 1995, and in 1994 broke the world record for her age group for the Indoor 3K. She still holds the age-group record for the Outdoor 3K. She ran her first marathon in 2000 in 3 hours 45 minutes, qualifying for her age group for Boston 2001. In 1999, she began competing in Adventure Races, and she placed 3rd in the corporate division in the New York Hi-Tec Adventure Race.

These days, if she's not writing, she's either out running, mountain biking, or looking for the next fitness adventure challenge. Or she's sitting beside the creek behind her house in the Sierra foothills enjoying the sounds of quiet.

ABOUT IDG BOOKS WORLDWIDE

Welcome to the world of IDG Books Worldwide.

IDG Books Worldwide, Inc., is a subsidiary of International Data Group, the world's largest publisher of computer-related information and the leading global provider of information services on information technology. IDG was founded more than 30 years ago by Patrick J. McGovern and now employs more than 9,000 people worldwide. IDG publishes more than 290 computer publications in over 75 countries. More than 90 million people read one or more IDG publications each month.

Launched in 1990, IDG Books Worldwide is today the #1 publisher of best-selling computer books in the United States. We are proud to have received eight awards from the Computer Press Association in recognition of editorial excellence and three from Computer Currents' First Annual Readers' Choice Awards. Our best-selling ...*For Dummies®* series has more than 50 million copies in print with translations in 31 languages. IDG Books Worldwide, through a joint venture with IDG's Hi-Tech Beijing, became the first U.S. publisher to publish a computer book in the People's Republic of China. In record time, IDG Books Worldwide has become the first choice for millions of readers around the world who want to learn how to better manage their businesses.

Our mission is simple: Every one of our books is designed to bring extra value and skill-building instructions to the reader. Our books are written by experts who understand and care about our readers. The knowledge base of our editorial staff comes from years of experience in publishing, education, and journalism — experience we use to produce books to carry us into the new millennium. In short, we care about books, so we attract the best people. We devote special attention to details such as audience, interior design, use of icons, and illustrations. And because we use an efficient process of authoring, editing, and desktop publishing our books electronically, we can spend more time ensuring superior content and less time on the technicalities of making books.

You can count on our commitment to deliver high-quality books at competitive prices on topics you want to read about. At IDG Books Worldwide, we continue in the IDG tradition of delivering quality for more than 30 years. You'll find no better book on a subject than one from IDG Books Worldwide.

John Kilcullen
John Kilcullen
Chairman and CEO
IDG Books Worldwide, Inc.

**Eighth Annual
Computer Press
Awards ≥1992**

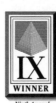
**Ninth Annual
Computer Press
Awards ≥1993**

**Tenth Annual
Computer Press
Awards ≥1994**

**Eleventh Annual
Computer Press
Awards ≥1995**

Dedication

With loving hugs to my parents, Richard and Roxy, who have always been there for me, telling me that anything I wanted to do and anything that I aspired to was within my reach. They nurtured and supported every step, as well as all my dreams and schemes — long before they became a reality. And with true love to my husband, Michael, who helps to keep me grounded and breathing. He is indeed my dream-come-true.

Author's Acknowledgments

It was over a steaming cup of "Calm" herbal tea on a rainy New York autumn morning that Mark Reiter, my International Management Group agent, asked me, "So what do you think about doing *Mind-Body Fitness For Dummies?*" Neither he nor I realized at the time we were all going to break new ground with such a compilation! So thanks go both to Mark as well as IDG's Stacy Collins for trusting me with this project.

Ralph La Forge, Duke University's clinical exercise physiologist and the book's technical reviewer, was actually more than that from the project's inception. A good three months before starting any reviewing, he became my advisor, mentor, guru, neutral overseeing eye, and all-around great guy and e-mail buddy. I could always count on Ralph to give me balanced opinions and a sane piece of unbiased advice, not to mention an occasional well-placed piece of mind-body humor. He was my anchor in what sometimes seemed like rough seas, and this project would not have been what it is without him.

Then come the legions of consultants and true experts in all of the areas I've covered who loaned me their advice, materials, opinions, instruction, as well as a willingness to fact-check instructions and let me bounce ideas off of them. They gifted me, and you the reader, with a valuable amount of their time and energy in order to meet my goal of making this project the best it could be. My biggest thanks (in the order their section appears in the book) to: Yoga experts Katie Carter, Deirdre Daniel, Georg Feuerstein, Jennifer Fox, Paul Gould, Richard Miller, and Larry Payne; Tai Chi Chuan teachers Manny Fuentes and David-Dorian Ross; Qigong masters and teachers Bingkin Hu, Ken Sancier, and Patricia Smith; Pilates educators Elizabeth Larkam, Maria Leone, Cathleen Murakami, and both Moira Stott and Alison Hope of Stott Conditioning; Feldenkrais practitioners Michael Purcell and Allison Rapp; Alexander teachers and authors Nicholas Brockbank and Robert Rickover; Laban teachers and authors Janet Hamburg and Virginia Reed; Inversion Therapy information source Hangups International; Body Rolling developer Yamuna Zake; NIA co-developers Debbie and Carlos Rosas; Chi Ball developer Monica Linford; as well as Juliu Horvath (Gyrokinesis), Jack Raglin, and Laura Sachs (E-motion).

Publisher's Acknowledgments

We're proud of this book; please register your comments through our IDG Books Worldwide Online Registration Form located at `http://my2cents.dummies.com`.

Some of the people who helped bring this book to market include the following:

Acquisitions, Editorial, and Media Development

Project Editor: Kathleen A. Dobie

Managing Editor: Tracy Boggier

Senior Acquisition Editor: Stacy S. Collins

Acquisition Coordinator: Lisa Roule

Copy Editor: Rowena Rappaport

Technical Editor: Ralph La Forge

Permissions Editor: Carmen Krikorian

Associate Media Development Specialist: Megan Decraene

Editorial Manager: Christine Meloy Beck

Media Development Manager: Heather Heath Dismore

Editorial Assistants: Jennifer Young, Alison Jefferson

Production

Project Coordinator: Leslie Alvarez

Layout and Graphics: Beth Brooks, LeAndra Johnson, Heather Pope, Jeremey Unger

Proofreaders: Laura Albert, Corey Bowen, Joel K. Draper, Susan Moritz

Indexer: Steve Rath

Special Help
Allyson Grove

General and Administrative

IDG Books Worldwide, Inc.: John Kilcullen, CEO; Bill Barry, President and COO

IDG Books Consumer Reference Group

> **Business:** Kathleen A. Welton, Vice President and Publisher; Kevin Thornton, Acquisitions Manager

> **Cooking/Gardening:** Jennifer Feldman, Associate Vice President and Publisher

> **Education/Reference:** Diane Graves Steele, Vice President and Publisher; Greg Tubach, Publishing Director

> **Lifestyles:** Kathleen Nebenhaus, Vice President and Publisher; Tracy Boggier, Managing Editor

> **Pets:** Dominique De Vito, Associate Vice President and Publisher; Tracy Boggier, Managing Editor

> **Travel:** Michael Spring, Vice President and Publisher; Suzanne Jannetta, Editorial Director; Brice Gosnell, Managing Editor

IDG Books Consumer Editorial Services: Kathleen Nebenhaus, Vice President and Publisher; Kristin A. Cocks, Editorial Director; Cindy Kitchel, Editorial Director

IDG Books Consumer Production: Debbie Stailey, Production Director

IDG Books Packaging: Marc J. Mikulich, Vice President, Brand Strategy and Research

◆

The publisher would like to give special thanks to Patrick J. McGovern, without whom this book would not have been possible.

◆

Contents at a Glance

Cartoons at a Glance

By Rich Tennant

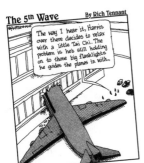

page 9

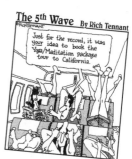

page 81

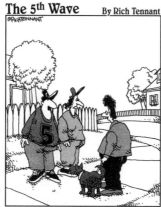

"We're really beginning to experience the Tao of walking, which is a good thing since we were also beginning to experience the Tao of potato chips and double fudge ice cream."

page 61

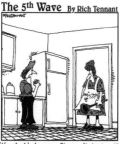

"You should do some Qigong. At least you'll unclog your energy channels if not the garbage disposal, the upstairs toilet and the lint trap in the dryer."

page 131

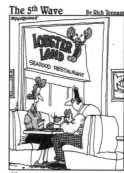

"Is there a way you can explain Pilates to me without using the carcass of your lobster?"

page 187

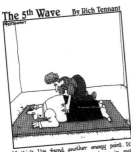

"I think I've found another energy point. It's at the end of an open ball point pen in my front shirt pocket."

page 235

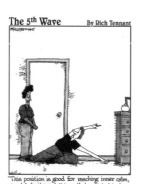

"This position is good for reaching inner calm, mental clarity, and things that roll behind the refrigerator."

page 303

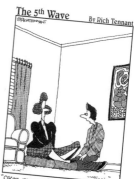

"Okay, your posture's very good. Now relax, concentrate, and slowly let go of your cell phone."

page 331

Fax: 978-546-7747
E-mail: richtennant@the5thwave.com
World Wide Web: www.the5thwave.com

Table of Contents

Foreword

. . . .

*O*ver the last decade, the term *mind-body* has pervaded nearly every facet of health, fitness, and medicine perhaps to the point of meaningless redundancy. When we talk about mind-body interactions, oftentimes we are also describing how kinesthetic sensations (for example touch, physical exercise) evoke changes in perception, attitude, and behavior. Mind-body fitness is a state associated with improved muscular strength, flexibility, balance, and coordination, but perhaps most importantly improved mental development and self-efficacy. Regular participation in exercise with a distinct contemplative component is one means of improving mind-body fitness. Much of what happens in mind-body exercise is therapeutic in that it promotes the therapeutic goals of integration, humility, stability, and self-awareness. These outcomes reach toward a farther horizon of self-understanding that is not ordinarily accessible through conventional exercise. When executed properly, Hatha Yoga, Tai Chi, Qigong, Pilates, and the many other forms of mindful exercise take qualities of mind and cultivate them internally so that the person's powers of self-observation are increased.

Therese Iknoian herein has written a text which is virtually unprecedented in fitness and health promotion — a practical and delightfully descriptive compendium of the major mindful exercise programs in the world today. This volume serves both as a useful resource for those desiring a brief overview and also as a guide to the essentials of mind-body exercise practice. Think of mind-body exercise as the sum of graceful movement, deep contemplation, and breathwork. Think of the output as creativity, clarity, and enriched physical and emotional health. Such attributes are catalysts for improving health and reducing the unnecessary emotional burden of chronic disease. May your life begin.

Ralph La Forge

Durham, NC

THE INFORMATION IN THIS REFERENCE IS NOT INTENDED TO SUBSTITUTE FOR EXPERT MEDICAL ADVICE OR TREATMENT; IT IS DESIGNED TO HELP YOU MAKE INFORMED CHOICES. BECAUSE EACH INDIVIDUAL IS UNIQUE, A PHYSICIAN MUST DIAGNOSE CONDITIONS AND SUPERVISE TREATMENTS FOR EACH INDIVIDUAL HEALTH PROBLEM. IF AN INDIVIDUAL IS UNDER A DOCTOR'S CARE AND RECEIVES ADVICE CONTRARY TO INFORMATION PROVIDED IN THIS REFERENCE, THE DOCTOR'S ADVICE SHOULD BE FOLLOWED, AS IT IS BASED ON THE UNIQUE CHARACTERISTICS OF THAT INDIVIDUAL.

Introduction

*F*itness has certainly evolved in the last four decades. From the jogging mania and high-impact aerobics classes all adhering to the mantra "No pain, no gain," to fitness walking and stretching classes promoting "Only do what's comfortable for you."

Not only have there been big changes in what the science gurus say you should do to achieve fitness, but also in the goals. Being fit a few decades ago just meant being thin. Thin and toned was The Big Ultimate.

Today, being fit takes on a broader meaning. It still includes fitness of your body, and now also includes how your body's fitness affects your physical health. However, the definition of fitness is slowly evolving to encompass the fitness and health of your *mind* also. If you bring your mind along for the fitness ride — in fact, ask it to join you in your routines — being fit suddenly becomes a holistic practice. And that practice leaves you feeling a whole lot better both inside and out.

In this book, I show you the future of fitness: Mind *and* body. Not one or the other. Both.

You may have a variety of reasons for wanting to try some of the practices or methods of mind-body fitness:

- ✔ **You're bored with traditional workouts:** You feel there has to be more that just breathing hard and pushing yourself to your physical limit.
- ✔ **You've never been comfortable with traditional workouts:** You've drifted in and out of fitness because your body wants something softer and more contemplative but you haven't known where to turn.
- ✔ **You're looking for ways to link your traditional workout with some ohmmmm:** You like both physical and mental practices but want to find a way to integrate them into your regular lifestyle.

Whatever the reason, you've come to the right place!

About This Book

I never questioned the ability to integrate both mind and body into fitness practices to achieve the best of both worlds. I never thought you had to give up one or the other to fully practice one or the other. I never once considered the concept of a book about mind-body fitness strange, funny, or unsettling. Then came the reactions from friends and colleagues.

Nearly every time I told someone the title of the book I was working on — *Mind-Body Fitness For Dummies* — the reaction was either a chuckle, an outright guffaw, or a dead-silent pause. Depending on the person's background, it was the combination of the words "mind-body," "fitness," and "dummies" that elicited the seemingly involuntary response. I felt either insulted or taken aback and was forced to puzzle over the reactions myself.

I concluded that non-mind-body enthusiasts often chuckled or laughed aloud because they were either unfamiliar or uncomfortable with the mindful element of fitness, and that mind-body purists usually responded with silence, because often they were aghast. They felt that the emphasis on a physical element could dilute their practices, or that the term "dummy" would lessen the seriousness of what they do.

For both groups, let me clear this up straight away: You are not a dummy for wanting to read this book. Nor are the methods portrayed for dummies. This book is for serious people who simply don't know very much about some of these methods — many of which can be very unfamiliar, scary, even feel unapproachable because of the customs and history. Some are just hard to find much information about.

This book then is my attempt — the first attempt ever it seems — to put all the major mind-body methods and a few not so major ones together in one text. I attempt to discuss both the mental and physical components in a way that retains the authenticity of each. I also attempt to break out of confusing or intimidating insider lingo to make each method accessible to everybody.

The Hazards of Forging a New Trail

As someone who has dabbled in all kinds of physical and mental practices since my late teens, I was like a babe in Toyland as I began to research this book. The concept allowed me to look into or practice many methods on a deeper level than I had before, or to learn something about or do more esoteric methods I'd only heard or read about.

Perhaps naively, I assumed that folks who practiced different mind-body methods would all support each other, and would in fact be divinely blissful to hear of such a consumer book linking them all together.

Well, suuuurrrrprise, suuuuurrrrprise, as my favorite TV goofball used to say (You like my Gomer Pyle impression?). What I found was that I sometimes had to walk as if on hot coals — and this was not a meditative practice, mind you, but one I was forced into as I frequently juggled words like a politician trying to remain a neutral party. Some methods didn't appreciate others. Some practitioners didn't relate to the philosophy of another, even of the same method. Philosophies of how to do, to practice, to combine, or to live the methods were as varied as the methods themselves differ in styles and teachers.

In the end, everybody seemed to accept the idea of one book with many mind-body methods as well as the link to fitness since it would introduce you, the eager consumer, to their worlds.

I share my experience so that you can be aware as you dabble. And so that you can be strong and unbiased in your personal search. If you find a practice you like, don't be put off by someone telling you that another method or style is better. That may be just his or her bias or personal preference. Know yourself and listen to what feels right to you.

Why You Need This Book

I cut a path through the mind-body forest for you so that you can more easily scamper from method to method with the help of this mind-body guidebook.

If you're a mind-body novice, the more easily you can make your way through the mind-body maze with this book — trying a little here and a little there as you read about philosophies and styles — the more quickly you can pick out the methods that suit you best.

Perhaps you're already experienced in one mind-body method and want to experiment with others you've heard about without committing yourself too deeply. This book can help you figure out your next mind-body destination.

This book makes it easy to dabble, whether you're a total novice or a more experienced practitioner, because it offers information about many different methods all in one place. You just don't find a variety of methods in one place, in one neighborhood, in one club, or in one studio. And they certainly aren't in one book anywhere — until now.

How to Use This Book

Do you ever go to a restaurant and just can't decide what you want to eat? Everything sounds so good — or at least worth a try. Ever wish you could order a plateful of lots of little bites of things to help you decide what you really want a full order of?

This book is like ordering a lot of little platefuls. It's an introductory reference book about mind-body fitness in general, as well as different types of mind-body methods and practices specifically. You can pick and choose as many as you want before deciding what you want as a full order. Or you can stay at the smorgasbord, taking a little of this, a pinch of that.

I could never be so vain or narrow-minded as to think that this book can satisfy your mind-body needs completely. In fact, I'd be terribly disappointed if it did. I want you to try these — as many and as much as you want — but I want you to want more. These chapters and sections are mere introductions. They don't begin to do justice to a full practice or a full knowledge of a particular method.

I hope to pique your interest to the point where you deepen your exploration and search for a more in-depth book, a video or two, a class at a local facility, or a practitioner or trainer who can help you go deeper into your practice.

At that point, this book can become a reference sitting on your shelf. I do hope you go back to it often to broaden your practice. Perhaps you didn't read about a couple of the methods the first time, but suddenly your neighbor mentions a class she's been to. So out comes the book again so you can refresh yourself about what it is, and whether that's something that would be good for you.

As Katie Carter, owner of Wild Mountain Yoga Center in Nevada City, California, in the Sierra foothills said: "Don't be afraid to flirt with your edges."

How This Book Is Organized

In this book, I lay out some introductory parts so that you can learn a little in general about mind-body and fitness practices, then give you several sections about different methods. In later chapters, I suggest ways you can combine various methods and use them in your life.

Part I: Setting Out on the Mind-Body Path

Before you start any journey, you need to explore various routes and what to take with you. In Part I, I give you definitions and guidelines as well as information about trends in mind-body fitness. I present a couple of tables for you so that you can more easily compare the features and benefits of different methods. You can also read about the basics that apply to all mind-body practices, such as breathing and posture. And of course you need to figure out how equipment and space fit in the picture, so I include that info, too.

Part II: The Science and Art of Mind-Body Methods

I try to build on the foundations with a touch of science. I lead you on a little journey through the scientific studies — what does exist — about mind-body fitness, and introduce you to some stories from real people who have found their lives changed, diseases healed, and pain gone for good. Sometimes, you see, anecdotal stories carry a lot of weight. I also discuss some of the general parameters of safely starting any fitness program.

Part III: Yoga Primer and Postures

In this part, I dive straight into one method: Yoga (Hatha Yoga, specifically). I choose Yoga as the first method to explore because it's probably the one Westerners are the most familiar with. You get a little intro into the different schools and types, the benefits you may realize, and ways to determine which branch is best for you. Then you get to try a series of postures, and read about how to combine them into sequences.

Part IV: The Flow of Ancient Chinese Mind-Body Arts

The ancient Chinese arts are often the basis for many other newer mind-body methods. I limited this part of the book to a discussion of Tai Chi Chuan and Qigong. These two give the basics and probe deeper into affecting the energy flow in your body, which, of course, I present. You can practice some basic Tai Chi forms, as well as some novice Qigong movements, and get tips on ways to combine them both into sequences.

Part V: Presenting Pilates

Compared to Yoga and the Chinese methods, Pilates is very young — only a few decades old really. But it is a contrast to the others with its exacting focus on alignment and less focus on energy flow. You find out what Pilates is, where it came from, and all about some basic movements, as well as how to string them together to fit your needs.

Part VI: Exploring More Mind-Body Methods

This is really the fun part! I introduce you to a dozen or so methods that are either fairly new or slightly esoteric. In the case of seven of them, you get short sections that discuss philosophy, history, as well as a few basic movements to try. For another dozen or so, I give you a short bit about what each method is and where it came from. I also introduce you to the names of another string of methods you may bump into, just so you're familiar with the names.

Part VII: Pulling It All Together

In this part, I give you pointers on how to make these methods a part of your life all the time, and how to use the benefits in small ways all day. Combining the methods — with each other or with more traditional fitness practices — may be the best way to at least start trying these methods, and I give you a primer on ways to put together routines with movements from various mind-body methods, and/or movements from more traditional fitness activities. The goal is to enable you to become your own teacher.

Part VIII: The Part of Tens

If you just want quick hits, turn to the Part of Tens. These Tens are by design a place to skim for quick hits of information. The chapters in this part introduce you in short order to reasons to do mind-body fitness methods, their benefits, times to get in a quick practice, questions to ask yourself to find the best method for you, and tips on tracking down a great class, studio, or teacher.

So many methods, so little time. . . . In the Appendix, I try to help you with the time crunch. A resource list gives you more places to turn for information, books, videos, Web sites, and equipment for each of the methods I present.

I encourage you to use the resource list as a way to explore any and all of these methods further. Poke around on a Web site, read a book that delves deeper into a method that grabs you, buy a video for some "live" instruction, or send an e-mail to ask about local teachers or practitioners. The information in the Appendix can help you take your stroll along the mind-body trail and turn it into a lifelong pursuit.

Icons Used in This Book

I use little icons throughout this book to draw your attention to points I think are interesting, useful, or valuable, and to highlight points I don't want you to miss. The following list explains what I use each icon for.

I use this to point out info that can help you understand the subject at hand, and to highlight interesting info that may give you a nice insight.

Everybody always has two cents to add. This icon points out particular experiences I've had that may help you on your journey, or gives you an insider tip that I found helpful when learning a method or movement.

When it comes to exercise and movement, your health is always a concern. So this icon firmly marks areas where you should be extra careful. It also points out when you would be wise to consult with a physician.

These bits are particularly noteworthy for helping you do better or absorb more. This icon also emphasizes text I don't want you to just skim over.

I don't want you to get baffled by bizarre words and terms. So when you see this icon, you know that some kind of jargon is imbedded in that paragraph. In most cases, I translate the lingo for you, so don't let this icon scare you off.

When you're concentrating on getting the movement down, it can be easy to miss the mindful elements behind benefits or different movements and their philosophies. But I want you to see each and every one. You find this icon when I note something particularly mindful or a tip about how to make it such.

Bottom line, this mind-body fitness stuff should be fun. Yeah, I believe in being serious. But you can't get so serious that you're blind to the humor in any situation or you can't joke about yourself or something you're doing just a little. So I'll leave you with this little bit of wisdom:

> If you're looking to find the key to the universe, I have some good news and some bad news. The bad news is: There is no key to the universe. The good news is: It's unlocked.

Part I
Setting Out on the Mind-Body Path

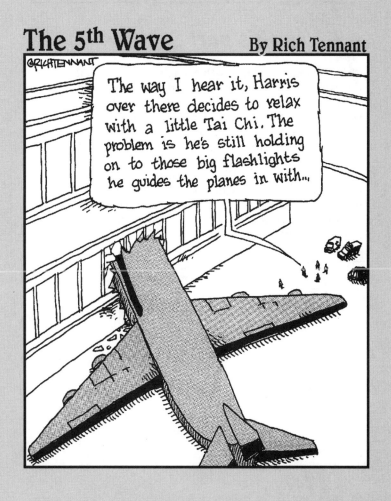

In this part . . .

*E*very journey starts with a single step, and so it is with your journey on the mind-body path. Figuring out what it all means, which route to take, which sights to see, what to pack, and how far to go are all part of the journey — and the chapters in this part help you with all these decisions. First of all, I give you some definitions and guidelines, then I point out some of the different roads you can take and why you may want to travel a certain path. I also provide you with all the vital stats — equipment, gear, space, and basic movements — so that you can start your trip properly prepped and packed in both mind and body.

Chapter 1

Making the Mind-Body Connection

In This Chapter

▶ Getting the lowdown on mind-body fitness

▶ Finding your type

▶ Adding mindfulness to all your workouts

▶ Revealing the methods in this book

*W*hen you think about exercise and fitness, what do you picture? Sweating a little? Breathing harder? Using and toning your muscles? Burning calories, losing weight, and thinning your thighs? Perhaps lowering your cholesterol or decreasing your risk of a heart attack or even some cancers.

Ever since the aerobics and jogging boom began in the 1960s, those images are what most people in the Western world connect with fitness . . . things that change the body in some way. So running, aerobic dance, lifting weights, swimming, bicycling, even walking were considered traditional Western fitness methods. Healthful they were and still are. They do wonderful things for your body.

But what about your mind? Doesn't it want to go out and play, too? And feel the benefits? Only recently did people in the world of traditional Western fitness begin to recognize, accept, define, and try to find a name for exercise and movement that wasn't just about calories, sweat, and the body. Those in that world have actually come a long way in a pretty short time toward not only accepting mindful fitness activities not of the traditional Western ilk, such as Tai Chi Chuan and Hatha Yoga, but also incorporating the mind into modern fitness methods that put the body in motion as well as use the mind, such as NIA. These days you can even find meditative components and conscious breathwork overlaid onto traditional physical exercise, such as running or cycling.

Although mind-body concepts may seem pretty new to many of us, many of the methods and components added to modern methods actually date back centuries. We latecomers have just stumbled across them. In fact, the Eastern world has had sort of a monopoly on many of these exercise forms, as you see when I take a look at forms like Yoga, Tai Chi, and Qigong. But these aren't the only mind-body forms. The entrepreneurs of today's world have used their own minds — and some of the basics of these ancient Eastern classics — to come up with hundreds and thousands of other methods that seek to balance our bodies and minds.

Defining Mind-Body Fitness

What is mind-body fitness? Maybe you already know and you picked up this book because of a new or continued interest. But maybe you're just dang curious.

I try to present a satisfying definition. Remember, though, that the mind-body fitness concept is so new and so loose that pinning down an exact and universal definition is a bit like trying to hold on to a water balloon — it just keeps slipping around and taking on new shapes. The definition I write now will continue to evolve as the fitness world debates what mind-body fitness really is and how to describe it.

For the exacting academics among you, this is how the Mind-Body Fitness Committee, established by IDEA, a California-based professional and educational association for fitness professionals, has nailed down the meaning. For now.

> *Mind-body exercise is physical exercise executed with a profound inwardly directed focus.*

Now, I interpret for the less academic among you who just want to, well, get it:

> *Mind-body exercise is a form of movement that increases fitness in some way — muscular strength, aerobic levels, flexibility, and balance but also enables you to engage your mind in a non-judgmental way and with an inward-directed focus that may become contemplative.*

What does that mean? In short, that means you ask your mind *and* your muscles to be present and accounted for and to stay intentionally connected to each other. "Inward focus" means you pay attention to what you are feeling in your muscles as well as to your breathing. Through this focus comes the contemplative state attributed to mind-body practices.

What is traditional exercise?

I use the term "traditional *Western* exercise" throughout the book because many of the Eastern mind-body methods I talk about are considered "traditional" in that part of the world. So what we consider alternative in the West is pretty dang mainstream elsewhere. You can also consider these mind-body methods and other forms of the West's traditional fitness and exercise to be complementary to each other's goals.

In addition, mind-body *fitness,* as compared to mind-body *exercise,* is an outcome and not a process. (Mind-body *exercise* is the process.) Mind-body movement focuses on the present, not the future. There is no goal, just a continuing practice, which in most cases leads to overall wellness.

So, compared to traditional Western fitness routines where your goal may be to lose 10 pounds or drop 3 minutes from a 5-kilometer running time, mind-body fitness routines are about just being there and doing them. Build it and they will come. Do it, and fitness will happen.

Presenting Three Classifications of Mind-Body Methods

You can find hundreds and thousands of methods and concepts to help you balance body and mind, or to increase your inner awareness and energy flow. Some methods are new; some are older. Some are a combination of several methods all mixed together, and some focus on improving how you do other activities, from everyday stuff like carrying a box to sports performance. I consider three categories of mind-body methods in this book:

- **Early Classics:** Some of these very early and well-respected methods are depicted on stone carvings or in ancient texts and date back centuries. Some have been handed down from family to family, or generation to generation, being taught and passed on by master teachers and their apprentices. They include, for example, the Eastern methods (Yoga, Tai Chi Chuan, and Qigong) and some ethnic dance forms (such as Afro-Haitian dance or Capoiera).

- **Modern Classics:** These forms date back 50–100 years or so. They tend to be very analytical, and so may help you do other things better, including other mind-body methods, because of their emphasis on focusing and becoming aware of very specific muscular movements. The concepts are often used by today's generation as it comes up with other contemporary methods. Modern Classics include Pilates, as well as Feldenkrais, Alexander, and Laban.

✔ **New Kids:** These mostly composite and contemporary forms draw from Early and Modern classic methods. They also draw on free-form movements and dance. Some are just a few years old. Some date back just to the 1980s or 1990s. New ones spring up each year all over the world to help satisfy one person's needs (who then sees the applications for others) or by a teacher to fill a need they see in his or her students' fitness. They vary in their focus on mindful involvement, breath, and movement. New Kids include NIA, Chi Ball, and Body Rolling, as well as many others that I introduce but don't go into detail on (E-motion, Tai Chi Chih, Gyrokinesis, and Brain Gym for example).

In this chapter, I lay down the foundation so that you can decide what kind of mind-body fitness house you want to build, what you want to put inside, and how you want to finish it.

Making All Exercise a Mind-Body Experience

You have probably heard of the runner's high that can come when someone doing traditional Western exercise, like running, gets so mentally caught up that he or she can "zone out" into a relaxed and euphoric state. That comes pretty close to being mind-body exercise. But not quite.

That's not to say that an inward focus during a step-aerobics class or on a fitness walk doesn't do great things for your mind. It can, and it does. And in later chapters I mention a couple of methods that seem like traditional exercise with added mindful components. In some cases, they are. The mind-body purist would argue whether they really fit the strict definition and quality of mind-body exercise. I'll leave that for you to try and decide.

Introducing the components of a true mind-body routine

To qualify as mind-body exercise, a fitness routine usually includes certain elements or specific ways of moving — or sometimes simply doesn't include particular components or styles.

A short history of exercise

Used to be that folks didn't have to think about keeping fit. They just did what they did everyday. And they stayed pretty dang well and healthy just from chores and farmin' and haulin' and carryin'.

Times changed in the twentieth century. As the people of the Western World got more and more out-of-shape and their minds lost touch with the importance of the health of physical exercise, the researchers began to poke and prod a bit. Ah-ha, Sherlock! Fitness. Movement. Heart rate! Of course, it took the world another few decades to figure it all out. At first, John and Jane Q. Public just watched the crazy loons jogging, which started the fitness trend in the 1960s — "Look at that weirdo, running on the side of the road! He could be driving instead! Should we offer him a ride?" Then fitness became more accessible to the masses with aerobic-dance studios popping up in all the malls, partly thanks to both Jazzercise and Jane Fonda. Women wearing matching pink leg-warmers, belts, and sweatbands jumped and kicked to upbeat and fun music. It may have hurt. It may have burned. But slapping the body into painful shape was *the* way to get fit, healthy, and happy, plus everybody saw results, which in this case meant weight-loss and muscle-tone.

As we approached the on-ramp to the information superhighway and technology that promised to save time and instead crammed us with even more to fill our allotment of daily hours, more and more people began to search for balance of body and mind, heart and soul.

Working out the ol' body was one thing — there was now proof for a whole truckload of physical and healthful benefits. What about our minds? And did this fitness stuff have to hurt? So the questions began to be asked louder and louder until the voices reached a crescendo.

Hey, balanced fitness wasn't just for those leftover hippies who still burned incense and sat cross-legged in rooms with calm smiles on their faces. Hmm, what are they doing in there that makes them look so peaceful?

So we all tip-toed closer. Those folks in tie-dyed clothing in there weren't really exercising, right? How can something called exercise make you feel calm and — for goodness sake — even bring a smile to your face! Getting fit was supposed to make you "feel the burn" so you'd get results. Forget how you get there. Just get there.

Modern-day mania, however, has led all of us to take a harder look at those folks "in there" *and* for those folks "in there" to come out to introduce us to their world of balance between body and mind. The IDEA organization — the international association of fitness professionals, which for years focused strictly on traditional Western exercise — formed a committee in 1994 on mind-body fitness to help advise the association on ways to help its members understand and apply mind-body fitness and exercise. IDEA's first conference on mind-body fitness was held in 1996. The demand continues to grow, and as it grows among instructors and trainers, so it trickles down more to you, the student.

Ralph La Forge, a physiologist at Duke University Medical Center and former chairman of IDEA's Mind-Body Fitness Committee, teamed up with several experts in various mind-body disciplines to create a preliminary classification of necessary components for a fitness routine to be mindful. As the definition I offered you earlier in this chapter continues to evolve, so do these components of the routine.

A mindful exercise should incorporate at least one — and preferably several — of the following components, as they now exist:

- ✔ **Mindfulness:** The mind is part of the routine in a non-competitive and non-judgmental way that is introspective and not goal-oriented, called *mentative*.

- ✔ **Body awareness:** Participants focus on sensing what the body and its muscles are doing in all of the movements, called *proprioceptive awareness*.

- ✔ **Breath focus:** The sounds and feeling of full and conscious breathwork as a centering activity, called *breath centering*.

- ✔ **Method-appropriate form:** Self-discipline allows the body to be aligned to conform to a method's particular pattern of movement, called *anatomic alignment*. Note that many forms, particularly some Eastern ones, put little or no emphasis on any specific alignment.

- ✔ **Energy flow:** A movement of your own personal inner energy helps achieve the centering, calm, and focus common to mind-body fitness, called *energy centric* or *bliss*.

In addition, research seems to indicate that the best mind-body awareness isn't accomplished during vigorous exercise, but rather needs a low to moderate intensity to be successful. That means if you rate your intensity on a scale of 0 to 10 (with 10 being very hard), it should not feel any harder than about a 6.

Finding your level of mindfulness

You can certainly take any type of non-traditional exercise and dump it into a barrel labeled "mind-body." That's fine if you prefer simplicity and don't want to get wrapped up with categorizing and rating. But you can also take a look at exercise programs at a deeper level, assessing the amount of mindfulness in a program to better choose one that will suit you.

I found three basic categories of fitness programming — one that lacks the mind-body component at all, one that has a level of focus and muscular sense, and a third that delves deeper into energy flow or spirituality. You find some methods can become either of the latter two methods or even somewhere in between, depending on how you practice them. Imagine a long line running horizontally across the page with three dots on it — one on each end and one in the middle — each representing one of these three levels described above. Every type of exercise — be it traditional or non-traditional — can be placed as a point on the line either next to a current dot that indicates a mindful level, or somewhere in between two dots, or mindful levels. Where you place your dot changes with your needs and tastes.

Because I'm talking about mind-body fitness, I limit my description of levels to the two Fs that fit these programs:

Focus

Many of the methods I introduce fall under this level. You begin to direct your mental focus internally and focus in a nonjudgmental fashion on what your muscles are actually doing. You allow yourself to become aware of the movement and its effect on your body. Sports psychologists sometimes call this *association.* You let your mind stay plugged in as you move so you actually don't dismiss what's going on — or miss what's happening — but instead you use it to let you progress better through the process. Feldenkrais and Alexander are, for example, "focus" methods.

This is about moving the muscles and using your mind.

Flow

Many may argue that you also flow doing routines that fall in the focus category. And, of course you do in some ways. But in pure focus methods, the intent doesn't go quite as deep into your internal spirit, nor does it tap into your energy pathways and chi (see Chapter 4). In these types of programs, you let the meditative aspect take over. The movement may become quite emotional as it stirs up your insides and brings on a sense of higher consciousness.

Taking traditional exercise to flow

The argument, whether the likes of running, walking, or aerobics can become a mind-body movement, continues. You may see mention of "mindful weight lifting" or "mindful water aerobics," and you may have experienced the zone that can come from getting so mentally involved with your traditional exercise that it feels like Meditation. Purists may tell you about one huge difference: whether the mindful element is primary or secondary. If the cognitive component is central to the process, it is a mind-body method. If it is secondary — that is, you tack it on to a traditional form — it may not be considered mind-body exercise. You decide. My opinion, for what it's worth: If you can discover something about mind-body movement, can apply it to what you do normally, and can grow in some way from that, that's a step in the right mindful direction.

This is where the meditative and breathing elements can lead to spiritual elements. Tai Chi Chuan, for example, can be a true flow method, even becoming kind of a lifestyle. Yoga, too, can be a flow method if you want it to become one. You can pull back to focus at any time, or even choose some mid-way level between focus and flow. Always your choice.

This level is about moving the muscles, using your mind, *and* accepting how it affects your physical matter.

Exploring Promising Mind-Body Methods

You're not the only one with a growing interest in what is now called mind-body fitness. Fascination and demand are spreading like wildfire. In this section, I share my list of the most prominent and developing mind-body practices, which are the ones I cover in this book in-depth.

Yoga-rific

I cover the basic elements of Hatha Yoga, which puts an emphasis on physical forms to help the mind. Added bonuses include increased balance, body awareness, alignment, strength, and flexibility. I don't cover styles that are purely spiritual, lifestyle-oriented, or all about Meditation — this is a book on *fitness* after all. A 2000 survey by IDEA, the association for fitness professionals, shows Yoga is among the top 10 programs being offered in health clubs and has nearly doubled in numbers in the four years prior to the survey, from a third of clubs offering it to two-thirds of clubs offering it. In addition, Yoga shows the third-highest rate of growth, coming in behind martial arts and boxing-based classes. (Boy, that's a big difference in methods!)

Three cheers for Tai Chi Chuan

Tai Chi Chuan, commonly referred to simply as Tai Chi, is an ancient, flowing method that stresses inward focus and moving slowly through forms that require great balance and control. It is beautiful to watch and peaceful to perform.

Tai Chi Chuan didn't make IDEA's top 10, but if you dig down the list, you see that the numbers are still climbing. In 2000, more than a third of clubs offered Tai Chi classes, up from about only 1 in 7 clubs four years earlier.

Queuing up for Qigong

Qigong is an ancient Chinese movement art that takes its lead from the energy pathways in your body and the energy, or chi, that runs through them. The goal is to free up your chi with slow, flowing movement, and to allow it to flow more smoothly without road blocks to wriggle through caused by stress or ill health. Better flowing chi, it is said, can lead to better health and happiness.

There are several styles, including a medical style that I do not cover in this book.

Practicing Pilates

Pilates is a structured method where participants move through exercises either on the floor or on various machines that emphasize mental focus on muscle control and alignment. Core strengthening — of the back and abdominals — is the real gem of this method.

Pilates offerings in health clubs have jumped wildly in the last couple of years. According to the 2000 IDEA survey, more than a third of clubs offer classes, where only 1 in 10 did three years earlier. Not only that, sales of the Reformer machine for Pilates exercises have more than doubled since 1998.

Limbering up with Laban

Laban is one of several methods that is less about fitness and more about function: that is, noticing how your body moves and becoming aware of that movement so you can function better in daily life. Movements are repeated, controlled, and analyzed.

Paying attention to Feldenkrais

Feldenkrais demands great mental discipline because you repeat very small movements and are then asked to simply think about how your body felt while doing them. Through the increased awareness — often additionally honed in personal sessions with practitioners — you can move more freely in daily life and other sports, and get over nagging injuries or pains.

Acting up with Alexander

Alexander is less of a series of movements you practice than it is a way to think about what you do all the time. There is a great emphasis on the placement of the head and its carriage by your shoulders and neck since many people carry so much stress in that area.

Flipping for Inversion Therapy

Going upside down — or even partly upside down — isn't for everybody, either because you may not be comfortable with the feeling or you have some illness or disease not recommended for the activity. If you can and like inverting yourself, you may like the relaxing feeling you can achieve as well as the way it loosens your entire back.

Playing around with Body Rolling

It's a marvelous thing to be given a ball and be asked to sit on it, lie on it, and roll around on the floor with it. In Body Rolling, you can be a kid again, while using a special ball to massage and work your muscles all over.

Rolling the ball in the Chi Ball Method

The Chi Ball Method uses a soft ball that you hold in your hand and pass around your body, or just hold while doing movements reminiscent of Yoga, Tai Chi Chuan, Qigong, traditional aerobics, or other mind-body methods. Scented with different aromatherapy aromas, the ball is something to play with while the scents can help create the feelings you want or need.

Discovering NIA

Free-flowing dance-like moves are the essence of the NIA technique. You use your voice, feel your feet on the floor, and do moves that resemble everything from modern dance and martial arts, to Yoga and Tai Chi. It can be quite aerobic, depending on the level of intensity you choose for your movement.

The mind-body trend will grow as Boomers, Gen Xers, and 20-somethings alike realize the powerful potential of even five minutes of movement that incorporates breathwork, muscular movement, and mindfulness.

Expressing yourself through other forms

I lightly touch on several other mind-body methods, such as those following.

- **Ethnic Dance:** a combination of martial arts and dance that requires mental focus and flow. Movement forms use vocalization and rhythm, and can be quite aerobic.

- **Walking Meditation:** not your mother's fitness walk, but a conscious and slow-moving progression where the focus is breath and focus.

- **Rosen Method:** a way to improve alignment and flexibility using breath-work and relaxation. Designed to supplement other routines.

- **Gyrokinesis/Gyrotonic XS:** a movement that is a combination of Tai Chi Chuan, Yoga, Qigong, swimming, and dance that coaxes the body through spiraling rather than linear forms. Gyrotonic XS uses a machine, while Gyrokinesis does not.

- **Tai Chi Chih:** a contemporary approach to Tai Chi Chuan-like movement but much simpler and less intense. Balance is particularly stressed.

- **E-Motion:** a composite method that brings the benefits of Eastern forms to Westerners in a way that is more comfortable in traditional health club settings. Includes an aerobic section for a full workout.

- **Brain Gym:** just like it says, a very mental and focused method said to enhance learning ability.

- **Yogarobics:** one of the earlier forms that brought Eastern Yoga to Western health club and fitness settings in a non-intimidating and more familiar style.

Chapter 2

Choosing Your Path

In This Chapter

▶ Discovering your mind-body bent

▶ Working it out around your time and life constraints

*H*ow do you begin to decide which mind-body method is best for you, or what to combine with other workouts you already do? And how does it all fit in with your fitness goals?

In this chapter, I help you answer those questions. Consider me the travel guide on your mind-body tour. My red umbrella is held high so you can see where I am in the crowd. Come along with me!

Figuring Out Your Goals

The beauty of mind-body exercise is that you and I can choose to do the same method for entirely different reasons. Yet we both do the same movements, take the same classes — focusing on different elements perhaps — and both get what we want.

To help you discover your mind-body fitness motivation and goals, I take you through some of the reasons other folks choose one method or another.

As a part of your quest, take a look at Chapter 23, a Part of Tens with questions to ask yourself about what you want to do and why. And don't miss Table 2-1, which gives you a quick way to cross-reference the benefits of the various methods I present.

As you look at Table 2-1, keep in mind that certain methods may be low in one area because that method's goals were never intended to be anything other than that level. This table does not assume 1, 2, or 3 ratings as better or worse. It only presents some averages to help you better choose. Put it all together, and soon you'll be heading down the right path knowing exactly where you're going.

Going for aerobic fitness

Many people start exercise programs to lose weight, which often means raising their heart rate in order to "burn calories." Increasing your heart rate helps get your heart and lungs more fit, too, which translates into all kinds of good things for your overall health. Take a look at Chapter 5 for the basics of good fitness and its health benefits.

You can make many of the methods in the table more aerobic, but the workouts will still be mostly at a low to moderate intensity. But even a lower intensity level burns calories and increase aerobic fitness. Methods like NIA and Chi Ball can be quite high-intensity. Even Tai Chi can be moderately high when you're strong enough to keep the forms low to the ground and you're knowledgeable enough to keep moving between forms.

Your primary mind-body fitness goal isn't to get aerobically fit. If, for example, your main goal is to lose weight or to enhance the performance of your heart and lungs, mind-body exercise alone isn't the best way to achieve your goal. Nevertheless, the low intensity of this work — as a cross-training tool with your other activity — can still give you a foot up toward your weight-loss or performance goals.

Targeting flexibility

The type of movements common to many mind-body methods requires flexibility throughout all parts of your body. So you can gain some flexibility from most any of these you choose. (Some that focus mostly on body awareness, such as Feldenkrais and Alexander techniques, may not increase flexibility. But that's not their goal!)

You can look at something like Yoga and see it simply as a great stretching exercise through which you can gain flexibility. Okay, it *is* a great way to get flexible, but if you practice Yoga just to stretch, you lose out on all the other mind-body benefits, including mental centering, focus, and clarity. Go for stretching, stay for mindfulness. And take a look at Table 2-1 to compare the different levels of stretch training involved.

Aiming for strength

Arnold wannabes won't fulfill their needs through mind-body workouts. Don't expect pumped-up muscles or beefed-up pecs. But you can get some of the leanest, and most toned muscles you've ever had — muscles that may not be big but are still very strong. You may be surprised how much strength the simplest of Pilates moves can build, or the repetitiveness of a Feldenkrais lesson can demand, ever so subtly. Table 2-1 shows which methods put more emphasis on the area of strength.

Strength is a good goal to have, especially if you want it, for example, for day-to-day functions such as lifting groceries, kids, or suitcases, to keep a chronic back injury at bay, or even to play another sport better. That's a useable strength compared to beefed-up muscles that just look big.

Increasing your relaxation

The whole world, it seems, is just too stressed out and overworked. Who doesn't need a restful island to go to once a week or even in the middle of every day? Finding a way to relax is an excellent reason to try mind-body exercises such as Qigong or Tai Chi.

Of course, the relaxation that comes from mind-body exercise isn't your typical zoned-out, nod-off-on-the-couch relaxation. It's much deeper and therefore longer lasting. What you find is that the peace and relaxation gained during even a few minutes of practice can, with experience, last many hours or even days. You find you get less upset or worked up over small things.

Working toward mindfulness

Mindfulness is the central point of many mind-body methods, especially the Chinese ones. Every discipline encourages you to be aware of what your body is doing both during your practice and after it. The mindful movement, the focus on your muscles, and the emphasis on steady breathing all help bring you to a state of centered calm.

The joy is that this centered state can last for a long time after you finish the practice.

Gaining body awareness

Certainly, being aware of what your body is doing, how you're moving, and applying that knowledge day-in and day-out are goals of many mind-body movement methods. For teachers of Laban or Alexander, increasing awareness is much of what the practice is all about.

Two sub-reasons for gaining more awareness of your body are:

> ✔ **Functioning in the day-to-day:** If you're a senior experiencing changes in the way your body moves, if you have a disease or chronic pain, if you're rehabilitating an injury, or otherwise conscious of mobility issues, body

awareness can produce better functional movement in all that you do. Heck, even if you aren't experiencing any limitations, you can develop more awareness day-to-day. Everybody can be better at balance, which you need every time you take a step.

✔ **Enhancing sports performance:** Forget that stuff about being able to function better day to day — you're an athlete at some level, whether you're a fitness enthusiast, a recreational athlete, or a seriously competitive one. Many mind-body routines can help you become more aware of your body's movement. That awareness can help your technique and, ultimately, your performance.

Seeking spirituality

Embarking on a spiritual journey may be the reason you want to try mind-body exercises. And, as with every aspect of mind-body fitness, the beauty is that you can take your practice to the upper tier, reaching toward new spiritual heights, or simply look to relax and become a little more focused. You can also start at one place and find your needs demand you move in a different direction.

Comparing the Benefits Side-by-Side

In this section, I offer you a way to compare basic mind and body benefits of different mind-body disciplines. I fondly call it Table 2-1. In it you see a rating for the benefits explained above, including aerobic fitness, strength and muscle toning, and flexibility. Of course, the table doesn't include all the methods that exist (since there are literally thousands of them!). It does include the disciplines I discuss in this book in depth, as well as a few I just mentioned in an introductory way without sample movement lessons. This way, you'll have more knowledge on which to base your own choices.

A low category rating for a method doesn't mean it's worse than one with a high rating in the same category. It's a matter of choices (for example, when you want more of a movement method) or goals (what that method sees as its goal). These aren't thumbs-up or thumbs-down ratings. Just classifications — again just so you can make a better choice.

The following chart explains the rating system I use in Table 2-1. For the purpose of the comparisons in this chart, I note the highest level or intensity you can reach with each method (Number 3 in the table). You almost always have the choice of lowering the level or intensity. The table itself lists mind-body methods in the same order I present them in this book.

Rating	Aerobic Fitness	Strength & Muscle Toning	Flexibility
3	Yes	all muscle groups	deep stretching
2	Yes	some muscle groups	moderate stretching
1	No	light to no strength-building	little or no flexibility work

Table 2-1		Benefits Comparison Chart		
Method **Early Classics**	**Aerobic**	**Strength**	**Flexibility**	**Other Info**
Hatha Yoga	Yes	3	3	Can be practiced at many mind and body intensities.
Pilates	No	2	3	Asks for mental, but not spiritual, focus to create muscular awareness.
Tai Chi Chuan	Yes	2	2	Meditative benefits are possible without high fitness enhancements.
Qigong	Yes	2	2	Much practice is needed to learn forms that can help you gain higher aerobic fitness. Spiritual aspect emphasized.
Body Rolling	No	2	2	Superb rehabilitative and function- or performance-enhancing method.
Chi Ball Method	Yes	2	2	A hybrid of Yoga, Pilates, Tai Chi and others, with an aromatherapy ball.
NIA	Yes	2	2	One of the most free-flowing aerobic, and fun of these methods. You can make it quite spiritual if you are so inclined.

(continued)

Table 2-1 *(continued)*

Modern Classics	Aerobic	Strength	Flexibility	Other Info
Feldenkrais	No	2	2	Asks you to think about what is happening to your body, without telling you any "shoulds" to avoid bias. Moves quite slowly. Great for injury rehabilitation.
Alexander	No	1	1	Very focused and small exercises — sometimes just a different concentration during normal activities — that demand concentration.
Laban	No	1	2	Focused movements that teach you to practice higher muscular and movement awareness to enhance the way you do daily tasks or sports activities. Often used by dancers and athletes.
Inversion	No	1	1	Can be dangerous if you have a heart problem, eye problem — even one you don't know about. Practiced by yogis and many others for centuries.

Others	Aerobic	Strength	Flexibility	Other Info
Meditation Walking	No	1	1	Not your average fitness walk, but a very slow and inwardly focused step-by-slow-step stroll. Contemplative, and forces balance.
Rosen Method	No	1	1	A very detailed method that creates more awareness for other activities.

Others	Aerobic	Strength	Flexibility	Other Info
Capoiera/Ethnic Dance	Yes	2	2	Free-spirited and fun. Can be very aerobically intense. A hint of martial arts with twirls and kicks.
Gyrokinesis	No	3	3	A hybrid of Yoga, Tai Chi and and Qigong that works on the the flow of energy in your body, as well as muscular awareness for good function.
Gyrotonic XS	No	2	2	A version of Gyrokinesis with a machine invented by its creator that allows for spiraling movements.
E-Motion	Yes	2	3	A method adaptable to fitness clubs because of a traditional class format, while still applying the techniques of slow movement, meditation, and energy flow.
Tai Chi Chih	No	2	1	A very soft and less-intense new version of Tai Chi Chuan. Not steeped in the history that Tai Chi Chuan is, but can be great for seniors or those seeking rehabilitation.
Watsu	No	1	1	A form of free-flowing and very embryonic movement in the water.
Brain Gym	No	1	1	Meant to create higher mental capacities through light movement.
Aqua methods	Yes	2	2	Water creates a low- to non-impact environment that envelopes the body, creating a soothing and often massage-like medium. Water's resistance can heighten the intensity if desired.

(continued)

Table 2-1 *(continued)*

Others	Aerobic	Strength	Flexibility	Other Info
Traditional + Mindful	Yes	3	3	Take what you do, add mindful elements, so you get a little bit of it all.
Five Rhythms	Yes	2	2	Another free-spirited dance-like

This table summarizes the highest level most participants could normally reach in a category. Many of these methods can range from 1 to 3, depending on the teacher or your own skill.

Of course, other authorities and enthusiasts may disagree with my ratings. But many, if not most, of these methods can easily fall at either end of the scale, depending on the form of the exercise, the teacher, and the skill of the practitioner. My ratings reflect what I think is typically the highest level achieved by average participants.

Determining Your Limitations

Everybody has limitations in life. They may be simple ones such as taking classes in the evening, or living in a small apartment, time-juggling issues such as with family and work, or more complicated ones such as chronic low back pain. I don't want you to ignore these limitations or to pretend they don't exist. I want you to embrace them, then determine how you can work with them to find the best mind-body method for you and your needs.

Many people embark on a fitness program without taking into account what they realistically can and cannot do. For example, you've always wanted to go to a health club and take aerobics. So you find one near your home, sign up, and walk away very excited about taking a class three times a week. One problem you didn't think about nor did the salesperson ask you about: The best time for you to work out is at lunch and your gym is near your home 30 minutes away. In the end, you can't get there regularly, you drop-out, and you feel like a failure.

Better planning — in this case, finding a gym near your office — can make you a success.

Table 2-2 lines up some of the more common limitations in a comparison chart to help you choose a method or combination of methods you can really live with. Some limitations you have control over, and some you don't. Just recognize before you embark on your program what you have to work with (or work around). Refer to Parts III, IV, V, and VI to read about specific methods and discover which one excites you. Then you can refer back to Table 2-2 to make sure it fits your lifestyle and needs.

Dealing with the day-to-day

These hurdles can be the hardest for many people. But with the right planning, you can get right over them and move ahead.

- ✔ **Finding space:** What kind of room do you have in your home or exercise space? If you have a teeny-tiny bedroom and no other space, deciding to buy a Pilates Reformer isn't your best bet. Nor is wanting to embark on a NIA program.

- ✔ **Wanting privacy:** Can you close a door and get away from family, roommates, or kids? Can you guarantee you won't be bothered? Does your club have a space that feels private and safe? Your program is your quality-time with yourself and you want to be able to focus on it to get the most out of it.

- ✔ **What about the kids:** Maybe your kids are always full of questions, need your help, or can't find something right in front of their nose. Or you may have young ones who need a lot of parenting. You may not be able to disappear for 30 minutes, but don't give up your mind-body workout. Schedule a time when they're in school or down for a nap. You may even be able to get them to join you! (Look, ma's a pretzel!)

- ✔ **Using a VCR or CD player:** I won't be so bold as to think you may not want to try an instructional video (I'd be disappointed if you didn't!) or may not want some background music even if I suggest quiet. Do you have these pieces of equipment handy in the room where you want to do your practice? Does the club where you may go have the atmosphere you prefer?

- ✔ **Finding storage:** Many mind-body methods don't require a lot of "toys," but even a mat takes up space. And, you may want to try bolsters, straps, chairs, and other equipment. Make sure you know the dimensions of stuff you have to store, and plan where to put them before you invest in space-consuming paraphernalia.

- ✔ **Working out outdoors:** Do you have access to a nice outdoor setting? A backyard, a nearby park, or a garden? These can be the best places to practice your mind-body movements: Trees, plants, and greenery can actually help you find and increase your energy. If you like the outdoors, you may also want to find a class offered outdoors, when weather permits.

Reckoning with your scheduling

Study after study shows that lack of time is the number one reason people give for not exercising. But, it's all about planning. Anybody can find 10–20 minutes a day a few times a week to practice a mind-body technique. If even that sounds like a lot of time all at once, know that you can gain nearly the same benefits even if you muster only three to five "time-outs" of a couple of minutes each. Those few minutes alone can help you find a lasting mind-body experience.

If you have trouble finding the time, read through the following list. I hope these tips can help you find your motivation.

- ✔ **Everybody starts with 168 hours:** That's how many hours you have each week. No more, no less. It's all about how you use that time. Take a few minutes and mentally walk through your typical weekdays and weekends — take notes if you need to — to discover when you can fit in your mind-body fitness routine.

- ✔ **Make a fitness appointment:** Just as you pencil in a doctor's appointment or a coffee date with your father, slot in a time for your exercise. If someone calls and needs something or wants you to go somewhere, just say, "I have an appointment." Your caller doesn't have to know that your appointment was a Yoga session in the backyard.

- ✔ **Find a buddy:** Sure, you're working out of a book, but who says you have to go it alone? Recruit a neighbor to join you after work, a colleague to take part at lunch, or your family to try it out with you on a weekend morning. Having a partner can help you stick with it.

- ✔ **Take a class:** A class with a good instructor can be motivating and challenging. You find out about new methods, new ways of doing an old method, and just get psyched up again from the energy of others around you. You also get personal instruction about your technique.

- ✔ **Get some clothing or gear:** This may sound trite, but there's nothing like embarking on a mind-body practice and really *feeling* the part in your new unitard or on your new sticky mat, which are fairly small investments. Plus, just putting on your outfit or rolling out the mat can help get you in the mood.

- ✔ **Take five . . . minutes that is:** Even a few minutes a few times a day can help you feel the benefits of mind-body. Avoid saying to yourself, "Why bother?" if you only have a few minutes now and then.

Considering your physical limitations

If you have physical disability, chronic disease, or injury, you can still do many of these exercises! Refer to the Real Life vignettes in Chapter 6 of those who have done just that.

First, however, do see a doctor to make sure you're choosing the right form of exercise and that there is nothing about what you're interested in that could aggravate your condition or make any injury worse.

If you use a wheelchair, you can still do much of the Tai Chi and Qigong, for example; just do them sitting down and work on your upper-body moves.

If you have a chronic illness such as AIDS, chronic fatigue syndrome, high blood pressure, heart disease, diabetes, or multiple sclerosis, listen to your body and take it easy, doing only a little bit at a time. Build slowly, and stop when you feel tired. Always consult with a physician first.

The same holds true if you haven't exercised in a long time or are very overweight. These mind-body methods can be a great way to get moving again.

If you have an injury — say a back problem or a sprained ankle — find a way to modify everything. Do what feels right to your body. And do what your doctor says can work for you.

Comparing the Limitations Side-by-Side

Because most of the possible limitations are so personal, it's difficult to rate them. So my rating system may seem especially arbitrary.

I include three primary criteria — space, equipment, and music — because these considerations may also help you ferret out your personal tastes and lead you to the best method for you.

As with the Table 2-1, these can vary widely depending on how you approach a method. I have rated it with what is most typical. And, as in Table 2-1, I present the info in the order I do in the book.

The following key shows my rating system to help you interpret Table 2-2.

Rating	Space	Equipment	Music
3	large, average living room size	Y/N (yes or no) rating only	Y (music is suggested) or N (music is not mandatory)
2	medium, small bedroom or 2-3 mats next to each other		
1	small, the size of a single mat		

Table 2-2		Additional Mind-Body Practice Considerations			
Method	**Type**	**Space Required**	**Equipment**	**Music**	**Comments**
Yoga	Early Classic	Small	None	None	When you start experimenting in a more in-depth way, you may look into additional Yoga "props."
Pilates	Modern Classic	Small	None	None	If you decide to do more more than mat Pilates, you need some large equipment and space to hold it, too.
Tai Chi Chuan	Early Classic	Small to Medium	None	None	This is the simplest of methods for which you never need much space or any gear.
Qigong	Early Classic	Small to Medium	None	None	Nothing but you and your breath and mind are needed.
Body Rolling	New Kid	Small	Yes	None	Do invest in the real Body Rolling ball if you're seriously interested.
Chi Ball Method	New Kid	Small to Medium	Yes	Yes	If you like a little variety, this method may suit your fancy. The aromatherapy Chi ball can enhance the workout.
NIA	New Kid	Medium to Large	None	Yes	Dance-oriented students like the movement, but you need a large space to really feel a higher aerobic intensity.
Feldenkrais	Modern Classic	Small to Medium	None	None	If you're left-brained and analytical, you may find a liking here.

Method	Type	Space Required	Equipment	Music	Comments
Alexander	Modern Classic	Small to Medium	None	None	Plenty of Web sites with movement samplers for this method. Sometimes just learning the concepts and applying it to all movement can help you.
Laban	Modern	Small to	None	None	You may need a partner for this work.
Inversion	Early Classic	Small	None	None	Just the floor and a pillow can get you started, as long as your doctor approves.
Meditation Walking	Ancient	Large	None	None	You can do this style of walking in a hallway if you don't have a wide-open area.
Rosen Method	Modern Classic	Small	None	None	An analytical method for creating true muscular awareness.
Capoiera/ Ethnic Dance	Modern Classic	Large	None	Yes	A group dynamic and music can help you whoop it up for this free-spirited movement.
Gyro-kinesis	New Kid	Small	None	None	A Yoga-like method, but less linear. The founder created it because of a personal back injury.
Gyrotonic XS	New Kid	Medium	Yes	None	Like Gyrokinesis but with a machine, so you have to go to a studio. Not too widespread yet.
E-Motion	New Kid	Medium to Large	None	Yes	Videos and audios can lead you through this workout quite nicely. More of a traditional workout.

(continued)

Table 2-2 *(continued)*

Method	Type	Space Required	Equipment	Music	Comments
Tai Chi Chih	New Kid	Small to Medium	None	None	Little space needed at all for these gentle movements, especially nice for seniors.
Watsu	New Kid	Pool	Yes	None	You gotta have a pool and some instruction to start.
Brain Gym	New Kid	Small	None	None	True analysis aimed at creating higher mental capacities.
Aqua methods	New Kid	Pool	Yes	You can use music	A pool you gotta have.
Traditional + Mindful	New Kid	Small to Large	Varies	You can use music	Take whatever fitness routine you normally do and make it mindful.
Five Rhythms	New Kid	Medium to Large	None	Yes	You're better off experiencing this dance-like art with a group first.

Note: For the purposes of this chart, I assume that you have at least a mat or carpeted area. In some cases, additional variations of one method using extra equipment is possible, but not mandatory. Plus, you may always use music if you like, but, unless it's integral to the concept, I said "None."

Chapter 3

Finding What You Need: Garments, Gear, Space, and Instruction

*B*efore you jump right into mind-body exercise, consider some of the gear, gadgets, gizmos, and garments you may need. You also need to take into account the space demands of certain workouts to help figure out whether that exercise is right for you. And, of course, as you find one or more disciplines that appeal to you, you may want to dig a little farther and find out more about that one method, or even find additional instruction via videos, Web sites, classes, or other books.

The Appendix can help you locate printed and electronic sources of information, including organizations, schools, teachers, and instructional tapes and videos. I also give you some tips on determining whether a teacher is right for you, rating a video, and navigating around the Web in your search to discover more.

Ah, but of course, the joy of all this is that — as with mind-body workouts themselves — the process is the important part, not the goal. Whatever teacher, club, video, or book you find, you'll be a step closer to fitness of mind and body your way.

So raise your sails, catch the wind, and see where the mind-body boat takes you next.

Dressing the Mind-Body Part

I'll never forget the first Yoga class I attended as an adult. I pulled on my thigh-length tights and a baggy T-shirt, left my long hair floating around my shoulders, and took my place on a mat. Well, it wasn't long before I ripped off that ol' tee (I thankfully had on a sports bra). With all those head-down postures, the shirt was hanging down over my head, caught under my arms, and basically doing its best to suffocate me every which way I turned. And my hair? That was another story. It flopped everywhere and got caught in all the wrong places. I learned quickly to tie up the hair and wear tight clothing that stayed put as I moved. One look at the instructor could have told me that!

Moral of the story: Take heed when you see people, especially the instructor, wearing certain items in a class, or you read recommendations for specific clothing. Nearly always, it's for a good reason.

Putting on the top

Both men and women should wear a sweatshirt or other top to and from a workout, even if it's in your living room. Usually as you cool down, your body core temperature starts to drop again and you may want to put on another layer to stay comfortable or use something to lay over yourself during your final stretching or relaxation.

Aside from that, gender differences dictate clothing differences, as the following sections show.

Choosing workout tops for men

For men, this is easy. A T-shirt. I know I said my baggy tee hung all over my head, but men, for some cultural reason, can't get away with wearing a sports bra! Can't imagine why.

Two ways to get around the suffocation thing:

- ✔ Tuck the T-shirt into your shorts or sweatpants (assuming you can get it to stay there as you stretch and reach in all directions).
- ✔ Wear a snug-fitting tank top or a stretchy exercise top.

Choosing workout tops for women

For women, what to wear on top is a little more complicated simply because women have more options. Plus, fashion trends can mandate all kinds of things as being right or wrong, particularly when it comes to breast support and how it looks. Of course, how it looks is moot if you're just in your living room by yourself.

First consideration is snugness: You want to be able to move, and to be able to see your alignment and body placement for better review and correction. Of course, in some methods, for example primarily the Chinese ones such as Qigong or Tai Chi that keep you mostly standing or sitting, you may actually feel better in loose garb. Look at some options:

- ✔ **Sports bra:** Just fine in many cases if you're comfortable baring your belly. Sometimes lying on the floor, a mat, or using one of the balls or other gadgets in some methods can pull on or stick to exposed skin though. And if you're in a public gym, it's considered bad manners to let your sweat drip all over the machinery or mats. So keep your method and location in mind as you choose. Or choose a waist-length version.

- ✔ **T-shirt:** Do try to tuck the T-shirt in so it stays put better, or choose one that isn't quite one of those one-size-fits-none humongous models. You can also start your workout with a T-shirt and sports bra on, then take the tee off as you get into the bending and twisting. For the Chinese arts, you may just then want to leave the baggy top on.

- ✔ **Unitard (short or long):** I know, this moves into an entirely new realm of revealing, head-to-toe, skin-tightness. But, there's a good reason many instructors wear these: They not only move with you, but stay put. No hiking up at the waist (or down at the waist) as when you have on two pieces. No need to be pulling and tugging as you work out. It just stays. Consider it. (Oh, these are sometimes called *catsuits,* probably because you feel all sleek and stretchy when you wear one. These may be less suitable for the Chinese mind-body arts and some Modern Classics.)

Pulling on the bottoms

One thing both men and women want to avoid: Pants that aren't elastic in the waist. Deep breathing exercises and other movements can often push the limits of non-elastic middles, plus the waistband can cut into you and inhibit your freedom of movement.

Otherwise, you can use my suggestions in the following sections.

Panting (styles) for men

Basically, wear whatever you're comfortable in, such as baggy sweats (as long as they stay put at the ankle), running or other workout pants, or the loose-fitting drawstring pants made for many mind-body workouts.

Many men aren't comfortable with tights on, especially in a public place, and that's okay. Consider them as an option.

One word of advice: Please, please don't wear short shorts if you are going to a public place. The baggy legs or loose liners make for some, er, revealing moments when you move or bend.

Panting (styles) for women

Same guideline as with tops: Think snug for some of the methods. Tights — short or long — are ideal. If snug doesn't feel right, then go with the same recommendations as for men. Try sweats, workouts pants, or drawstring-waist pants.

The dilemma of short tights or shorts versus long tights or shorts is not easy to answer. Usually either will do. It may be more a matter of personal taste, because having your legs stick to a mat isn't much of a problem.

Consider a unitard or catsuit for some methods. (See the previous section, "Choosing workout tops for women.") No crawling up, no hiking down, no slipping and catching. It really could be the best of all worlds.

Sporting fine footwear

Actually, usually nothing! Most mind-body methods want you to feel the ground, and that means being barefoot. In some cases, if you're outside doing Tai Chi or Qigong, you may want a lightweight shoe or rubber-soled slipper.

If you're inside doing a class — at home or in a gym — keep socks handy since your feet may get cool as you finish up with relaxation or meditation. Nothing spoils a good deep relaxation more than icicle toes!

If you're in a public place, you may want a pair of slip-on sandals or shoes to get to and from the studio, from a locker room, or your car. Good manners prohibit bringing dirty feet or dirty street shoes onto a clean floor that you and your exercise buddies will be lying on. Plus, slip-ons are just a heck of a lot easier to get on and off for your workout!

Tying up your hair — or not

If you have long hair or long bangs, you definitely want a rubber band (best option) or small clip to get the hair out of your way. First of all, many workouts involve stretches and head-down movements. There's nothing more annoying than having hair get in your mouth or caught everywhere. Second, some workouts, like Pilates, may involve equipment that can catch your hair and, well, sorta rip at it. Pain doesn't help you stay mindful.

You want to avoid:

✔ Hats of any sort that can fall off (even backwards baseball caps) or have a brim that can get in your way.

✔ Large hair clips that stick out of the back of your head, such as those spring-loaded ones with big handles. You can't lie down with your head back and properly aligned with that kind of monster on your head. Even clunky flat metal clips pinned right on the back of your head cause a strain in your neck as you align yourself when you're lying down.

Assembling Other Odds 'n' Ends

The things you really need to have comprise a pretty short list. The list can grow longer as you find out what makes you more comfortable, helps you feel more successful, or generally adds to your enjoyment of the workout.

Collecting the basics

Generally, mind-body workouts are relatively inexpensive. Most of the clothing and gear you need is stuff you already may have around your house. This section sticks to the must-haves for nearly every mind-body method.

✔ **Mat:** You really want something to cushion your body and bones from floors (and, if you sweat a lot, to protect the floor from your perspiration). The kind of mat you need depends on what you do.

- **Yoga mats** are commonly called *sticky mats* because they're thin and actually feel like slightly sticky human flypaper. They make it a lot more comfortable, and even easier, to do postures where you use your hands or feet against the floor. They roll up into small, storable bundles.

- **Regular exercise mats** provide cushioning and protection. Some come with double or tri-folds, so they don't take up a lot of space.

You may eventually want both these kinds of mats, alternating with the type of workout you choose.

✔ **Towel:** Either to toss over you to stay warm at the end of a workout, or to fold up to cushion either your head (like a small pillow) or some other bone, such as a knee or elbow. You can also use it to sit on in seated hamstring stretches done in several methods if your hamstrings are very tight and keep you from having the best alignment. You can also fold it and lay it across your eyes to knock out distractions if you want to relax.

✔ **Water bottle:** You may be moving slowly in some cases, but you're probably still perspiring. Stay hydrated by drinking 1 to 3 cups of water an hour. Remember, as soon as you feel thirsty, you are already dehydrated.

✔ **CD or cassette player:** You may likely want to listen to workout-appropriate music. It keeps you motivated and entertained, and may help you become more meditative or mindful, depending on the music.

✔ **Strap, belt, or long towel:** Many of these methods involve some kind of stretching. If you aren't very flexible, having a strap, belt, or towel to help you reach a foot, ankle, or other body part can help you experience the stretch and work on your flexibility in that position.

Gathering method-specific gear

As you get more experienced, or decide you want to get more involved in certain advanced methods of some workouts, you may want to consider some additional equipment. Refer to the Appendix to find resources for equipment and other accessories.

Some methods I discuss have their own specialty gear. In each section where this is the case, I offer makeshift objects to use — usually common household items — or alternate ways to do something so that you don't have to open your wallet before first trying a workout.

Look briefly at some of these categories of workouts and the gear you may want to use for them:

✔ **Pilates workouts:** Besides the basic mat you need for the simplest workout, you may also want to use other, large pieces of equipment for other workouts, ranging from the size of a stool or a chair, to the size of a small sofa. (I explain these pieces of equipment in Part V.) The Reformer is the largest piece, and is no small expense since it ranges in price from about $800 to several thousand dollars. You can also check out the Wunda Chair and the Cadillac, not to mention various other benches, bars, and stools that you can use in other practices.

✔ **Yoga and other stretch workouts:** Straps, blocks, bolsters, and bags: The Western world has come up with quite a selection of things to use to help people past their lack of flexibility in practices that involve stretching.

• **Straps:** You can get away with a belt or towel, but a webbed strap is sturdier. You wrap the strap or belt, for example, around the ball of your foot while you're sitting down, then hold the other ends with your hands so you can stretch your upper body lower even if you can't actually reach your foot. Consider straps akin to arm extenders!

- **Blocks:** Made of foam or wood, blocks can help you reach the floor when leaning over, for example, even if you aren't flexible enough. That means your body positioning is better because you aren't straining.

- **Bolsters:** These can make for better body positions, or cushion or support for some body part, or you can sit on them in forward-leaning stretches. That takes the pressure off your hamstrings and helps you stay better aligned during the stretch.

- **Eye bags:** These can help you ignore outside distractions for better relaxation or meditation and sometimes have fillings that offer aroma therapy. They're also much nicer than a folded towel.

✔ **Aquatic workouts:** A pool. Seems sort of simple, so I apologize for that. But do realize that when I discuss aqua versions of any method, I mean for you to do it in a pool, not in the shower or a sprinkler! The resistance of the water as you move against it helps build strength, too.

Choosing Your Room to Move

Part of choosing your workouts also depends on how much room you have available. When you read about each method, it probably becomes pretty clear that you don't need a huge room to do a stretch workout, for example, but you may need more room to perform standing Tai Chi Chuan forms. Check out Table 2-2 in Chapter 2 for space requirements for the mind-body methods I cover in this book.

Note that some of the workouts in the chart have ranges of space needs, because how much space you demand depends on either how you do the workout or what kind of equipment you choose.

Also note that most of these methods don't need much more than a small space, with a couple of exceptions, which is good for those of you who don't have huge rooms to spread out or a backyard or park handy!

Where Oh Where Does My Practice Lie?

Health clubs and fitness facilities aren't the only places to take classes or get further education. You can find all different ways to broaden your education after you choose your method. The following list gives you a few of the places you may find yourself able to move mindfully:

✔ **Working it out at home:** Instructional videos and tapes can help you continue your workout routines and increase your knowledge without venturing out of the house.

✔ **Working it out in classes:** Many studios, community centers, and adult education facilities offer drop-in rates or short-term classes of four to eight weeks. You can simply pop by when you want to get some personal instruction during a class to make sure you're progressing in the right direction, or to get a little group motivation and challenge. Or a short-term weekly series can give you the push you need to the next level.

✔ **Working it out in specialty studios:** Yoga studios tend to have their own place they call home. Sometimes they'll also offer related methods, such as Pilates or Tai Chi Chuan.

✔ **Working it out with a private instructor:** Some methods, such as Feldenkrais, Alexander, and Laban, require that practitioners take in-depth study and complete apprenticeships of hundreds of hours. These teachers usually have private offices for lessons. If you poke around a bit, you may even be able to find a teacher who can come to your home and give you private instruction — for a fee, of course.

Be open-minded! I found a totally free Tai Chi and Qigong class at a senior center. I'm not a senior, but anybody was welcome. Check the listings for workshops in your local newspaper.

Investigating Instructional Info

It would be nice if this book were enough for you to discover what you're looking for. But I think I'd actually be a little disappointed if it were! What I'd really like is for you to treat this as kind of a get-to-know-you sampler menu. Then you can figure out what method suits you best and what you'd like to learn more about so you can do more. Also, watching or listening to a live person can help you take the next step and find out even more about your favorite method.

Finding out even more, of course, means more information gathering from classes, private instruction, books, videos, or Web sites.

Where to go? Where to look? You can start with the Appendix, which provides resources for instruction, teachers, equipment, print and electronic instruction, and Internet sources. But you also want to poke around a little yourself. Who knows what treasure you may discover down the street! And sometimes you can actually discover a teacher-down-the-street by surfing the Web, no matter how worldwide it is.

Finding a teacher, trainer, or class

Think locally. Even if you start that search globally.

- ✔ **Local health clubs:** If you belong to a health club or gym, you may find a class right in front of your nose. Many fitness centers are mixing mind-body classes with traditional offerings these days. That also includes a community center, adult education school, or senior center.

- ✔ **Inquiries with those you know:** Ask around. Some of your friends may be taking classes and want to share their finds with you! Try asking at local sport stores or even health food or alternative stores, or read their bulletin boards.

- ✔ **Let your fingers do the walking:** Try the phone book (print or electronic version). The trick is discovering where to look in your local phone book. It may be under Yoga, Wellness, Fitness, Health Clubs, New Age, Mind-Body, or other such listings. You may also find that names of centers could be misleading — one may call itself a Yoga Club, but if you call you may find out the center also offers Tai Chi. Many of these mind-body methods are crossing over, given that one who does one practice is often interested in doing others. So ask.

- ✔ **Referrals from national associations:** Contact a national organization or association (either by phone or on the Web). Many maintain lists of teachers you can research by area. Even if the group doesn't list someone in your area, ask further. The number of teachers is changing so quickly that groups often can't update printed or electronic lists fast enough.

- ✔ **Recommendations from area teachers:** If you find a teacher or class, but the location is a bit too far from you, ask that teacher if he or she knows another class or teacher located closer to you. Each method tends to have a network, and teachers know who is where and doing what.

- ✔ **Browsing the Internet:** Input your area of interest and see what comes up. You can narrow the search by putting in your city if you want, and may be able to find local instructors and classes.

Locating a certified instructor: Should you insist on that?

Now, what about certifications? What do they mean?

If you have any familiarity with traditional exercise, you may recall seeing claims at clubs, by teachers and trainers, or in advertisements stating the importance of "certified" personal trainers, or "certified" water instructors, or "certified" step instructors.

But with these mind-body methods, no such advanced system of certifying instructors exists . . . yet. Some methods, such as Yoga, are beginning to grapple with the needs of a certification program as demand for classes increases. But this won't likely be in place for a number of years. It took traditional exercise, such as aerobics, a decade or more to get to that place, and that industry is still upgrading and modifying the needs of educational demands. In conflict with this attempt is the fact that some mind-body methods stem from ancient forms that require apprenticeships and years of study. As such, it's difficult to certify an instructor, and it's even more difficult to force them to do continuing education to keep their certificate, as is necessary in the Western way.

What you may find are *certificates,* which claim that an instructor has taken a certain workshop or class from some guru (usually referring to a well-respected master or long-time instructor). For that workshop attendance, instructors receive a certificate saying they took blah-blah course from so-and-so. That's all. They may have listened and learned. They may not have. But usually if someone takes the time and money to attend a workshop, they pay attention.

Even if an instructor you find claims to be "certified" or "certificated," you may find a better one who is *not.* So it pays to look around and *feel* what an instructor has to offer, and to listen to what that instructor not only says, but doesn't say. Bottom line: If you like a teacher, go for it. Take a look in Part VIII for my tips on finding a good teacher.

Viewing the stars of the small screen

These days you can find a wealth of information on videos and the Internet. Without getting into an entire lesson on how to search the Web, just start your search by entering the name of the method you want more information about into your favorite search engine. You will get back sites to peruse. I promise.

In some cases, you can just enter: www.methodname.com and find one site right off, such as www.feldenkrais.com. Some of the Asian arts are a bit more difficult to find because spellings, spaces, and placements of apostrophes can confuse a search engine. Plus, if certain non-English words can be spelled several ways, most engines only know one spelling. For example, Qigong can also be spelled Chi Kung or Qi Gong, but may have been entered with only one of those spellings into the search engine's database and is tagged with only one of those names on the site itself.

Videos may be more difficult because, again, nobody screens a video and approves its production. If someone can push a button on a camera, they can have a video made. Try legitimate video sources, not only for mind-body arts but also for exercise videos (some of those carry the non-traditional alongside the traditional now). Read the package cover to see what kind of credentials the instructor has. See whether the catalog or store has a "satisfaction guaranteed" warranty so you can take it back if you want.

Take a look in Part VIII for my tips for picking out videos.

Also refer to the Appendix to get started finding video sources on and off the Web.

Reading more about it

You can always find something else to read, can't you?

Your next step may be to find a specialty book going into more depth about your chosen method or methods. Once again, see the Appendix to get started.

If you take a class, ask the teacher for recommendations for reading material. Even if you don't take a class, call a local club and ask for recommendations.

If you choose to go to a bookstore, don't pick out the biggest or flashiest book you see. Decide what you really need (more explanation? more pictures? more definitions? detailed instructions?) and look specifically for that feature in a book. And, as with videos, read the author's credentials.

With all this information, you can't go wrong as you move forward on your travels in search of a mind-body method that works for you.

Chapter 4

Bringing You All the Movement Basics

As you read about, experiment with, or wonder about all of the different types of mind-body exercise I cover, you'll hear a lot of do's and don'ts about what you're supposed to do with your body and brain. Although each method — be it Eastern or Western — has its idiosyncrasies, a whole sewing basket of common threads ties them all together.

So instead of harping on you to "stand up straight" every few pages (I'll leave that to your mother), I just go over each of the basics or fundamental concepts in this chapter so you can refer back and review them as you need to. Oh, I touch on them again here and there, especially as different movement forms emphasize various degrees of the basics.

But you can always be comfortable coming back home here to figure out if you're tucking and tightening, straightening and standing, bending, or breathing the mindful way.

Throughout this chapter, I also point out distinct places where one mind-body method or another actually contradicts these basics in some way. Unfortunately, mindful work can appear to be a bit contradictory: I may say "tighten your abs" in one chapter then tell you to let them relax in another.

Or I may tell you to move your muscles with focus for one method, but suggest you not even think in another. But because mindful exercise is a process, not an outcome, every way helps you attain your mind-body fitness.

Turning Off Your Gray Matter

This concept is easy and difficult all at the same time. It sounds easy, but is terribly difficult for those of us raised in the Western, competitive, technologically advancing world.

The point of mind-body exercise is not to analyze every muscular move, critique yourself in the mirror, compete with your neighbor, or worry about whether you're doing it right. The point is just to do it. Feeling the way your body moves is the ultimate goal. Letting your limbs and muscles move in a way that feels good and can make the difference between a good mind-body workout and an unsuccessful one.

In other group-exercise classes or individual sports like running or cycling, it's way too easy to fall into a competitive and judgmental trap. (Picture those step-aerobics classes with everybody moving in unison in front of a mirror.) You may find yourself peeking out of the corner of your eye at the person next to you to compare how you stack up to his or her movements. Or, if you run, you may start timing your routes or trying to beat your best time or your companion.

In a mind-body class, the most productive thing you can do is to turn off your gray matter, and simply feel the workout, letting yourself flow through it. Avoid passing judgment or grading yourself (leave that for your second-grade teacher). Go inside yourself to achieve an *inward focus,* and listen to what your body tells you about how far, how fast, or how low you should go. Your body talks to you — you need only listen. You can hear it if you let it talk.

Mind-body fitness is about the process, not the outcome or a goal. It is not a means to an end, but simply a means. There is no *there,* only *here.* And you can achieve your "here" with your mindful exercise program.

One exception is Pilates-inspired movement, which requires inward focus, but also demands exactness in its movement. A Pilates instructor may correct you if you have your spine or leg placed in a position considered incorrect. Sure, there are modifications and alternatives to movements if you aren't flexible or strong enough to do a move a particular way. That's not being "wrong," just a modification to let you continue.

Breathing Deeply and Easily

Breathe? As if you need to be told to keep breathing? Am I serious?

Well, yes. If you ever sit back and watch a group of people in an exercise class or in a weight room, you may be surprised to see how many people hold their breath while they're trying to accomplish a movement. Yet that very action marches them toward failure (and injury) more than many others.

If you've ever taken a group-exercise class, you probably remember the instructor constantly saying, "breathe!" Perhaps you've heard it so much that you tune it out.

Now's the time to tune in that voice, but make it your own in your own head instead of someone outside issuing commands.

If you're having a problem accomplishing a strength move, or stretching as far as you'd like in a flexibility posture, a simple focused breath often brings you over the line to a moment of personal success.

That's the first part, just the simple process of keeping air going in and out of your system for more success, safety, and comfort. The flow of oxygen also helps to *center* you, or bring you into the moment. Some forms of Yoga and Qigong may advise you to breathe loudly or with a sound for particular cleansing or meditative reasons. But that's usually reserved for more advanced practice.

The second part is that some methods, such as Qigong, use breathwork for more than just managing muscular or flexibility moves. Breathing consciously develops and facilitates a better movement of energy through your body. In fact, some mind-body forms may hold classes strictly in breathing to help clear people's energy pathways. So do you need to take a class in it? Oddly enough, many people do. Even if they *do* breathe, they often breathe so shallowly, never fully inflating their lungs, that exercise, energy, or feeling good in movement remains a stranger.

A full inhalation moves all the way down your abdomen and inflates your belly a little without causing your chest to move upward much at all. If you're like many people, the breaths you take make your chest and ribs puff upward and then just stop there without moving down into the belly at all. If that's true for you, try inhaling again, letting the inhalation move your belly out.

A breath can be rejuvenating. Sometime if you're just feeling a little stressed, turn your focus inward for a moment. What do you wanna bet you'll catch yourself holding your breath? (Confession: I do too; it's just become second nature to remind myself to breathe deeply.) So before you get into a habit of holding your breath, put yourself into a habit of breathing deeply when stress builds.

Then, there's the matter of which way to breathe. What, you ask? There's a wrong way? In a true and serious practice of some methods, how an instructor asks you to breathe differs. Some disciplines want you to exhale through your nose and inhale through your mouth, others want inhalations and exhalations through both nose and mouth, and some want you to breathe through your nose. I don't get too wrapped up with these differences in this book.

You also need to be aware of whether to inhale or exhale at certain times during particular movements. Although there may be some differences (even between different schools of one method), you generally exhale when you are exerting, bending forward (flexing) or sideways — such as on the curl-up of an abdominal exercise or a forward-bending stretch — and inhale when you are bending backward (extending) or during relaxation. But not always. Again, I don't get too wrapped up in this in this book. Just breathe in and out the way that feels good to you as you try everything.

If you take a Pilates class that follows the authentic tradition of Joseph Pilates (turn to Part V for more information about this method), the breathing pattern may be the opposite. Also, Pilates-inspired routines encourage very little belly expansion and more expansion of the ribs to the side and back.

So, in sum, I can state the three main concepts about breathing pretty darn simply:

- ✔ Breathe consciously
- ✔ Breathe fully
- ✔ Breathe with the movement

That's really about it. So why do I spend so much time talking about it? Because most of us don't breathe deeply or consciously.

Relaxing Those Muscles

Like turning off your gray matter, relaxing your muscles can be oh-so-easy and oh-so-difficult, partly because of its contradictory nature.

You have to contract muscles to accomplish a movement. How do you lift a leg in a Yoga balance or place a foot in a Tai Chi bow stance if you don't contract a muscle to get it there?

Okay, okay, you don't just flop like a fish. Still, you can use your muscles in one of two ways:

> ✓ **Gripping:** Muscle use often accompanied by clenched teeth, a clamped jaw, or clenched, white-knuckled fingers. Not to mention all the surrounding muscles also getting tight even when they don't need to. This builds tension and usually stops conscious breathwork.
>
> ✓ **Contracting:** Using a specific muscle without involving your entire body and all the muscles not involved in that movement — including your clenched jaw. This usually allows relaxation and continued full and deep breathing.

Have you ever floated on your back in water? If you fight the water, flailing and splashing, you can't begin to float. But if you just relax and breathe, you can float effortlessly — even though, of course, you do use some muscular contraction.

That's what you need to do in most of these mind-body exercises — float effortlessly, using only the muscles needed in a mindful and focused way and leaving the others to come along for the ride.

Warming It Up and Cooling It Down

You've probably heard about warming up before you start an activity. If you don't remember the recommendations, I remind you here: Do 3 to 5 minutes of low-intensity activity that engages the muscles you will be using and allows the tissue to soften and your body core temperature to rise slightly so that you can challenge your muscles and body more fully. The cooldown is just the opposite, going from higher intensity to lower level activity.

In traditional exercise, that usually means moving through space in some way using large muscle groups — like cycling before you lift weights, or walking before you start your run.

Mind-body exercises are all a little different in their warm-ups. You usually have little or no large-muscle movements through space because with many mind-body exercises you focus inwardly and are meditative, which leads to softer movement. So big, high-level movements just don't quite fit a smooth Yoga session.

Some aerobic mind-body methods encourage light activity that moves through space. But this movement resembles soft, low-impact moves rather than large intense ones.

Mind-body warm-ups usually start with less demanding movements — often gentler versions of the movements in the exercises I outline in Parts III through VII that you do in a more challenging way. Warm-up movements get your body's fluids and oxygen moving to the right places to prepare your body for the main exercises. Your blood moves into the muscles and makes them softer and more pliable, which helps decrease the chance of injury, and your *synovial fluid* (a lubricating fluid in your joints) increases so your joints can move without grinding or otherwise harming the bone.

Remember to use the movements I present to help you warm up safely for each method in Parts III through V as well as the order presented in sampler combinations of various methods in Part VII. If a movement, such as a full-stretch posture in Yoga, calls for a cold start, avoid pushing that stretch to your limit. Keep your movements moderate until you start to feel a little warm, then you can start pushing yourself more — if that feels right.

The same applies for the cool-down. You don't actually get cooler. But you do move more slowly, press less hard, and let your mind settle down. You need to walk away from a mind-body workout feeling peaceful; not in pain or stressed out.

A warm-up is just as much for your mind as it is for your body. So make sure you have enough time to tune out the day and bring your mind into the moment so you can fully enjoy what you're about to do. I've been to classes where I've rushed in with my mind so fully occupied with what I have to do that it took me half the class to disengage and focus on the movements rather than on my to-do list.

Striking the Perfect Posture

For many mind-body workouts, how to achieve an aligned spine and tall posture are the first things you find out. Achieving a great, tall, yet relaxed posture can in fact be the foundation of doing many mind-body exercises in the best way.

The basics of good posture are those you've heard all your life, but I review them here. I put them in some technical terms, too, so when you bump into them later, they'll be familiar.

Start simply by checking your current posture: Stand with your side to a mirror and your feet about hip-width apart so you can see your entire body. Wearing snug clothing, or shorts, helps you see your alignment, too.

1. **Stand as you normally do. Now take a look at the curves through your spine.**

The natural curves of your spine should remain — they enable your spine to be more forgiving of impact. But are the curves overemphasized? Ask yourself these questions as you scan your posture:

- Is the curve in your low back too deep, forcing your belly to hang out?

- Are your shoulders sort of rolled over to the front, forcing your chest to sink in?

- Are your head and chin kind of protruding to the front so that if you dropped a line from your ear lobe to the floor the line would fall in front of your chest?

2. **Now straighten up as much as possible by following the points below:**

- Your chin and neck should be pulled in so that your ears are over your shoulders.

- Your shoulder blades should be rolled back and open, but flat on your back. This position causes your chest to lift tall and open wide. That doesn't mean your rib cage is puffed up, it's just lifted so you can breathe better. Oh, and do breathe as you stand there!

- Your abdominals need to be pulled in tight with your pelvis and spine in "neutral." Uh-oh, what's this neutral stuff? Read on. . . .

Achieving a Neutral Spine

In this section, I talk you through what a *neutral spine* should look like and how to get into it. You want to achieve a neutral position with your spine and pelvis so you don't fall into postures both painful and harmful. Yes, painful. The spine is meant to curve in one direction or another, to one degree or another, in different places along your back. Having more or less curve can mean that your spine doesn't handle impact well (think of the curves as kind of like springs), your vertebrae have more pressure put on them, or certain muscles and ligaments are pulled tighter or looser and can offer more or less support than you may need.

You see, achieving a neutral spine isn't just about putting your body in a different place. Most folks either tuck their buttocks under too much, eliminating the low back curve, or sag their bellies out to the front, over-emphasizing the curve. Years of either posture can lead to injury, especially basic low back pain or strain. If your body is used to standing around with less-than-perfect posture, your muscles have adjusted to your stance by becoming either tighter or looser than they should be. You may have to work on stretching and strengthening the muscles first to get yourself re-aligned. So be patient with yourself. This is about process, as always.

Barbie Doll versus Neanderthal posture

Think of Barbie Doll and Neanderthal as visual ways to describe two typical incorrect postures. These names were dreamed up by Cathleen Murakami, Pilates instructor and owner of Synergy Systems Studio in Encinitas, California, and I bet your mind is already busy picturing what they look like.

You're practicing Barbie Doll posture if your chest is puffed out, your back is swayed, and your buttocks are sticking out behind you. That usually goes along with shoulder blades pulled back too far. High heels can contribute to this posture, and standing and walking in this position can put pressure on your lower back and tighten the front of your hips.

You're practicing your best Neanderthal if your chest is caved in, shoulders rounded forward, and buttocks tucked under you. That usually goes along with your head poking forward in front of your chest. This posture can flatten out the curves in your lower back, making it more susceptible to impact injuries.

Follow the steps below to help you get to the right place eventually.

1. **Rock your buttocks back to create a big curve in your back.**

   You may likely stick out your chest to compensate for the weight shift, kind of like Murakami's Barbie Doll posture (see the sidebar on this page.)

2. **Tip your belly forward and try to tuck your buttocks underneath you.**

   You may sink your chest to compensate for this move, much like Murakami's Neanderthal posture.

3. **Rock back and forth between these two exaggerated positions, allowing your shoulders to move in response, but not focusing on their action or making it any larger than required by the pelvis shift. Slowly lessen the swing until you find yourself coming to rest sort of in the middle to a neutral position that doesn't over-curve or -flatten anywhere.**

4. **Test your position.**

   Place your hands palm down on your belly, with the base of your palms on your hip bones, your thumbs reaching inward, and your fingers pointing toward your pubic bone.

   Your hands should be perpendicular to the ground. If your fingers are farther ahead of your thumbs, your hips need to tip backward a bit more. If your thumbs are farther forward than your fingers, you need to tighten up your abs and pull under a bit more.

5. **When you find what seems to be neutral, take away your hands and see how this feels.**

   Are you feeling forced to bend your knees or do you feel as if you are straining to stay in position? If so, you need to work on your leg and hip flexibility to help you along. You may also need to work on low back or front-of-hip flexibility to help you stay there, too.

You can experiment with this neutral spine position anywhere: sitting in a car, walking through the grocery store, or standing in line at the bank. Just working into it can help you stretch and strengthen a little. You'll feel taller and statelier to boot!

Instructors of Yoga, as well as of the Chinese mind-body practices of Tai Chi Chuan and Qigong, not only don't talk about neutral spine, they actually instruct you to "just be." They don't want you to pull in your abdominal muscles or worry whether your shoulder blades are sliding down on your back to open your chest. But, if you practice these methods, you do find that your posture gets taller and your abs get stronger just from the practice and muscle use.

Carrying a Powerful Center

Contrary to what many people believe, your legs don't power you through movements, nor do your arms power you. Your brain isn't even what powers you. Your physical (and mental) power center is in your core. Right smack in the center of your body, basically around your belly button and abdominals; that's your *core* and that's where your *power center* is. These terms are used interchangeably in most cases because they're the same in location and function.

If you try to walk, balance, stand up from sitting, reach to a cabinet or any kind of common sports or daily-life movement, without your core engaged, you aren't able to move smoothly or strongly. No matter what you do, imagine its movement stems from your center, your power center, and not from the limb doing the action.

Try this little game:

1. **Stand up, and pick up one foot so that you're doing a stork imitation.**

   Contrary to your previous instruction on neutral spine and aligned posture, let your abdominals hang out and your whole body sag. Toppling over, are you?

2. **Pull in your abdominals and turn on all circuits in your power center by focusing all your energy right to your core. Balancing is easier, yes?**

   That's the importance of using your core.

Physically, dancers and other movement artists use their core's power to allow them to perform sensational feats. Mindfully, your *core* is the fountain of all your body's energy and, according to the theories of some mind-body practices, the core must be worked and massaged so that you can break free of pain, fill yourself with positive energy, successfully complete a move, or find the true meaning of bliss. To accomplish these goals, you don't just need that central place for power, but you need that central place for energy and healing. I discuss the concept of the power center and the core, specific to both Tai Chi and Qigong, in Part IV on the Chinese mind-body arts. But I touch on this concept in the following section, too.

Finding Energy Central

No matter the level of a mind-body workout, each one has its link to focused energy flow. Rather than gripping or clenching and stopping the energy flow — sort of like a kink in a hose — if you breathe, loosen up, and let the movement happen, you can "unkink" your energy hose and feel the healthy and healing power flow through your body.

Pretty esoteric stuff. But go with me as you read not only this, but through the book, especially as you see more of this concept in Parts IV and VI.

You hear everything from the term *chi* (which translates loosely to "life energy"), to power, to intrinsic energy, to vital life force, to breath of life, to prana, to . . . the list goes on.

All mean one thing, no matter how esoteric or concrete the term: Everybody is born to this Earth with a life force or energy central in their core and in their body. Many people throughout life block that energy because of cultural or physical reasons. It's just not okay in some cultures to feel much, let alone discuss something so ephemeral as energy flowing in the body because it isn't scientifically proven. Some people in these cultures are raised to not trust their feelings and to just move through the world sort of from the skin outward. There is some thought — although again not scientifically proven — that not admitting to or recognizing feelings can actually cause some diseases. I leave this for you to choose to believe or not.

Feeling the energy flow can be a very emotional and even healing experience — and a very scary experience. This energy flow may not be the experience you seek immediately. That's okay. Just move your body through these samplers, and as you begin to feel those movements, you may become more comfortable with your physical power center. When you become more comfortable with your physical power center, you can slowly become more curious and more comfortable with your mindful power center and a potential release and flow of its energy.

I touch briefly on energy or chi throughout the book, particularly as it relates to specific mind-body practices. For more advanced reading and practice, you can peruse the resources in the Appendix.

For now, you've got all the fundamental concepts down . . . turn off your brain, breathe and relax, while you warm up and cool down with great posture and a neutral spine, while using your power center to stimulate your energy central.

Healing my hard drive . . . with energy

I was a mere 12 days from the final deadline for this book. Out of town on business, I had some sections to finish writing before I returned home. My computer had a different idea. When I went to boot it up on one of my first evenings away — after having worked quite fruitfully that afternoon — I got the rather frightful message, "Operating System Not Found," on a dead-black screen. Now, if you know anything at all about computers, you know that this is not a good thing. In fact, it's a really, really bad thing — one that has driven good men (and women) to drink. I spent the next four hours trying everything technical — turning it off and on repeatedly, fiddling with my setup, unplugging it and shaking it around a little and, yes, even kinda whacking it a few times. (Okay, I was desperate.) That wasn't so technical. It still kept telling me, "Tilt," in its lovely computer-speak. As a last resort, I turned to my chi, my energy central. It certainly couldn't hurt, I thought.

I planted the soles of my feet flat on the ground so a strong energy-gathering point could gather chi from the earth. I sat up straight, and positioned my palms (where another strong energy point resides) on each side of the dear ol' laptop facing in and allowing the energy to travel between them and through the computer, which was now off. You're laughing. Really, I did this. Next, I meditated for a minute or so to try to get everything flowing.

Then I opened my eyes and calmly hit the on button again. Yup, you can guess what happened. It booted up just like nothing had ever been wrong. I'm not kidding. This is a true story. Really.

Part II
The Science and Art of Mind-Body Methods

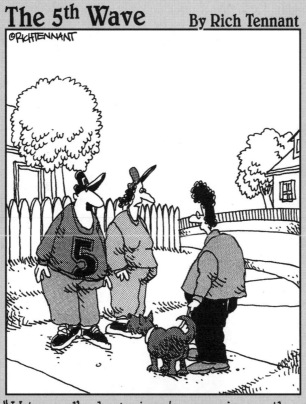

The 5th Wave   By Rich Tennant

"We're really beginning to experience the Tao of walking, which is a good thing since we were also beginning to experience the Tao of potato chips and double fudge ice cream."

In this part . . .

In this part, I show you how to prepare for your workout — give you questions to consider about your physical and mental state. I summarize what traditional exercise scientists say you should do for fitness and health. I also take a quick march through the science — where studies have been done — as well as through some stories and personal experiences highlighting the benefits of various mind-body methods.

Scientifically proven facts are not the riches behind the art of mind-body. Sure, some studies have been done — particularly in the areas of Tai Chi, Hatha Yoga, and Qigong. But Western science doesn't always accept the results of studies unless those studies use all the right controls and methods, and not all research into mind-body benefits uses Western standards. Beyond studies, anecdotal evidence abounds, and although this anecdotal evidence doesn't pretend to be definitive, it's very difficult to ignore.

Part of the beauty of mind-body fitness methods is that the sometimes mystical aspects are the very qualities that can lead you to better physical and mental health.

Chapter 5

Getting Your Mind and Body Fit and Healthy

....

....

*Y*ou probably want help getting your mind and body more fit. And that's exactly what I try to provide. But before you dive in, you need to be sure you're ready for the routine — and doing so involves more than just plopping open the pages of a book. You need to make sure this journey is safe, sane, and smart. Before I talk about how much working out to do, you need to assess your physical fitness to determine how fit and healthy you are currently and whether you need to see a doctor before starting to work out. You also need to assess your mental fitness to make sure that you can keep an open mind and listen to your intuition.

Prepping for a Safe, Sane Workout

One of the keys to a good workout is first laying the groundwork for overall good physical and mental health. This section is all about finding the path to start your journey so that yours is a long and fruitful venture full of discovery and health.

Evaluating your physical fitness

Many mind-body programs are so gentle that nearly anyone can do them without fear. But to be on the safe side — and that's always a smart thing when it comes to movement — take a few moments to assess your current fitness and health using the questionnaire in the next section.

Assessing your general fitness level

If you answer "yes" to any of the following questions, see a physician before starting an exercise program, especially a program that raises your heart rate and puts any additional stress on your heart or other systems. Even if the program doesn't raise your heart rate, it may involve bending or twisting that may aggravate your blood pressure or any joint problems that you already have or may be inclined toward — also good reasons to be safe with a physician's visit.

If you don't answer "yes" to any of these questions, but if you are age 40 or older, or haven't exercised regularly in a year or more, you should still see a physician to check on your overall health and to discuss any medical conditions that may run in your family. If at any time an answer to one of the questions below changes to "yes" during your exercise program, you need to see your physician.

Don't let any of these warnings scare you off from movement! It simply makes good sense to see a physician once a year anyway.

- ✔ Are you currently not exercising regularly?

- ✔ Do you have a personal or family history of heart disease or chest pains, especially before age 50?

- ✔ Do you smoke or have you been a smoker in the in the past two years?

- ✔ Do you have any joint problems such as achiness or stiffness that get worse when you move in certain ways?

- ✔ Do you have high blood pressure, diabetes, high cholesterol, or high blood sugar?

- ✔ Are you taking any medications for any of the above conditions that may change the way your body responds to exercise?

- ✔ Are you considered very overweight or obese? (I'm not just talking about those annoying 10–15 pounds here. If you think you're overweight, you probably are.)

- ✔ Do you know of any other reason why you should not do physical activity?

Taking count of your heart rate

Take a moment to measure your *resting heart rate* (that's the speed at which your heart beats when you're doing nothing, preferably taken first thing in the morning before any activity or caffeine) so you can track it as you begin a routine or activity. Doing so can help you sense any abnormal spikes in your heart rate while you're moving that may indicate a problem, and let you see whether your heart rate declines as you get fitter. (The latter maybe a good sign of your body's fitness and health.) This measurement may be especially important if you plan to combine any mind-body methods with traditional aerobic exercise because most mind-body methods don't put a lot of emphasis on heart rate or its changes. This is more for your awareness and safety. You have a couple of options to test your resting heart rate:

> ✔ If you have a wireless heart rate monitor, you can put that on first thing in the morning before you get up, drink coffee, or start thinking about stressful deadlines or other stuff that keys you up.

> ✔ If you don't have a wireless heart rate monitor, put your two middle fingers (not your thumb) either on the inside of your wrist, or beside your Adam's apple. Relax and count beats for a minute for the most accurate reading. You can also count for less time and multiply to get the beats-per-minute reading.

Your resting heart rate is probably somewhere between 60 and 90 beats per minute — lower if you're already fit or have a genetic tendency to have a lower heart rate, higher if you are less fit (or already stressing for some reason).

Measuring your mental fitness

Okay, this is a *mind*-body book, so what about your mental state and attitude? In Chapter 4, I address certain principles basic to all mind-body practices. But you need to do other mental preparation, too.

Listening to your body

This ain't no competition, especially when you're in your own living room or backyard (as if the dog cares). Always listen to your body and stop if anything hurts, feels uncomfortable, or otherwise just isn't pleasant. This exercising — be it traditional or mind-body — is about feeling good.

Following your muse

Forget deciding to do Pilates-inspired movement just because "everybody else is," "my neighbor says she loves it," or "I just read an article in the newspaper about it." Try a practice that sounds like it's something you will like *and* stick to. Who cares if Madonna does Yoga or Drew Barrymore is dedicated to Pilates. This is the time to be selfish and think about you.

Taking heed of your gut feelings

If I recommend something, that doesn't mean it's etched in stone. If an exercise or movement doesn't feel right to you, forget it. Move on. Leave it out. Change it. Try a different method. Go find a teacher or class to see if you're doing it right. Take action. But don't ignore what your gut feelings tell you.

The next section looks at a couple of levels of low-to-moderate exercises. Exercise scientists call this an exercise prescription, but that name sounds about as palatable as cod liver oil. It's just your way to go.

Trying Aerobic Exercise

Aerobic exercise, is activity that raises your heart rate (see Chapter 2 for a more complete discussion). In this section, I talk about different ways of doing just that. Some mind-body methods may not be a way to raise your heart rate, but that's not the only reason to choose a fitness program. Still, for a well-rounded routine, you need to consider some aerobic exercise.

Going the traditional way

The traditional exercise model still stands as a recognizable way to improve aerobic fitness, lose weight, or get better physical performance, which may sometimes work with a few mind-body methods. The traditional regimen requires exercising:

✔ 3–5 days a week

✔ For 20–60 minutes at a time

✔ At 60–90 percent of maximum heart rate (moderate to vigorous)

That percentage can be pretty intimidating, especially because heart rate is hard to understand and even harder to measure during exercise for many people. The range of 60–90 means moderate to pretty dang hard.

Taking a softer, gentler approach

In 1995, the exercise powers-that-be came up with recommendations for another way to get healthier. This way requires exercising:

✔ On most days

✔ For 30 minutes at a time

✔ At low to moderate intensity

No, you won't lose oodles of weight or be able to compete in next weekend's 10K race. But this approach recognizes not only less intense forms of activity (such as some mind-body methods), but also non-traditional activities, such as walking the dog or vacuuming. It also recognizes the need to accept less for good health, such as lower blood pressure or lowered risk of heart disease. This approach also does not require you to check your heartrate. More is still better, the experts add, but a little is better than nothing.

Getting a Hold on Strength Workouts

Strength-building routines also offer a traditional prescription and a less-than-traditional prescription. The traditional meant too much time in a sweaty gym for many people.

Going the traditional way

The idea was to increase your muscle strength and endurance with the following workout pattern:

- 2–3 days a week
- 8–10 muscle groups each time
- 8–12 repetitions per muscle group
- 1–3 sets of repetitions

But the traditional idea was to do at least two, if not three, sets of repetitions, which could take 30 to 40 minutes for a workout. Time became an issue.

Taking a softer, gentler approach

So, in 2000, following a huge review of all the literature, the exercise gurus found that you don't have to do quite as much to improve your overall health! The new statement advocated an exercise regimen that includes:

- 2–3 days a week
- 8–10 muscle groups each time
- 8–10 repetitions per muscle group
- 1 set (only one!) of repetitions

Lo and behold, one quick set provides all the same healthy benefits such as lowered blood pressure, a stronger heart, lowered risk of heart disease, and so on. And this approach requires only about 10 minutes a couple of times a week, and even many mind-body methods give you a push in this direction. And you don't have to pump iron; you can yank on elastic tubing, do pushups, or other activity. That's doable. Once again, though, the experts say that more can be better for even more strength and fitness.

You may ask how this approach applies to mind-body fitness. Some of these mind-body methods do incorporate strength work like pushups and abdominal work. Don't neglect it if it's a part of the method. You may also question whether some of this less intense activity helps your aerobic health. It does: In a smaller way, but it does. But that also means that if you choose a truly non-aerobic mind-body fitness method, or do one so low level that it doesn't have an aerobic element, you may want to consider adding walking, cycling, or other cross-training to your week for well-rounded fitness.

As you begin to plot what you want to try, take these concepts of what fitness means into consideration so you get healthful exercise. If you have not been exercising at all in a long time, 10 minutes of Tai Chi — even as a very gentle movement — may be a lot. That's okay. Build slowly and add more or make it a little more intense as your body is ready. Pretty soon, you'll be ready for the longer and more intense routines or methods. In Chapter 19, I talk about how to combine some of these methods for a balanced mental and physical program.

Chapter 6

Managing Your Health Mindfully

• •

In This Chapter

▶ Examining the benefits of mind-body fitness

▶ Considering your environment

▶ Applying the benefits to your situation

▶ Reading real stories from real people

• •

I use the word "health" in this chapter title in the loosest sense — health of body, health of mind, health of spirit, all wrapped up in one package and not as separate pieces. Not just stand-alone physical health, like your dear ol' doctor says about your heartbeat sounding good through that cold stethoscope or your blood pressure being under the prescribed numbers. That looseness somehow seems fitting for this book on mind-body fitness, where the use of the word "fitness" is also in the loosest sense — fitness of body, fitness of mind, fitness of spirit, all in one grand package. Not stand-alone superficial fitness, like your health club may prescribe based on buff muscles, a tight tush, and curvaceous calves.

The problem is, researchers just haven't turned out enough quality, air-tight, peer-reviewed, placebo-controlled, statistically significant scientific studies to make the kind of broad conclusions that you and I would like to make — and some practitioners do make — about what you can gain from these mind-body methods. So many of the claims remain kind of loosey-goosey.

But it's not as if the researchers don't want to find a way to do a study that is sound or that they want to disprove the mind-body methods. It's just that for many of these methods, finding a truly scientific and air-tight way so that subjects won't know what a study's goal is can be very difficult to achieve. If subjects know the study's hypothesis, it taints the results and makes them not worth much. So without pages of scientific proof mind-body practitioners make all kinds of curative claims — some less than reputable, some purely anecdotal, but perhaps not so far-fetched.

You know what? Science doesn't have all the answers yet. And you know what else? Science probably never will have all the answers when it comes to mind-body practices. You will never find the "perfect" Yoga study or Qigong study or Alexander study, because removing all possibilities of bias by subject or researcher is next to impossible. And perhaps we don't need the "perfect" study.

You may find it interesting, however, that even the U.S. government has taken an interest in mind-body methods. The National Institutes of Health has a branch called the National Center for Complementary and Alternative Medicine. Its goal is to spark and fund research in these areas. So who knows what kind of great science we'll see five or ten years down the road? I'll stay tuned. You should, too.

For now, my recommendation is this, for whatever it's worth: Read a study citing some results. Take them at face value. They can prove interesting and even motivating. (I cite some in the next sections myself.) But don't be afraid to listen to anecdotes from your teachers or the books you read. Sometimes those stories of injuries-gone-away and diseases-that-disappear can mean more to you than some laboratory research done by planting electrodes on someone's body.

None of this information should make you dump your doctor and try something like curing liver cancer through meditation. Instead, consult with your doctor to see whether alternative practices are appropriate for you. Perhaps your doctor can make some recommendations specifically for your case. Read up on non-traditional healing methods. Perhaps supplementing your traditional medical care with, for example, some nontraditional Chinese moving meditation may help you feel better.

And who knows, it may even open your mind, make you more relaxed, and help you reduce stress, too.

Weighing the Variables

After you consider all the studies and their results over the years, three variables stand out in both quality research from reputable journals and questionable reports lacking true quantifiable criteria. If these three variables exist within a method, that method — often Yoga is the method of choice for study, but a few others have been, too — can produce health and fitness results. Again, remember that some of these health results are proven, and some may still only be hinted at in the science.

> ✔ **The method is mindful.** You aren't just cranking out postures or positions that make you work your muscles. Instead, you are using your mind in a meditative and inwardly focused manner during these positions and exercises.
>
> ✔ **The method emphasizes full and deep breathing.** Exhaling and inhaling fully as you do the movements is a key component to the method. Instructors and books prompt you to breathe during and while holding positions.
>
> ✔ **The method incorporates some muscular work.** It doesn't have to include high-intensity pushups and jumping around, just so long as you are using your muscles in some way, even lightly.

Stating which of the mind-body methods fit those three criteria is impossible because, well, you need to take some other factors into account, including:

> ✔ What style or school you choose
>
> ✔ How much exercise you do
>
> ✔ The intensity at which you do it

And even if science begins to see these three variables as key, the researchers don't really know to what degree each variable needs to be present in each method.

Remembering Your Environment

Sometimes even the environment in which you choose to practice can have a spectacular effect on what you get out of it. Try doing your meditations in the common room of a dorm. Hmm. Maybe in the living room while your kids are watching cartoons? Weeeeeell. How about in your Los Angeles apartment's courtyard facing a smoggy street with heavy traffic? Oh yuck. Now, you may not be able to sit in a beautiful forest every day. But you can still create a calm and focused atmosphere in a corner of your home or yard. Doing so can mean the difference between successfully managing your health with mindful work and not being so successful.

Light a candle. Hang a lantern. Put up a screen. Play a tape of restful water and bird sounds. Plug in a fountain so you can hear the peaceful sound of water tinkling over rocks. All these things can help create an environment for success. Refer to the Appendix for a few suggestions about where to find such accessories.

The ever-hopeful mind

Perhaps you've heard of the placebo effect. The effect comes into play when, for example, researchers give patients a sugar pill and tell them it will make them sleep better. The mind overpowers the body, and the people do indeed sleep better. The same idea applies with mind-body methods — you join a Qigong class because you hear it relieves arthritis pain. Several weeks later, you indeed have less pain.

The question is, is the possibility that the placebo effect occurred a bad thing? If you really are fitter, healthier, or pain- or disease-free, did you do yourself any harm? The mind has been shown to have a powerful effect on the body, whether spiritually or just optimistically. Mind-body methods take that power and actively applies it. So whether you believe in the mindful benefit, the spiritual benefit, the healing energy pulsing through the body, or, well, you just believe, you may indeed find what you want or need.

Sizing Up the Benefits

Depending on what method researchers use and whether they incorporate the right combinations of variable, studies have shown you can get a variety of positive physical benefits from mind-body fitness. Those benefits include

- Better cholesterol levels
- Decreased blood pressure
- Decreased chronic pain
- Decreased depression
- Decreased falls (particularly in seniors) due to better balance
- Decreased risk of cardiovascular disease
- Decreased stress and anxiety
- Increased aerobic fitness (stronger lungs)
- Increased endurance
- Increased immunity (less sickness)
- Increased muscle strength and flexibility
- Increased relaxation
- Less asthma
- Less low back pain

Now, that's quite some laundry list of possible health benefits! Keep in mind that some of these benefits apply only to certain methods, and some depend on the type or intensity of exercise you choose.

Of course, some of these benefits aren't fully proven by recognized scientific studies. Of the studies that have been done, some haven't excluded bias by subjects or researchers, and the findings of other studies haven't been replicated, which means the results haven't been repeated. (*Replication* is key for the scientists to know that the results weren't just chance.) Still, as you can see, this mind-body stuff ain't chicken feed in terms of what it can do for you.

Making the Benefits Work for You

In this section, I take you on a little stroll through what the literature shows about the physical benefits of mind-body fitness, citing some research as backup. Just for fun, I occasionally throw in a personal story from someone who has been-there, done-that, or felt-that. Remember, this isn't some thorough and exacting scientific review — c'mon, I'm not writing my thesis! — but instead a pleasant tourist trip where you can you can see a few sites and draw a few conclusions for yourself

Overcoming stress, anxiety, and other related maladies

"Related maladies" means depression, obsessive-compulsive disorder, and even heart disease because too much stress can increase your risk of developing any one of those conditions, too.

Living with success over stress

A slow and prolonged *exhalation* (the breathing out part of breathing) has been shown to enhance a reaction in the body that causes overall muscular relaxation. Chanting, singing, or breathing techniques can promote that slow and prolonged exhalation. If you are more relaxed, you handle your stress and your emotions more easily, and you may even sleep better.

One study specifically compared moving Tai Chi Chuan practices to walking and found that reactions in the body during Tai Chi were similar to the reactions caused by moderate fitness walking in reducing anxiety and increasing vigor. Of course, researchers even pointed out that people may have been biased after hearing of the wonderful relaxing effects of Tai Chi Chuan.

Success over stress

More than two decades ago, Larry Payne was an overworked, overstressed advertising sales executive for a major women's magazine based in tumultuous New York City. Low back pain was a part of his daily anxiety-ridden life. He consulted every medical professional and physical therapist known to man (at least to an overworked executive-type man) but got no relief. Then one day, a colleague dragged him — literally — to a Yoga class. "I will never forget it," said Payne. "I couldn't do a lot of the poses. But at the end of class during the relaxation, my back problem disappeared for the first time in three years. I knew I was onto something." Immediately after that, Payne took off on a two-week de-stressing, healing retreat, then he took a year-long sabbatical that led him to Yoga teachers and healers in 11 countries, including India. Payne, who is now a respected Yoga teacher and authority in Los Angeles and the co-author of *Yoga For Dummies,* has devoted himself to spreading the word about Yoga and its healthy lifestyle ever since.

The only study that actually used the NIA technique compared women who did NIA with women who just did traditional aerobic dance. Lo and behold, the NIA group had less anxiety and generally felt better. (I give you the lowdown on NIA in Chapter 17.)

Even non-aerobic methods like Feldenkrais and Alexander (both detailed in Chapter 16) may have tension-reducing effects that can leave you feeling better in your everyday life.

Lowering the risk of heart disease

When you aren't bound up by stress and anger, you just feel better on a day-to-day basis. But living without stress and anger may also cause decreases in your blood pressure, bad-cholesterol level, and other factors that can raise your risk of heart disease.

One recent journal article reviewed research about meditation and relaxation techniques (although not specifically mind-body exercise) and found a reduced risk of coronary artery disease. Yet another article, which also looked only at related areas such as relaxation breathing, found fewer secondary heart attacks after five years in patients with cardiac disease.

Controlling obsessive-compulsive behavior

One study recently found that simple breathing techniques had as much positive effect on people with obsessive-compulsive behavior as drugs did! That means the obsessiveness and compulsiveness decreased and allowed the people to live better day-to-day . . . without drugs.

Managing chronic disease

Chronic disease can mean any number of medical conditions, such as asthma, hypertension (high blood pressure), arthritis, *fibromyalgia* (a muscle disease that causes ongoing pain), or even cancer.

Dealing with high cholesterol or high blood pressure

One of many studies using simple, very low-intensity Qigong — in this case, Qigong walking — compared results from three groups: one that did meditative Qigong walking, one that did regular walking, and one that did nothing. The group that did Qigong walking, which is so slow that it doesn't really raise your heart rate to the level of any kind of aerobic workout, still ended up with lower heart rates. A lower resting heart rate can mean a stronger heart. A stronger heart can mean fewer problems with cholesterol and blood pressure.

Chronic disease: Real-life triumphs

Patricia Smith and Monica Linford had lives as different as night and day. Patricia, who was disabled, worked as a hospital administrator when she discovered that she had breast cancer. Monica, on the other hand, was "fit" (in the traditional sense) but extremely stressed by her work as a group-exercise instructor in England. She pushed herself from class to class until one day when she collapsed from utter fatigue and disease, later diagnosed as Chronic Fatigue Syndrome.

Patricia turned to all kinds of doctors for chronic pain — she even spent a couple of years on crutches, had surgery to block the pain, took strong painkillers, and underwent therapy for her depression. Then came the breast cancer with its chemotherapy and radiation. While recuperating from cancer treatments, Patricia discovered Qigong — the mind-body art known to heal — and began practicing, although at first she was still in great pain. Within about three weeks, however, the pain began to subside and for the first time in a decade, she cut back on the drugs. In three months, the pain and depression were gone. The cancer never returned. She

had reclaimed her life. Patricia became a Qigong instructor and is still practicing and teaching Qigong in Santa Cruz, California.

Monica wasn't really sure where to turn after the "fit and healthy" life she thought she knew collapsed around her: "Having ignored all the warning signs that my entire body was in crisis, I was finally brought to a complete standstill by an enormous abcess behind my left knee." After it was drained in an emergency room, a doctor appeared in the room: "You have a hole in your leg 1½ inches deep and 2 inches wide. It has taken us two hours to drain it. Whatever you are angry about, go and sort it out." That experience jolted Monica and prompted her to rethink her life. A Chinese medicine practitioner diagnosed her with — in simple terms — having sucked dry her "chi," or her body's energy. Monica then turned to Yoga, Meditation, Qigong, and other alterntative arts. Not only did the England-based instructor heal, but she also developed the Chi Ball mind-body fitness method, which combines many mind-body practices, because of her desire to share her healing experience with others.

Other proof shows that methods such as Yoga and Tai Chi can lower high blood pressure.

Coping with cancer

In no way am I telling you to practice a mind-body technique instead of seeing a regular physician, especially when it comes to treating a life-altering disease such as cancer.

That being said, there are people who give mind-body methods at least some credit for helping them manage chronic conditions. Some folks go even farther: My first Tai Chi teacher said he started practicing two to three decades earlier when he was diagnosed with a brain tumor. The brain tumor went away, and no operations were scheduled. He attributes the tumor's disappearance to his Tai Chi and Qigong practice. Proof? He has none. Except the fact that he's still alive and healthy.

Combating the effects of asthma

Enter the positive effects of breathing again. Practicing full and deep breathing stimulates the lungs and can cause positive increases in the amount of air you can get into and out of your lungs. If you can get more air in and more air out, you may be able to diminish the effects of asthma or other breathing ailments.

I know that if I breathe deeply and stay relaxed, I don't have the coughing fits I sometimes get due to exercise-induced *bronchospasm* (another way to say "coughing fits with exercise"). It's almost as if I do a little meditation when I start to feel my lungs tighten so I can mentally relax them.

Relieving arthritis and other chronic pain

People with arthritis or other kinds of joint pain know that every move can hurt, so they tend to move less. And that reduced movement causes the muscles and tendons that support their joints to get very weak.

Over the years, studies have shown that simple, gentle movements help relieve the pain and allow people with arthritis to function better day-to-day. Tai Chi, Qigong, and some Yoga exercises have been used as the gentle movement needed to stimulate the joints and free up movement to relieve pain. Mind-body exercises can also help alleviate pain. I'm talking about chronic pain here — the kind of pain that doctors often can't figure out but that causes diffuse problems. Sometimes this pain is due to chronic fatigue syndrome, fibromyalgia, lupus, or other related ailments.

One of many hundreds of studies done in China required two groups of pain patients to take Qigong classes. One class studied with a "real" master who is known to be able to "move energy" and heal with his energy. The other class was led by someone who could do the movements but wasn't known to be a healer, otherwise called a sham master. Pain decreased in both groups — researchers think because participants just believed — but pain symptoms in the group with the real master went down twice as much!

Beating pain at its own game

More often than not, back pain and injury stories surface as reasons people give for trying mind-body methods. Oh, other reasons are plentiful, too. Feet, hips, ankles, and the like all may bring one person or another to a mind-body method, too. But backs are one driving force.

Take, for example, the story of Tai Chi Chuan instructor Manny Fuentes from Louisiana. Fuentes wasn't new to Chinese movement when he started doing Tai Chi. Since college, he had been practicing combative arts such as Tae Kwon Do. Then — luckily, Fuentes can now say with a hint of sarcasm — he suffered a back injury that doctors later diagnosed as a nerve impingement. Traditional doctors gave him strong medications and told him to rest. But the injury continually flared up, causing debilitating back spasms. Frustrated at being unable to continue combative martial arts, Fuentes discovered the mindful martial arts. "My back responded very well to the training, and I am now also able to run, lift weights, and perform other physical activity," says Fuentes. "Doing Tai Chi has been very helpful in loosening the area and strengthening the surrounding muscles." Apppropriately, Fuentes now specializes in teaching Tai Chi to chronic pain patients and seniors.

Sometimes even health professionals have injuries that force them to rethink what they're

doing. Yamuna Zake, a longtime New York-based Yoga teacher and massage therapist, came up with her Body Rolling technique after she ripped up her left hip muscles when she had a baby at age 25. She ended up dislocating her hip because it didn't have the muscular support it needed. Depression struck. So did tears when she saw how that side of her body had started to atrophy. Later, while living in Spain with no one to give her massage, Zake began to experiment with a ball to work the deep muscles on her own. Now she teaches her technique to massage therapists, personal trainers, osteopaths, and other health professionals. (And her hip is just fine, thank you.)

Then there's Moira Stott, program director of the Pilates-inspired Stott Conditioning program. When she was in her late twenties, Stott had to quit her career as a professional ballet dancer with the City Ballet of Toronto. For years, she had ignored horrible foot pain in her quest to keep dancing, even when she broke her foot. Finally a doctor told her bluntly: Either you quit or you won't be able to walk when you're 35. Now, she and her husband, Lindsay Merrithew, co-own the international company that she orginally started to help other injured dancers recover. Stott now teaches and trains fitness professionals and has rediscovered her former self-esteem. And, at 39, she can still walk quite well.

Healing injuries

Sometimes people turn to mind-body methods temporarily to make a muscle feel better or to make an injury go away. The funny thing is, they often stay and become devoted followers after they see how much the movements can help.

I, for one, took to Yoga — actually, I went back to Yoga after doing it in college — when years later, as a competitive athlete, I ended up with chronic ankle sprains. I came for the rehab that the balance and strength training helped speed up; I stayed for the focused calm I left with after each class.

The physical balance that you can hone through the movements in many of these mind-body practices — such as Yoga, Tai Chi, or Qigong — can train the *proprioception* of the nerves and muscles (basically the muscle sense). When the muscles and nerves can sense correctly how and when to contract or fire, you don't fall or get hurt. Staying upright can help decrease not only sports injuries, but also broken hips in seniors. Core (abdominal) training emphasized in methods like Pilates also can help keep you from falling on your nose and getting hurt, too.

Broken hips and other bones caused when seniors fall cost the health care system heaps and heaps of money. And they cause the seniors who fall mountains of despair because the injuries often take from them any semblance of independence. Maintaining strong bones that can withstand a bump here and there is vital, but being able to stay upright can mean the difference between living in a nursing home or your own home.

Tai Chi, in particular, has been found to help physical balance. Its emphasis on slow, flowing movements mandates core control and one-legged balance throughout the practice. You may not actually hold a balance for a long time, but rather you move through it. To achieve the smooth flow of Tai Chi you must have balance, perhaps more so than to perform a more traditional exercise well.

Many studies have also shown that people who practice mind-body methods can have less chronic low-back pain. One study compared people who did a modern offshoot of the ancient practice of Tai Chi Chuan, called Tai Chi Chih, to a group that did not do the practice. What happened? Pain diminished in the Tai Chi Chih group and did not in the control group.

Because 8 out of 10 of us will have back pain at some point in our lives, mind-body methods may be an option worth considering.

Modern classic methods: Helping you reach your goals

When it comes to overall muscle and aerobic fitness, the Modern Classics you read about — Feldenkrais, Alexander, and Laban — don't generally do a whole lot for you. But don't just ignore them. Their focus on releasing muscle tension, improving posture, increasing movement efficiency, and improving how you perform certain tasks can help you do other things better that also make you more fit! Of course, doing other "things" may mean just lifting a baby without back pain or bending over to pick up something you dropped, but it could also mean running faster or jumping higher. Remember, fitness is a well-rounded picture, not just a toned body.

Rediscovering fitness and health

Rediscovering fitness and health can mean a lot of things, from a physical awareness to mental happiness to a greater meaning in life. Consider these two stories as motivation for you:

Nanci Conniff, a longtime fitness professional in Palo Alto, California, always prided herself on her fitness. Then at age 40, she had a baby, and due to complications had to stop all activity for the last 3½ months of her pregnancy — something she hadn't done in two decades. A few weeks after giving birth, however, she set out on her own reconditioning program, going to a private Pilates exercise studio. Mentally, she was ready, but she discovered that her body was not the same one she knew before having her baby. She had so little ab strength and had gained so much weight that she couldn't even begin to raise her hips off the ground while lying on her back. "I just started to cry," she admits, because exercise had always been so easy and enjoyable for her. But within a few weeks, as she also combined meditation with her movement, she started feeling like her old self again. And she even went a step farther because she now works as an aerobics instructor at Stanford University in California and also teaches Pilates classes.

As a young girl, Debbie Rosas, the co-developer of the NIA technique, had learning disabilities that left her with very low self-esteem — that is, until she discovered movement as an expression. Rosas became a successful aerobics instructor and studio owner in Northern California. But she felt that her life still lacked something. High kicks and jumps just weren't doing it. She and her fellow teacher (and future husband), Carlos Rosas, questioned the speed and style of aerobics. So in 1983, they changed all their classes, took off their shoes, began to dance and encourage feeling and flow, and started incorporating Eastern and Western mind-body methods into their routines. Considered forerunners in the fitness industry for their introduction of mind-body fitness long before it was truly recognized, it still took them years to get their method accepted. They now know that fitness is more than just a toned body, which is the message they work to spread through NIA.

Fostering function and fitness

Do you just want to get in and out of a low beach chair more easily? Do you want to make sure that you don't fall and break a hip when you get older? Do you want to run a marathon, or ride a bike better up hills? Mind-body methods may help you achieve all or part of those goals.

Honing muscle strength and flexibility

Particularly in elderly people, even the lowest-intensity forms of mind-body exercise show a cumulative effect on the muscles. Now, if you really push that Yoga class, NIA movement, or Tai Chi practice, you can challenge your muscles' strength and flexibility as much as with any other traditional Western exercise. Okay, science hasn't proven this idea. But you try it and see how you feel. You may be able to carry more bags of groceries due to more arm strength, or pick up something off the ground without pain because of greater low-body flexibility.

Rediscovering function

Want just to feel better each day? Following are the stories of two people who do:

In high school and college, Michael Purcell was a successful distance runner. But after that time he began to realize something was askew with his posture, partly because he was tight from all his running. He discovered the Feldenkrais method. "The strain and pain I had encountered was, as I came to see it, through my own misinterpretation of what I was supposed to do (with my body)," he says. Four years later, he trained with Moshe Feldenkrais and became a practitioner. Purcell also served as the Northern American Feldenkrais Guild president. "My previous self," he says, "is only a dim recollection."

Within a few weeks of starting to take an Alexander course, Robert Rickover says he grew an inch. Actually, he learned to stand up straight and take the pressure off a sway back. "I had a lot more energy," he says, "and my breathing seemed somehow easier." Soon Rickover quit his job as a research economist and went on a three-year trek to England to learn Alexander. "I believe," he adds, "the Alexander technique is one of the most powerful methods of self-discovery and self-transformation available."

Mind-body practices can also help you maintain flexibility, which people naturally lose as they age. Sometimes the idea of plopping on the floor for a stretch after the daily walk is just so, well, tedious. But if you incorporate stretching into your fitness practice — just all those forward bends and upward reaches — it's a lot easier not to ignore the healthful stretches, and they bring results, too.

Increasing aerobic endurance

Think that these slow-moving forms of mind-body exercise don't give you the aerobic pump that you need or want? Think again. Even a slow but steadily paced class or routine can produce about two-thirds the benefits of traditional aerobic programs, such as running or group exercise.

Promoting anti-aging

Researchers are beginning to realize that many of the conditions society has always attributed to "just getting old" are really the result of leading an unfit, sedentary life. So if you if you wrap up all the benefits cited in this chapter in one big box and tap into them all, guess what? You probably won't get old — or what the public perceives as old — as fast.

Part III
Yoga Primer and Postures

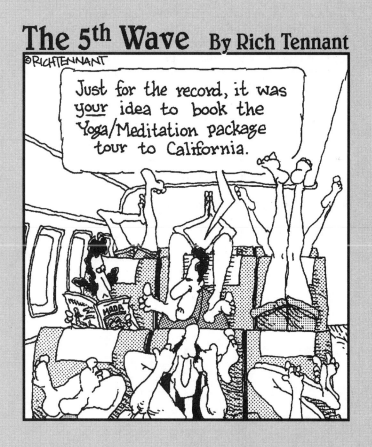

The 5th Wave   By Rich Tennant

Just for the record, it was your idea to book the Yoga/Meditation package tour to California.

In this part . . .

*I*n your quest to find out more about mind-body workouts, Yoga has to be the first method that comes to
mind. What is mind-body fitness without Yoga? What is
Yoga without its mind-body component? No matter what
your reason for practicing Yoga — as a meditative, spiritual, or physical art — the important thing is that you try it.

In this part, I give you the foundation you need, whether
you're trying Yoga for the first time or looking to increase
your exposure to this discipline. You can read about the
different types of Yoga, its benefits, various reasons to
practice it, and ways to determine which type is best for
you. I introduce you to a series of basic Hatha Yoga
postures with detailed instructions, as well as ways to
mix and match those postures in a workout depending
on your tastes, needs, and time constraints.

Chapter 7

You Go, Yoga! The Basics and Benefits

In This Chapter

▶ Discovering Yoga basics and styles

▶ Personalizing the benefits

▶ Sorting out equipment options

Although Yoga has been around for centuries (after its birth in India) as a spiritual, mental, and physical practice, the Western world can probably thank the hippies of the 1960s for bringing it to a wider audience. In the era of Woodstock and Haight-Ashbury, teens and twenty-somethings were looking for anything anti-establishment or anti–Western culture that helped them explore their own and the world's inner meaning. What better way to turn their back on their parents' world of *Father Knows Best* and canned-tuna casseroles than to sit cross-legged on the ground, burn incense, and meditate?

I find it intriguing that the interest in Yoga, which faded slightly in the last decade as baby boomers needed to work and raise kids, has now suddenly spiraled upward just as baby boomers are getting older but want to continue to exercise without pounding themselves into the ground. Even boomers who never exercised are looking to mind-body fitness like Yoga as something they can do successfully without pain and with both physical and spiritual gain. And why not? The benefits can't be beat.

To Ohmmm or Not to Ohmmm

For Yoga to be Yoga, you have to pay attention to the spiritual or meditative side of the practice. If you ignore that, Yoga becomes mere stretching with a funny name or an unfulfilling and perhaps funny-looking series of calisthenics abruptly placed one after the other.

Because I present mind-body *fitness* in this book and not purely devotional practices, I address the branch of Yoga called *Hatha Yoga,* which is the one that focuses on physical practice. (Refer to my list in the next section that introduces the different branches of Yoga.) If you want more devotional or extremely spiritual practices, you can use this introduction as a jumping off point.

You don't have to practice Hinduism or abandon other personal religious beliefs if you decide to experience the meditative, inner-calming, and physical powers of Hatha Yoga as a fitness activity.

Note, though, that I do use Sanskrit names — those derived from the classical Indic literary language and commonly used for names of Yoga postures — alongside their English translations. I believe it is important to fit the practice of Yoga — or any other art — into the culture from which it came to fully experience it, thus the inclusion of the Sanskrit names for postures and practices. A Taco is a Taco, not a flattened-cornmeal-pancake-filled-with-meat-and-cheese. Brie cheese is Brie cheese, not cheese-that-is-soft-in-the-middle. To ignore the Sanskrit names would be like having a BLT sandwich without the B. There'd just be something missing.

Long story short: As I move along using Sanskrit names and discussing meditational and deep-breathing aspects of Yoga, I may ask you to try a little "ohmmmm" a couple of times, but you don't have to if you don't want to. If you want to just get physical, you can do that, too. Keep in mind, though, that the more you open yourself to all the benefits Yoga and other mind-body methods offer, the more you can receive.

Connecting the Branches of Yoga to One Trunk

Just as the branches on a tree are all connected to the same trunk, so the many different Yogic disciplines all connect at a common root. And as you try the physical branch called Hatha Yoga, you may become intrigued enough to shimmy up the tree and explore other branches, too. Each branch itself then also has smaller leaves and twigs sprouting off it that represent various Yogic schools.

If you know a little about Yoga already and notice some differences from what you are familiar with as you move through this section and into the postures and sequences, remember that Yoga has innumerable schools and styles. Every one of these styles — sometimes a combination of several branches or schools where the teachers have studied under different or several mentors — has its own little niche. Consider this analogy: Your best friend likes peppermint ice cream. You like chocolate chip. You meet a third person who likes peppermint chocolate chip. And do either you or your friend think that the mint-chippy person has bad taste? Nope. Just a different flavor for a different taste. Same goes for Yoga. Keeping an open mind is always a good thing with mind-body practices.

Even though I don't go into detail about all the branches of Yoga in this book, of which there are at least eight depending on how you classify them, knowing a little about each helps you fit your own practice into the picture and gives you tips as to which branch you may want to move toward.

The following list introduces you to the basic branches of Yoga:

- **Bhakti:** a practice of devotion. Bhakti followers place devotion to a supreme being ahead of all else and may include offerings — physical and mental — to that being. The heart is the focus.

- **Guru:** a practice of dedicating yourself to a master. A follower dedicates him or herself to one enlightened master.

- **Hatha:** the disciplined physical practice. Hatha attempts to balance body and mind and to bring the ultimate goal of all Yoga branches — enlightenment — to fruition through disciplining the body. Followers believe the body must be prepared, strengthened, purified, and fully aware before enlightenment can be achieved. (I explain a little bit more about different schools of Hatha Yoga in Chapter 8. Ashtanga Yoga, popular today because of its athleticism, is a style of Hatha Yoga, as is also Bikram Yoga, where followers practice very physical postures in rooms that swelter in temperatures near 100 degrees Fahrenheit.)

   Whichever branch you ultimately follow, a true Yoga follower (called a *yogi* if he's male and a *yogini* if female, and *yogis* for more than one of either gender) finds healthy living and taking care of the body important components of the practice. A true yogi/yogini, for example, doesn't go to class and then stop for lunch at the closest Beef and Fries Hut and follow that with a double beer chaser.

- **Jnana:** a practice of wisdom. The goal of followers is to look beyond the wisdom accepted as reality and — through meditation and contemplation — begin to understand Truth. Instead of thinking through a Truth, though, all of what is commonly thought to be true is questioned. Enlightenment occurs by going inside yourself and discovering the divine Truth.

- **Karma:** a practice of self-transcending action. Karma followers are all about working for the good of society and acting unselfishly, because they recognize that every action has far-reaching consequences.

You may also sometimes find a branch called Kriya, used in the same breath as Karma, because it also involves action, but in this case more spiritual action.

✔ **Mantra:** a practice of powerful, sacred sound. This is another branch of Yoga that you may not always find on the tree because the use of sound can be a part of the other branches, too. You use sound to bring the body and spirit into harmony. Mantra followers receive a personal *mantra* (a syllable, word, or phrase) from their teachers that they, and only they, know and use in their practice. For some Westerners, any word that sounds good and vibrates in your body can work to experiment casually with Mantra Yoga.

✔ **Raja:** the Royal practice. This is the classical practice with its eight-step (or "eightfold") path to enlightenment and true ecstasy. It becomes very esoteric and your best chance to understand it is to explore it very thoroughly.

✔ **Tantra** (also known as **Kundalini**): the practice of continuity. This branch is all about customs and rituals, and although folks have connected the principles of Tantra to sex, it is certainly not just about sex. The rituals and visualizations that followers practice are immensely detailed and demand great focus.

Realizing the Benefits, Whichever Branch You're Out On

What you get from a regular Yoga practice can vary with the branch you decide to go out exploring. But no matter which branch suits you, you experience certain basic benefits across all the branches.

Take note of the word "regular" describing "practice" in the first sentence of the preceding paragraph. Doing Yoga once a month isn't regular, and you won't reap the benefits that are possible if you practice Yoga or another mind-body method several times weekly or even daily. That would be like going on a diet one day every couple of weeks and expecting astounding results. Won't happen.

That's not to say that if you're looking strictly for physical benefits (such as more flexibility) that mesh with other types of traditional workouts you also do, that you won't get these benefits. You will — in some minor way. Then Yoga becomes that fancy stretching class. And if you are clear that's what you want and are honest with yourself about what you're getting, go ahead. Just know that the omnipresent calm or meditative powers — and most certainly the enlightenment that yogis talk about — doesn't come home with you with this kind of practice.

Spelling out the ABCs of Yoga benefits

The following sections talk about the areas where you can make the most important personal gains with regular Yoga practice:

A for awareness

Awareness doesn't just mean being more aware of, say, a car down the street or other material things. It means being more aware of the smallest things, from a tiny sound in the distance to a gentle twinge of energy in one part of your body. Because of Yoga's demand for concentration, you train yourself to be much more attentive to yourself, your feelings, and your surroundings.

B for breathing

Breathing keeps cropping up as I talk about mind-body fitness, and I keep bringing it up throughout the book because it's such an important component of almost every mind-body practice. Different methods involve different ways of breathing — something you and I take for granted. In Yoga, a true follower breathes through his or her nose both on the inhalation and exhalation. Yogis fill the abdomen deeply and fully without worries about keeping the belly pulled in and flat.

The most concrete benefit of a conscious and continuous breath is that it can increase the function of your lungs and the muscles that support your breathing, such as the abdominals and diaphragm. That can maintain strong and steady breathing, even as you age. A few simple solid breaths, not to mention regular deep breathing overall, can release stress and anxiety and promote relaxation, too. (Check out Chapter 6 for more information about the benefits of mind-body fitness, including breathing practices.)

C for calming and concentrating

Ever have a day when you feel utterly scattered and can't seem to concentrate on the smallest task? We all do. And perhaps that's one reason you're interested in mind-body fitness — to gain some focus in a distracting world.

Yoga is one method that can help you find out how to calm yourself in a fast-paced world and life and can also help you after you posses that calm to concentrate and focus more. How does Yoga do that specifically? In the physical practice of Hatha Yoga, your calming concentration is brought into power along with your awareness and breathing (the first two of the ABCs in this section), which have to be at full power as you move your body through different postures. If you don't concentrate and breathe, you may fall over, fall out, or tip over . . . which can of course still happen as you discover a new posture or refine your Yoga practice.

Enjoying other beneficial perks

In Chapter 2, I talk about overall benefits of mind-body fitness, but I want to quickly review the ones that apply to Yoga specifically.

✔ **Reducing stress:** Even without the pluses of a regular practice that brings an awareness of body, soul, and earth, you can achieve a reduction in your stress and an increase in your relaxation. Just taking the time for yourself each day to do some deep breathing can help you get there.

✔ **Gaining flexibility:** Whether you choose to practice Hatha Yoga as a purely physical endeavor for fitness or as a path to enlightenment, you can still find the benefit of greater flexibility from elbows to ankles, hips to hands. Greater flexibility can mean fewer injuries overall.

✔ **Building up your strength:** Most people don't imagine that Yoga is a path to greater muscular strength, tone, and definition, but it is. Some powerful moves involve not only *dynamic muscle contractions* (where you move your body through space), but also *isometric contractions* (where you don't move a limb through space but still actively contract your muscles).

✔ **Developing some endurance:** *Endurance* is the ability to do an activity steadily over a period of time without stopping. Marathon runners, for example, have great endurance! But yogis can also develop great endurance, by combining postures one after another in a quickly moving power Yoga sequence that pushes their limits and their heart rate.

✔ **Improving posture:** With Yoga, you will use your arms, back, shoulders, and abdominals in very aligned positions. That means you'll strengthen those muscles that are so key to being able to stand tall with good posture and without fatiguing. Also, having a good, strong, aligned spine can decrease or eliminate low back pain.

Using Yoga Your Way

If you read through the first part of this chapter, where I review the eight branches and their philosophies and I take a look at the basic benefits of Yoga, you probably already have a good idea how you can or want to use Yoga . . . or if you will. The reasons and benefits in this section may give you ideas about other ways to use Yoga.

Tuning in to Yoga relaxation and meditation

You may choose to use only the meditative and relaxing postures of Yoga, or focus on awareness and breathing. These aspects of Yoga can help you both calm down and de-stress, which means that Yoga may become more of a pre-bedtime meditation or a relaxing cooldown for you after other exercise or activity.

Practicing Yoga for fitness and as sport

You'd rather not get all wrapped up with enlightenment; it's the muscular toning and flexibility that intrigues you. A practice for you is purely physical. Sure, you breathe and focus, but that's not the top priority. The fitness training is. Or maybe Yoga is cross-training for your other activities or as a pure sport itself.

Working with Yoga for therapy and rehabilitation

One of the ways I've used Yoga over the years is as injury rehabilitation. Although I frankly believe the injuries served more to remind me that I'd fallen off the wagon, so to speak, and would feel a heck of a lot better if I got my behind back into a Yoga class. The flexibility, strength, and balance training can stretch and tone parts of your body, such as your back, hamstrings, or ankles, so you don't hurt them as often.

Finding Yoga as a way to manage chronic disease

More and more, Hatha Yoga is recommended by the medical community as a way to manage diseases such as coronary disease, anxiety disorders, high blood pressure, and muscle and nerve diseases such as fibromyalgia. Refer to Chapter 6 for more detailed information about the medical benefits of mind-body fitness, including Yoga.

Practicing Yoga as a path to spiritual awakening

Maybe it really is the spiritual and meditative discipline that rocks your world. You can focus purely on that aspect and train yourself to work more with your mind, perhaps even moving toward becoming comfortable with calling yourself a "yogi" or "yogini."

Making Matting (And Other Equipment) Decisions

Look at Chapter 3 for more of an overview of all the different kinds of stuff you may need for a mind-body practice such as Yoga, including pointers about your clothes, hair, and feet. But here I list a few specialty items.

Yoga is a simple mind-body practice. Bottom line is, you really don't need any stuff. Okay, okay, if you don't have any carpet in your house, you probably need a remnant of carpet or a few thick towels to cushion your bones on some postures. But you don't really have to go out and buy a mat.

If you decide to buy a special mat, look for a *sticky mat*, which I describe in Chapter 3. Maybe even two mats are good if you have prominent hip bones or *vertebral spines*. Those are the bony ends of each vertebrae running all up and down your back.

Beyond that, you need nothing else to start (except your energy and a water bottle). Other props come as you develop your practice. I mention in the instructions (in Chapters 8 and 9) a few places where you may want to use a prop in some of the postures, depending on your own abilities or preferences. These props include:

- ✔ **A strap, belt, or long towel:** You use these to help you hold onto a limb that you can't reach as well with your hands because of some inflexibility.

- ✔ **Blocks of wood or hard foam:** You use these in places where, for example, you would normally put a hand on the floor but you can't reach the floor yet. They act as "floor extenders," so to speak. (But a short stack of books will do.) You also use them to sit on to enable you to do hamstring stretches better. (But a short stack of blankets will do, too.)

- ✔ **Bolsters:** You place these cushions under your back, knees, buttocks, or head, either as a cushion or to help the body into a position. You can also use simple pillows to see if you like them.

- ✔ **Eye bags:** These can block out light and help you move more easily into relaxation or meditation. But a towel folded over your eyes will do, too.

As you get more and more into Yoga, you find all kinds of other stuff you may want to try. Take a look at some of the resources in the appendix for places to shop or other ideas.

Now, however, it's time to get moving!

Chapter 8

Preparing Yoga Postures

In This Chapter

▶ Tuning in to Yoga types

▶ Discovering Yoga principles and postures

▶ Hastening to Hatha

▶ Practicing the postures

*I*n some mind-body exercise methods, I go right to the punch line in the movement section, immediately explaining the basic concepts and jumping right in to give you an exercise sampler. Well, with Yoga, you need a little introduction before you can dig right in. You may want to read a little bit about the Sanskrit terminology, since I use these names, so you can understand more about the movements as you go along. I particularly believe there is something about the sounds of these Sanskrit words that really puts you more in the mood. Okay, that's one woman's opinion, but see what you think as you move through this section.

First of all, yogis tend to call the movements *postures* in English, versus exercises. I suppose you could call them exercises if you're just, umm, exercising. But if you add any of the awareness or concentration basics, then they aren't just exercises, in the way that a pushup is an exercise. You may also hear the movements called *poses*. Some people prefer one term and shun the other; some interchange them.

Speaking the Language of Yoga

In Sanskrit — the language of Yoga — the accents are not in the traditional English positions of second or third syllables, so watch your automatic responses when you say these aloud. You may hear these said different ways, but try to let the words sort of roll off your tongue in one fell swoop without a huge emphasis on any syllable. And let all the syllables lengthen gracefully rather than grind or swell to stops as is common in English.

Now, where was I? Oh, yeah, postures. . . .

- **Asana** *(ah-sah-nah):* This literally means "posture." A posture can be standing; it can be sitting, but it is a stationary posture. In Yoga, a descriptive Sanskrit word is tacked onto the front of the word "asana" to create a specific posture. For example, one you see early and often in this book is "tadasana" *(tah-dah-sah-nah).* In Sanskrit, *tada* means palm tree, which is a tall, stately tree. And that's what tadasana is: a tall stately posture (called *Mountain Posture* in its English translation).

- **Chakra** *(tshah-kra):* Actually spelled "cakra" despite the common English addition of an "h," a chakra is a center of energy between the top of your head and the base of your spine. Chakra literally means "wheel." Think of these centers of energy as little pinwheels. If the wind stops or you hold an end of one tip, it stops turning or turns very slowly. Same with your energy centers, which are thought to be wheels that whirl actively — unless your energy is blocked. In Chapter 18, I talk about some methods to ground and center yourself that work well anywhere. These methods subtly use the energy from the chakras. Refer to Chapter 4 for more detailed information about your energy centers.

- **Mudra** *(moo-drah):* A mudra is normally a hand gesture added to a posture. However, it's not just any hand gesture, but rather one that is said to "seal" or "lock" the life energy inside the body. It is said that when the life energy escapes, it can cause ill health and unhappiness. "Namaste," (see the following bullet) is a mudra.

- **Namaste** *(nah-mah-stay):* Whether you want to find a spiritual balance through Yoga or you just want to work out, you use *namaste.* It is a simple prayer-like position with your hands in front of your breastbone, thumbs touching the breastbone, fingers and palms pressed together, and elbows high. Many asanas or vinyasas (see the last bullet item) start or finish with a position that includes namaste. Perhaps you've been in traditional exercise classes where everybody applauds at the end? Well, in Yoga, you find a quick moment of quiet with your hands in namaste, then all students bow slightly toward the teacher and say, "Namaste" as the teachers also bows slightly in return saying, "Namaste." It translates loosely as "May the divine light be with you" or "I salute the divine light within you." A nice parting word, blessing, and thank you, don't you think?

If you don't have a lot of flexibility in your forearms, even putting your palms and fingers together may be a painful stretch. Don't force it! Instead, just interlace your fingers in some way at your chest so you can still get the energy connection. You can also lower your elbows with your palms together, too.

- **Pranayama** *(prah-nah-yah-mah):* As one word, this means "breath control." Controlling your breath (see Chapter 7) helps you concentrate and boosts your health. This word stems from "prana," which means "life force" or "life energy." You help your life force and energy flow smoothly without hurdles and bumps by using good breath control.

> ✔ **Vinyasa** *(vee-nyah-sah):* This means "sequence" and is used quite a bit in certain styles of Hatha Yoga where smoothly linking together asanas into a vinyasa is a basic tenet of the practice. No matter what style you practice, try linking together your asanas (postures) for flow.

Recognizing the Key Principles

To properly master Yoga and attain some or all of the benefits, you want to keep a few principles tucked safely under your sticky mat for safekeeping. I describe these principles in this section.

Three basic benefits of Yoga are awareness, breath control, and calm. (See Chapter 7 for more about these basic benefits of Yoga.) These basic benefits are also among the basic principles — here I present a way to put them into action:

> ✔ Be aware
> ✔ Breathe
> ✔ Stay calm and concentrate

So keep these principles in mind as you move forward.

Breathing

I talk about breath a lot because I can't talk about it enough. Every mind-body method preaches the importance of breathwork in successful and energizing movement. In every mind-body method, and especially in Yoga, the motto is: Keep breathing, and breathe deeply and consciously.

Keeping a good attitude

Look for an open and dedicated attitude that allows you to find an inner quiet as you explore different movements and what they make you feel inside and out. Check negative attitudes at the door — for example, doubt about your abilities or judgment about your looks. Yoga demands openness, and you may discover characteristics that don't work well for you, or ones you thought did work but suddenly don't sit right.

Grounding yourself

Whether you are standing or sitting, on one foot or two, make sure that you're firmly planted on the ground with all edges of your feet (or legs or buttocks) feeling the surface. Try not to float on top of the earth as if someone just plopped you down there. Rather, feel as if you are a true part of the earth, as if you are a tree growing out of the ground.

Aligning yourself

Check out your body and put it in not only correct spinal alignment (not swaybacked or stooped shoulders, for example), but also in a position that feels good. In your Yoga positions, you should feel long, strong, powerful, and energized, not as if you're hanging there all sloppy. You should feel a powerful breath flowing through you and a strong center with good alignment and posture. If you can't breathe comfortably, check your alignment. (Chapter 4 has a section on how to achieve good alignment and a neutral spine.)

Modifying poses when necessary

Don't be afraid to alter a posture so that it feels good. If I say to turn your knee out a certain way, but you stare at the book like I'm crazy, then don't! Listen to your body and place yourself in such a way that allows your energy to flow. You shouldn't be grunting and straining and in pain. Yikes, is that ever contradictory to the principles and concepts of Yoga practice!

Accepting the mind-body connection

After you get into the position or modification that feels right to you, accept it. Yoga is not a competition with a goal and a finish line. Like other mind-body methods, it is a process, not an end. So accept where you are right now as perfect. Tomorrow may be different. But that'll be perfect, too. Until you can accept, you may have difficulty making those steps to a mind-body connection.

Releasing your tensions

Let go of clenched teeth, fisted hands, curled toes, hiked-up shoulders, and other tension in your body when you are in a pose. Relax into the posture and see whether that modification or position still works for you. If that gripping is what kept you there, perhaps another modification is in order.

Meditating

No, no, we haven't come to the "ohmmmm" word. Yet. But in each posture, allow yourself to pause, breathe, and settle into the position. Turn your focus slightly inward and relax. Take a few moments to just be. That can be pretty hard. I know, because normally I am the queen of ants-in-her-pants — until I get to a Yoga session and I let myself "be" and settle into that moment. Try some breathing and concentration to keep yourself in a meditative or contemplative mindset.

It Hasta Be Hatha

Many of those who now teach Yoga or other mind-body practices took it up when they were trying to heal themselves in some way, physically or mentally. Traditional exercise or healing disenchanted them. Then they found Yoga. But they weren't happy with one cookie-cutter version. They had to carve out their own pattern with slight changes to sequence, breath, or other mechanics, based on a combination of teachings from different mentors, gurus, swamis, masters, or sages.

A little Yoga humor: How many yogis does it take to screw in a light bulb? One. But 99 others will do it differently.

The physical form of Yoga — Hatha Yoga — has numerous styles, and you may find that some classes are blends of those styles, sequences, and postures. Don't let that alarm you! No one can tell you that one path is correct and the others incorrect. Remember, it's all a process. Just do what feels right to you, and you're on the road to discovery.

The following list gives you a few of the names for Hatha styles you may see, and the primary emphasis of that style. This list just helps you get familiar with some names you may stumble across as you move along your personal path:

- **Ashtanga**: Ever heard of Power Yoga? It's not some fitness guru's concoction, but the teachings of a real yogi, born many decades ago, by the name of K. Patthabi Jois, who originally studied under Krishnamacharya. This is athletic stuff that can challenge your muscles and turn your sticky mat into a slippery (with sweat) mat. Not really for beginners unless you're already extremely fit.

- **Bikram:** Rumor has it that a Bikram class leaves you grinning ear to ear. Whether that's true or not, it is another highly powerful style that isn't for beginners. But if you want Yoga for the Stars, this be the style done by the Hollywood trendophiles. Bikram, which has become quite popular lately, is very physical, very strenuous, and is taught in sweat-box studios with temperatures reaching 100 degrees Fahrenheit or so. Not for the weak of heart . . . literally, or for anyone with back problems or most chronic diseases.

✔ **Integral:** Another disciple of Swami Sivananda, Swami Satchidananda, developed this form, then became a part of new age history with an appearance at Woodstock in 1969. He's probably responsible for all those hippies who started practicing various forms of Yoga, chanting "ohmmmm" . . . and getting on their parents' nerves.

✔ **Iyengar:** You can thank B.K.S. Iyengar for popularizing the use of blocks, belts, bolsters, and other Yoga equipment that can help you achieve a perfect asana. These aids make it possible to practice Yoga postures even if you're not as flexible as you'd like to be or have other physical limitations. Posture perfect is one of the key terms here. You see a lot of Iyengar being practiced in the West.

✔ **Kripalu:** A three-step program well-suited for Western needs and progressions, partly because it breaks down breathing and alignment in very clear ways. A good place to get your feet wet.

✔ **Kundalini:** Originated by Sikh master Yogi Bhajan, Kundalini style uses postures, breathwork, meditation, and chanting to awaken the "kundalini" or "serpent power" within. Your energy with this style is directed through the *chakras* or energy centers along the spine. (Refer to Chapter 4 for more on energy centers.) The style places an emphasis on the integration of several breathing techniques. Headquarters of this very separate branch are in Los Angeles.

✔ **Sivananda:** If you want a pure Yoga book, consider the beautifully illustrated classic, *The Complete Illustrated Book of Yoga,* by Swami Vishnudevananda (Crown Publishers, 1960), a disciple of Swami Sivananda. Don't be put off by the 1960 original publication date! This is a very comfortable practice, with sequences you can feel at home with. This book is out-of-print, so to obtain a copy, check your local library or ask your favorite bookseller if they can do a search for you. You may be able to find it through an out-of-print specialty shop, or you can search the major bookstores online for out-of-print books. Or check out a Yoga studio near you that has it and is willing to loan it to you.

✔ **Viniyoga:** This is a slower, flowing, and more sequenced approach that you see in many clubs today, but was originated by Shri Krishnamacharya. Asanas coordinate with the breath, and practitioners are encouraged to breathe into a stretch, moving just a little farther on an exhale. Great for beginners because of the slow approach.

You can choose from literally thousands of postures, or *asanas,* not including all the variations on a theme concocted by one swami or another. I introduce you to a dozen or so basics, starting with some warm-up asanas (yes, even yogis warm up). I go through some strength, flexibility, and compensation (or resting) asanas, then show you some meditative or relaxing ones.

But don't just open the book and go through the entire menu of postures your first time out. In fact, people probably never just go through the entire list, one after the other. You may even try some postures that you'll just never do again because they don't feel good to you or they hurt your knees, back, or neck. That's okay. I want you to be wise in your choices. Yoga is not about pain, but all about gain.

Working through the Three Parts of a Yoga Session

Just as you wouldn't randomly toss furniture into a room — a bed here, a stove next to it, the workbench over there — you don't want to toss the parts of the basic Yoga menu together whimsically. I discuss mixing and matching your Yoga lineup in Chapter 9, but look here for the explanations of the postures.

The following list explains the three parts of a Yoga session. Remember to breathe into and with the pose.

- ✔ **Warm-up:** You want to massage your muscles and do some movements to raise your body temperature so you are safely prepped for more active movement and deeper stretches to come. Breathing helps your body warm up better.

- ✔ **Posture-pacing:** This is the middle section where you "find your pace" and move through the asanas actively. You also apply so-called "compensation" postures to rest muscles whenever you need to as you pace along. Again, breathe fully and deeply to help you achieve the postures comfortably.

- ✔ **Home stretch:** This consists of two sections to make up the final third of a session:

  - **Stretching:** After thoroughly warming up and moving, your muscles are now ready to stretch more deeply and always with a conscious breath.

  - **Relaxation:** Man, this is like the butter on the bread. Did you do all that work to just get up and walk away? Time to relax, breathe calmly, and meditate.

Getting into It: 22 Asanas to Try

Warm-up postures in Yoga are less of the jumping-around type — or the type of warm-up you do in a traditional Western exercise session — and more about gently telling your body that you're going to be moving more. You can do some warm-up postures during a session, too, but in a session, you probably want to do them with a bit more intensity or push the stretch a bit farther.

Use the warm-up to help you begin to focus and breathe mindfully.

Warming up

Take these as gently as you need to as you begin to move. You're warming up your sides, waist, hips, upper back, arms, and shoulders, as well as your neck.

Side Stretch

Shown in Figure 8-1, the Side Stretch, appropriately enough, works your sides. Try Side Stretch during your warm-up or stretching sections.

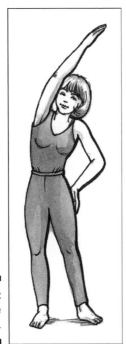

Figure 8-1:
Side
Stretch.

1. **Stand tall with your feet about hip-width apart and your arms hanging comfortably at your sides.**

2. **Lift your right arm out to your side and straight up, turning the palm up as it goes higher than your shoulder and reaches overhead.**

3. **Let your left arm hang palm-down against your thigh.**

   If you feel any neck, spine, or low back tension, you can widen your stance, bend your knees, and rest your left hand on your hip or thigh to take pressure off your lower back. Also, modify the stretch so you are only stretching upward and not to the side.

4. **Turn your head to look down over your left shoulder and reach your right arm up and out, rather than over and down.**

5. **If you are comfortable with that, also turn your head so you are looking into your right arm.**

   If you feel any neck tension, continue to face front and relax.

6. **Return to the start position and repeat on the opposite side.**

What to avoid:

✔ Tension in your neck

✔ Hiking your shoulder up to your ears

✔ Sinking in your back

Cat and Cow

You may also hear this called a Cat and Dog stretch. Choose whichever name suits your animal fancy! This pose helps massage and warm up your back muscles, as well as wake up your abdominals, and is shown in Figure 8-2. Try Cat and Cow during your warm-up phase.

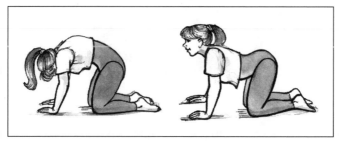

Figure 8-2: Cat and Cow.

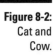

This is a particularly nice posture for pregnant women because it can help relieve low back pain. Just don't force your lower back to move beyond your comfort zone and do consult with your physician to be sure it is suitable for you.

1. **In an all-fours position, place your hands directly below your shoulders and your knees directly below your hips. Even though you are kneeling, think "tall" by lengthening your spine and keeping your neck strong and not drooping down.**

2. **Inhale, then exhale and round your back up like a mad Halloween cat. Allow your head to drop and your tailbone to pull underneath you. Pull your abdominal muscles in.**

3. **Inhale and arch your back like an old gray mare, lengthening your neck so you look slightly upward.**

   If this hurts your neck, keep your head neutral — facing the floor.

4. **Repeat this in a flowing pattern several times, allowing the breath to continue its pattern.**

What to avoid:

✔ Letting your abdominals just hang there

✔ Over-extending your back when you arch it

✔ Compressing your neck when you look up

Knee to Chest

You warm up your hips and hip flexors, gluteals, and hamstrings with this warm-up, shown in Figure 8-3. Try Knee to Chest during your warm-up or posture-pacing sections.

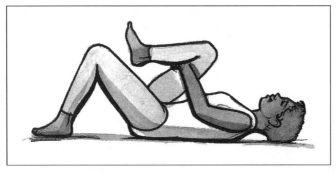

Figure 8-3:
Knee to
Chest.

1. **Lie on your back, keeping good alignment and focus.**

2. **Bend both knees so that your feet are on the floor.**

3. **Lift your right knee to your chest, grasping either your shin or behind your knee.**

   If you are lying comfortably with your hips firmly on the floor, you can begin to straighten your left leg away from you. If your neck, back, or hips start to peel off the floor, stop and return to the position that keeps you aligned. If you're flexible, you may be able to extend the leg completely.

4. **Hold this position and breathe comfortably for a minute, then return the right leg to the floor and repeat on the opposite side.**

What to avoid:

> ✔ Lifting your hips off the floor
>
> ✔ Dropping your head back
>
> ✔ Holding your breath

Lying Hamstring Stretch

You can do this stretch as a continuation of the preceding Knee to Chest posture. You get a good stretch of your hamstrings in the back of your lifted leg, and of your hip flexors in the front of your support leg. Try Lying Hamstring Stretch during your warm-up or stretching sections.

1. **Lie on your back with both knees bent and your feet on the floor. Your arms remain at your sides for now.**

2. **Raise your right knee to your chest, grasp the back of your thigh with both hands, and lift your foot toward the ceiling, holding your foot in whatever position is comfortable.**

   You should be able to straighten the leg that you're lifting overhead. If not, lower it slightly. If this is comfortable, you can slide your hands to where you can hold your shin, ankle, or even foot. You can also try flexing your foot, so the sole is facing toward the ceiling, for a deeper stretch.

   If you are much more flexible, you can also try this posture with an extended bottom leg. But only if your hips don't curl up off the floor. You must be able to keep your spine long and your buttocks down.

3. **Hold this position and breathe comfortably for a minute, focusing on the muscles that are working, then lower the leg and repeat on the other side after a short rest with both knees to chest.**

What to avoid:

> ✔ Lifting your buttocks up off the floor
>
> ✔ Bending your leg that's up
>
> ✔ Reaching forward with your shoulders

Standing and forward-bending asanas

These asanas are combinations of postures that you can use in the flowing sequences called *vinyasas* or as simple stretches. You can repeat each asana several times as is comfortable for you.

Mountain Posture — Tadasana

You may think it easy to just stand there, but this posture pushes the envelope of easy if you do it correctly and mindfully. Practice Mountain Posture a lot because you can do so much with it, as well as return to it during sequences and between stretches to rest. Also, Mountain Posture, shown on the Cheat Sheet in the front of this book, is the basis for the stability and balance you need to master other standing asanas. Try Mountain Posture during your warm-up, posture-pacing, or relaxation sections.

1. **Stand tall with your feet slightly narrower than hip-width apart and your hands hanging down at your sides, palms turned toward your thighs.**

2. **Imagine a string at the crown of your head, pulling you up tall. Practice a good aligned spine and open chest and shoulders, without adding any tension to the posture.**

3. **Breathe deeply and bring the focus inside. Sense how everything relaxes, yet stays stable and balanced.**

If you are comfortable here, you can also close your eyes. Careful! Balance is much more difficult with your eyes closed because you don't have visual landmarks to help you. You have to use the muscles and nerves in your feet and ankles more to sense your body's position in space.

4. **Feel your weight centered on your feet, with your arches lifted. Relax your face, eyes, and jaw.**

5. **When you are ready, step out of the posture and shake out your arms.**

What to avoid:

✔ Slouching

✔ Caving in your chest

✔ Putting your weight on your heels

Standing Forward Bend — Uttanasana

This asana, shown in Figure 8-4, is another one that sounds easy enough but actually takes continued work. You stretch your hamstrings in the back of your legs, your calves, Achilles tendons, and, of course, your back also. Try Standing Forward Bend during your posture-pacing or stretching sections, after you are thoroughly warmed up.

Make sure you have a doctor's clearance if you have back problems. Also, because this is an introductory version of an inversion posture, talk to your doctor first about whether you have glaucoma or any other eye disorders, or high blood pressure. Placing your head below your heart can put a strain on the blood flow or strain overly tight back muscles, for some people. (Refer to Chapter 6 for tips and cautions on how to use mind-body methods for various medical benefits and in certain circumstances.)

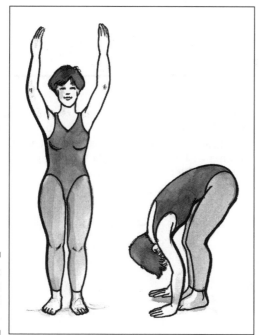

Figure 8-4:
Standing
Forward
Bend.

1. **Start in Tadasana (See "Mountain Posture" on the Cheat Sheet).**

2. **Inhale and lift your arms forward and then overhead.**

3. **Exhale and bend forward from the hips, folding your body from the hips (not the waist) toward the ground. When you start to feel tightness in your back or the back of your legs, bend your knees to allow yourself to hang lower. Keep your weight forward on the balls of your feet.**

4. **Relax your neck and let your head just hang loosely. Touch the floor if you can. Breathe.**

   If you can't touch the floor, put a block in front of your feet and rest your hands on it, or, if that is uncomfortable, place your hands on your thighs for support as you hang there.

5. **When you're ready, roll up, one vertebrae at a time, feeling as if you are stacking your vertebrae one on top of the other, with your head the last to come up, and your arms returning loosely to your sides.**

   Note: if you are strong enough, you can come up from your position in Step 4 by sweeping your arms out to the side and using your abdominals to lift yourself up from the hips as your arms continue overhead and your torso lifts out and up to standing. But don't try this unless you're strong, particularly in your abdominals and back, and an advanced Yoga practitioner!

What to avoid:

- ✔ Forcing your knees to straighten
- ✔ Tightening your neck muscles

Triangle — Trikonasana

The triangle, shown in Figure 8-5, feels a bit quirky at first and it takes some balance to hold the posture. But when you get use to it (and get your butt tucked in!), you find it feels graceful. You stretch your hamstrings, Achilles tendons, back, sides, and hips with this posture. Actually, if you do the posture fully, you also work the shoulders, neck, and arms. Hmm, what else is there? Try Triangle during your posture-pacing or stretching sections.

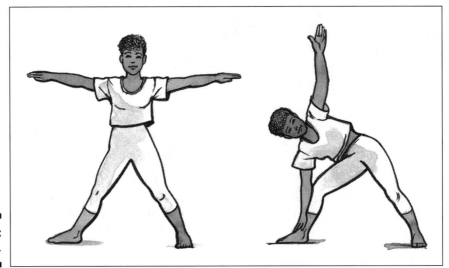

Figure 8-5:
Triangle.

1. **Start in the Mountain Posture (refer to the Cheat Sheet). Spread your feet about 3–4 feet apart, or about the length of one leg.**

2. **Turn your right foot out about 90 degrees, so that it points straight out to the right.**

3. **Turn your left foot out between 30 and 45 degrees (whatever's comfortable for you).**

   To check the position of your feet, imagine drawing a line starting at the toes of your right foot, and going straight through that heel toward your left foot — the line should meet your left foot at the arch.

4. **Lift your arms out to shoulder height at your sides, palms down, remembering to lengthen through the fingers by feeling as if your arms are getting longer from shoulder to fingertips. Think strong.**

5. **Inhale, and shift your pelvis to the left as if you were trying to nudge someone out of your way with your hips. Then exhale and reach your right arm down to the right shin. If you're comfortable you can also grab the ankle or even put your hand on the floor.**

This part of the posture is another good place to have a block handy if you can't reach down very well. Placing your hand on it can relieve tension in your back. Feel free to bend that knee until you become more comfortable with the posture.

6. **Reach your left arm up toward the ceiling with a strong hand, not a dangling one. If it's comfortable, look up toward that hand; otherwise, look down.**

7. **After you find the position, try to flatten your body as if you were doing the position with your heels, buttocks, and shoulders flat up against a wall behind you.**

8. **Hold the posture and breathe, then return to tadasana by bending your front leg and lifting your torso. After repeating this posture several times, do it on the other side.**

What to avoid:

- ✔ Sticking out your buttocks behind you
- ✔ Letting your elbow and hand soften
- ✔ Straining your neck

Warrior — Vira Bhadrasana

Shown in Figure 8-6, the Warrior posture is a traditional Yoga posture seen commonly in most classes. The beauty of it is that you can modify it, so as a beginner, you can still do it and feel strong, while if you are more advanced, you can use the identical posture and still challenge yourself by, for example, sinking lower with your legs. You stretch your entire hip and groin area, including the inner thigh, and you also strengthen your hips, thighs, arms, back, and shoulders, not to mention your warrior mind. What a deal of an asana! Try Warrior during your posture-pacing section.

Try to feel the graceful power and strength the warrior posture can transmit to your inner soul. Your heart is open, but your lower body is planted strongly. Avoid letting your eyes wander around the room; instead, set your eyes on one fixed spot in front of you.

1. **Stand in Mountain Posture (see the Cheat Sheet). Step back with your left leg about 3–4 feet, or the length of one leg.**

2. **Turn out the left foot so the toe is facing toward the left wall, but make sure it is right behind you and not out to the left side. The right foot remains pointing straight ahead.**

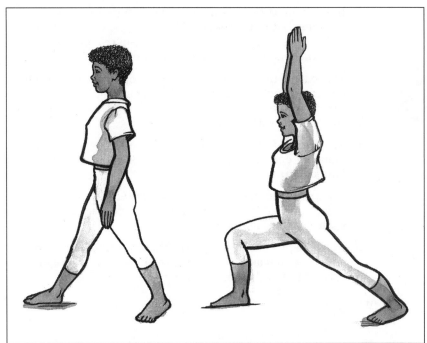

Figure 8-6:
Warrior.

3. **Turn your hips so both pelvic bones are facing the front like two headlights. Use your abdominal and torso muscles for this action, which means you may have to bring your left foot closer to you.**

4. **Inhale, then exhale and shoot your arms, palms in, straight out in front of you and upward over your head, as you bend your front knee.**

Make sure your front knee is over your foot and not sticking out unprotected in front of your toes. If it is, widen your stance a little more or lift your hips higher.

5. **Hold this position and breathe. Try to deepen the stance, bringing your groin and hips closer to the ground as you advance further in strength and flexibility.**

6. **Hold the posture for several breaths, then straighten your front knee, lower your arms, and return to Mountain Posture.**

7. **Repeat on the other side.**

What to avoid:

✔ Arching your back and leaning backward with your shoulders.

✔ Letting your hands and elbows droop.

Downward Facing Dog — Adhomuka Shvanasana

Like a dog sniffing the ground, this posture, shown in Figure 8-7, pulls your face toward the ground. It stretches the backs of your legs, Achilles tendons, back, shoulders, arms, and wrists. It also strengthens your upper body and pumps blood to your brain. Try Downward Facing Dog during your warm-up or stretching sections.

As with Standing Forward Bend, make sure you have a doctor's clearance if you have back problems. Because this is an introductory version of an inversion posture, talk to your doctor first if you have glaucoma or any other eye disorders, or high blood pressure, because of the pressure it can place on your blood flow.

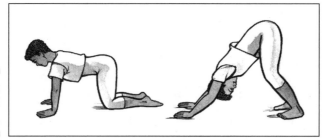

Figure 8-7:
Downward
Facing Dog.

Yogis call this a rest posture. I suppose after a hard vinyasa, it seems like rest, but normally hanging there in down dog, as you also hear it called, is plenty of work on its own. So don't be concerned about needing to take breaks from it with one of the compensation postures I discuss later in this chapter.

You can start this posture any number of ways — from a Standing Forward Bend, from your hands and knees (the easiest), and even from the strength posture called the Plank (explained later in this chapter). I describe it here from a hands-and-knees position. But in Chapter 9, I combine it with a preceding Cobra posture, as well as from a Plank and also from the Warrior.

1. **Start on your hands and knees.**

2. **Inhale and curl your toes under against the floor.**

3. **Exhale and push your hips up and back so your body is now in an upside-down V position. Your arms are straight, not locked, and you are trying to put your heels on the floor.**

4. **Relax your neck so it hangs easily between your shoulders.**

5. **After you find the position, try to push your weight back onto your feet, lift your tailbone, and arch your back slightly to press your chest toward the floor.**

Take your time! You can also bend your knees to release any pressure on your hamstrings or back so you can continue to hold the posture.

6. **Return to your hands and knees.**

You may want to drop your hips back after this into the compensation posture called Child's Posture, described later in this chapter.

If this hurts your wrists, you can rest your weight on your knuckles with your hands in a fist and your wrists straight. Or you can hold onto the handholds of a small set of dumbbells to free your wrists and allow them to not bend backward so sharply.

What to avoid:

- Staying in the position too long at first
- Letting your abdominal muscles flop out

Balancing, basically

Many of Yoga's teachings involve balance in life and energy, work and spirit, earth and sky. Balance asanas teach you to stand firmly on the ground while becoming empowered and strong so small winds cannot push you over.

There are many balances in Yoga, some of which require a lot of strength in muscles as well as spirit and mind. They are beautiful to experience. I show you only the most common posture of the many available.

The Tree — Vrikshasana

Feel as if you have roots that are extending into the ground below your feet. The taller and stronger you imagine yourself and the clearer you are in mind, the easier this is. You of course strengthen your lower body, including your feet, ankles, and legs, but you also strengthen your torso, including your abs and back. Depending on how you use your arms, you also strengthen your arms and shoulders. Figure 8-8 shows the posture, and I offer two modifications as well. Try The Tree during your posture-pacing or relaxation sections.

1. **Start in Mountain Posture (Tadasana).**

2. **Inhale, then exhale and slowly lift your left foot, toes down. Turn out the leg, then place the sole of the foot against the inside of your right leg where you are comfortable. When you first try this balance, your foot may be on the inside of your ankle, but your goal is to place it against your inner thigh between knee and groin.**

Never put pressure from your foot against your knee — always protect your knee joint.

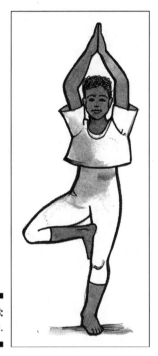

Figure 8-8:
The Tree.

3. **Fix your eyes on a point ahead of you. Lift tall through your chest and breathe.**

4. **After you find your balance there, inhale, then on the exhale, raise your arms overhead, turning the palms in and place your palms together over your head.**

5. **You are now a tree. Think rooted. Think tall. Think focused. Breathe.**

6. **When you are ready, lower the foot, lower the arms — all slowly please! — and return to Mountain Posture.**

7. **Repeat with the other foot.**

    One side may be wobblier than the other. After you discover that weaker side, try forcing yourself to do the posture on that side first.

What to avoid:

✔ Hiking up one hip or poking out one hip

✔ Tensing your shoulders upward

✔ Not breathing!

A beginner modification is to keep your hands at your sides or on your waist. Or you can try raising them to shoulder height. Or try this intermediate modification: Try to straighten your elbows while your arms are overhead and to pull your arms slightly behind your head.

Sitting pretty with seated asanas

You can just sit, or you can sit while you bend or stretch. This section introduces a couple of postures that involve bending and stretching.

Butterfly — Baddha Konasana

If you have tight hips, this asana may strike you as impossibly hard. However, some people may feel at ease from the first moment in this asana, even if they haven't ever practiced flexibility before. Everybody's hip joints are positioned differently — more to the front or more to the side — which may mean the ease or difficulty is genetic.

Use a folded blanket or a block to sit on so you can sit more comfortably and with a tall spine. This posture, shown in Figure 8-9, stretches your hips and inner thighs, as well as strengthening your back. After you fold over, you also stretch your back and ankles. Try Butterfly during your warm-up or stretching sections.

1. **Sit on the ground and bend your knees to bring the soles of your feet together in front of your groin. If you can, bring your heels closer toward your body, but only as far as you can while still sitting up with a tall, straight spine.**

   Forget flapping your knees up and down like everybody used to do in this kind of position. That does nothing for your flexibility, and makes you look kind of silly, too; sort of like a gooney bird trying to take off.

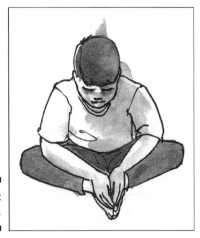

Figure 8-9: Butterfly.

2. **Inhale, then exhale and lengthen your spine out and forward by reaching, not just collapsing downward. For beginners, just sitting tall will do. As you get more flexible and in control of your body, you can fold over more and more.**

3. **Use the exhalation of each breath to relax your muscles, your back and your hips, and let yourself lean over farther.**

What to avoid:

✔ Collapsing in your chest to reach downward over your feet

✔ Holding your breath

Seated Forward Bend — Pashcimottanasana

This asana may look familiar to anyone who has ever done any traditional exercise, but with the mindful and awareness elements added, it may feel a lot different. You stretch everything up and down the back of your body, including your back and the backs of your legs. Figure 8-10 shows you how. Try Seated Forward Bend during your warm-up or stretching sections.

If you're not flexible enough to do this comfortably, sit on folded blankets or a block to ease your hamstrings as you do this posture.

1. **Sit tall on the floor with a straight back and with your legs extended in front of you and your arms at your sides.**

2. **Inhale and lift your arms overhead, palms facing in.**

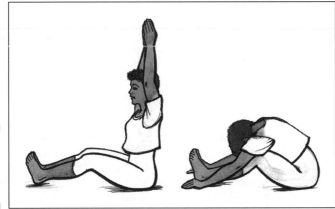

Figure 8-10: Seated Forward Bend.

You can choose between lifting your arms to the front, or sweeping them out to your sides. Pick a version that feels best to you and which you can accomplish with good form and control.

3. **Reach your arms and chest forward and out as you begin to lean forward from the hips over your legs.**

   Until you are more flexible, you can bend your knees so you don't strain your back or hamstrings. You may only end up a few inches forward with your hands resting on the floor beside your thighs. That's okay.

4. **Breathe and use the exhalation and your mind to let your muscles relax and help you come farther forward over your legs.**

5. **Release back up to a sitting position.**

6. **Bend your knees and shake out your legs to relax the muscles before you do it again.**

What to avoid:

- ✔ Collapsing through your chest
- ✔ Bending forward from your shoulders rather than your hips

Taking it lying down . . . with asanas on the floor

This section introduces a few postures that take you parallel to the floor. No, you aren't lying down yet, nor are you relaxing. Not quite yet. You're still working hard in these. You'll also see all of these resurface as a part of the vinyasas (sequences) that I put together in Chapter 9.

Plank

The plank posture looks exactly as it sounds: You're straight as a board (therefore the plank analogy) in a push-up position. Sounds easy? Wait 'til you hang out there a few minutes and then try to push back up or out. You strengthen your entire upper body, as well as your toes, feet, and legs, with this posture, shown in Figure 8-11. Try Plank during your warm-up or posture-pacing sections.

Plank is usually not done in isolation (although no ancient Yoga rule says you can't!), but is most often done as a part of a flowing vinyasa, such as a Sun Salutation. The Plank isn't a warm-up posture you want to jump right into to start a routine, but it works well toward the end of a warm-up or when you find your pace in the middle to help raise your core body temperature to prepare it for deeper stretches.

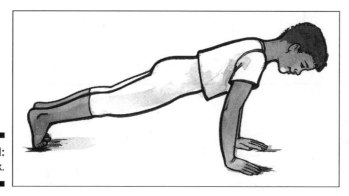

Figure 8-11:
Plank.

I put you into this from a stationary position just so you can get the feel for it. Usually you are moving into it directly from another posture, as you see in Chapter 9.

1. **Start in Mountain Posture (see the Cheat Sheet).**

2. **Follow the instructions for the Standing Forward Bend, earlier in this chapter, bending your knees so you can put your hands on the ground in front of your feet.**

3. **Walk your hands forward, keeping your abdominals tight, until your hands are below your shoulders. Keep your arms straight, fingers pointed straight ahead. Your neck and shoulders need to be relaxed, but still hold them straight out in perfect alignment as if it's a continuation upward from your spine. You have become a plank!**

4. **Hold this posture for a few seconds. (Breathe, please!)**

5. **Release by simply lowering your knees to the floor and then your whole body. Or you can (get ready for this) inhale, then on your exhale push your hips back strongly into a Downward Facing Dog position, then return yourself to a Standing Forward Bend.**

You find lots of ways to use the Plank posture and lots of ways to get in and out of it, using one leg or two, dropping down, forward, or back up. I frankly love it for the feeling of balanced strength and the connection between earth and sun. When you're in Plank, feel as if you are widening across your upper back. Spread the area between your shoulder blades rather than sink into it. Try to push your heels back and straighten your knees.

A modification, if you are a beginner, is to drop your knees to the floor, still keeping your body straight from knees to head.

What to avoid:

- ✔ Dropping your head
- ✔ Bending your knees while in a full Plank
- ✔ Tensing your shoulders

Caterpillar

This position isn't usually taught separately. Yet I for one find it a difficult one to grasp because the body position is very unusual for Western minds that are not used to Yoga, because your butt is up and your chin and chest are down like, well, a caterpillar wiggling across the lawn. I go through it step-by-step, and Figure 8-12 illustrates it. The position also appears in the flowing sequences as the posture after a Plank. Here, you also strengthen your entire upper body. Try Caterpillar during your warm-up or posture-pacing sections.

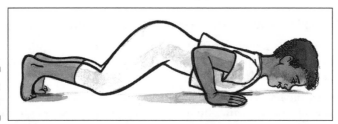

Figure 8-12:
Caterpillar.

Look for two more advanced modifications at the end of these instructions.

1. **Start in the full Plank posture with your knees off the ground.**

2. **Drop your knees to the ground without altering the placement of your feet or hands.**

3. **Keeping your elbows close to your ribs, bend them while you lower your chest, chin, and nose to the floor. You keep your buttocks up in the air.**

   It sort of feels as if you dropped something that rolled under a chest of drawers and you're on the ground trying to look under the chest to find it.

4. **Hold the posture and breathe (this posture can be a nice rest from the Plank). Release your body to the ground or your buttocks back into a Child's Posture (see the section, "Compensation Asanas," later in this chapter).**

For an intermediate modification, put your knees down, but lower your chest, chin, and nose so they are just hovering over the ground.

In an advanced modification, keep your knees straight and lower your body by bending your elbows until your entire plank-like body and the chest are hovering a couple of inches above the ground. Your buttocks are still slightly lifted, but not sticking up in the air.

What to avoid:

- ✔ Dropping your head and chin down.
- ✔ Letting your abdominals sag
- ✔ Turning your fingers in or out

Cobra — Bujangasana

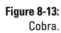

Cobra is a beautiful posture that everyone seems to know of or perhaps even do as a part of traditional exercise. But it is one with which to be very careful — avoid it if you have back problems, or modify it if you experience any pain in your back or neck. You stretch your back and open your chest with this posture, shown in Figure 8-13.

Westerners spend a lot of time bending forward while seated (think about sitting at computers, hunched over steering wheels, or plopped on couches), so bending backwards into what is called *spinal extension* (the opposite of bending forward) needs some patience and slow work.

I start with the simplest Cobra and give you a more advanced modification. Choose the one that works best for you, even alternating one posture as you tire of another. Try Cobra during your posture-pacing or stretching sections.

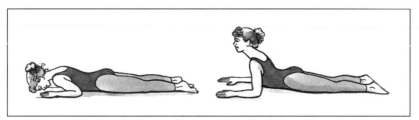

Figure 8-13:
Cobra.

1. **Lie on the ground, stomach down, forehead on the floor.**

   This position is called a *prone* position. In any mind-body exercise, unless you are simply doing a deep relaxation, your abdominal muscles are still engaged and tightened even when you're flopped down on the floor. Nobody can see them, so it's all up to you to use them so your back stays supported.

2. **Place your hands palm down against the floor, on each side of your face about even with your temples.**

3. **Inhale, then exhale and push against the floor with your forearms as you raise your upper body off the floor. Stop when your upper arms are unfolded, but your elbows and your hip bones are still on the floor. Feel as if you are lengthening your back out and up.**

   Avoid collapsing at the back of your neck; instead feel as if you are lengthening your neck up and out, and you are still looking forward.

4. **Hold the posture and breathe. When you're ready, exhale as you lower your upper body back to the floor.**

   This is another good place to add a compensation posture called Child's Posture. (See the section, "Compensation Asanas" later in this chapter.)

Try these intermediate modifications:

- ✔ Lift your chest and head up, as described in the preceding steps, but go farther to where your elbows come off the floor, still keeping your hip bones down.

- ✔ Place your hands closer to your shoulders and lift your chest, as described in the preceding steps. Although your elbows come off the floor again, they remain a little bent and your hips still stay glued down.

Try to keep your gluteal muscles (your buttocks) relaxed as you lift up. Recent theory has it that this conscious action can help take strain off the lower back.

What to avoid:

- ✔ Pushing beyond the flexibility of your back and lifting your hips up
- ✔ Dropping your head back
- ✔ Relaxing your abdominal muscles

Spinning around with twisting asanas

In Yoga, you can twist and shout all night long, but these are difficult for our locked-up Western spines. So here I introduce two simple twists for you to try.

If you have any back problems, you should also consult with your doctor before trying twisting moves because they may place strain where it is not good for your back. As always, you should always listen to your body and go no farther than feels good.

Simple Seated Spinal Twist — Maricyasana

You may already do a version of this when you feel as if your back needs a little break. This stretches your spinal muscles, as well as opens your chest and strengthens abdominals, if you do it correctly (shown in Figure 8-14). Try Simple Seated Spinal Twist during your posture-pacing or stretching sections.

1. **Sit on the floor as if preparing for a Seated Forward Bend. (See earlier in this chapter or refer to Figure 8-10.)**

   As in that asana, if your hamstrings are tight, sit on a blanket to help you sit up tall.

2. **Slide your left foot up along your right leg toward your belly button, keeping the sole of that foot on the floor. Stop when you can't move your foot any farther without slouching or straining. Try to keep your right leg straight.**

   Relax your right knee slightly if that helps you sit taller.

3. **Hold your left knee to your chest with your right hand. Your left hand is palm down on the floor behind your left buttocks.**

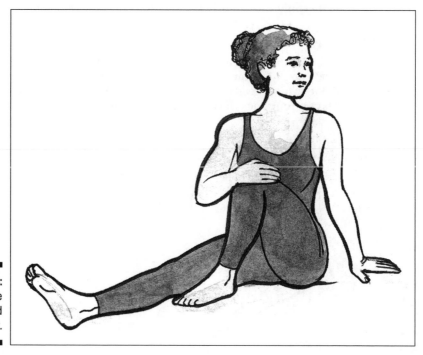

Figure 8-14:
Simple
Seated
Spinal Twist.

4. **Inhale and then exhale as you open your chest and twist your right side toward and even beyond your left knee. Try to lift your abdominal muscles as you open to that side. Turn your head gently, and look as far over your left shoulder as you can.**

5. **Hold the posture and breathe. Release smoothly, sliding your left leg out to join the right.**

6. **Repeat on the right side.**

Variations include:

✔ **Office Spinal Twist:** Do the same twist, but stay seated in a chair and hold onto the back of the chair or the arm — instead of your knee.

✔ **Intermediate Modification:** Do the twist as instructed, but place your left foot over the top of your right knee so that the sole of your foot is on the floor on the outside of your right knee.

What to avoid:

✔ Rounding your back and slouching

✔ Twisting only with your head and not your torso and spine

Bent-Knee Twist on Your Back

This posture is a simple starter spinal twist while lying down. I give you an intermediate modification also. You stretch your hips, back, and spine, while you also open your chest and shoulders. Figure 8-15 illustrates it. Try Bent Knee Twist on Your Back during your stretching section.

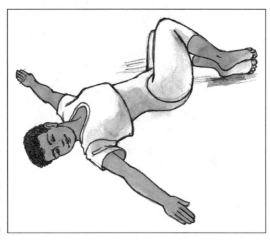

Figure 8-15:
Bent-Knee
Twist on
Your Back.

1. **Lie on your back with your knees bent and your feet flat on the floor, knees about hip-width apart.**

2. **Place your arms out to your sides at shoulder-height, palms down.**

3. **Inhale, then exhale and slowly lower your bent knees to your left. At the same time, turn your head and neck to look to the right. Lower your knees only as far as you can go without lifting either shoulder off the floor.**

4. **You can either remain in the side-lying position for several breaths, or inhale and bring your back to the center position.**

5. **Repeat to the right and several times on each side.**

I like to hold this position to the side and feel as if I am exhaling into any tight muscles, feeling them relax as it becomes easier to stay in the twisted position.

What to avoid:

✔ Letting your ribs and chest pop open and up

✔ Allowing your shoulders or head to come off the ground

✔ Tensing your hands and arms

Resting with compensation asanas

You can do rest or compensation postures any time after a more difficult position to rest your back or your mind. These postures become second nature after awhile. Just listen to your body to know when you should do one. Use these asanas at any time you feel a need for a break, during any section of your session.

Child's Posture — Balasana

You're going to love this position, and you may find yourself doing it ad lib in the evening or around the house. It's a beautiful way to relax your back and return circulation to your entire body. Look for one modification, and the illustration in Figure 8-16.

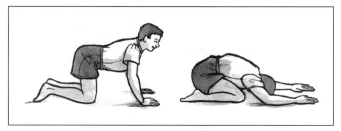

Figure 8-16:
Child's
Posture.

1. **Start on your hands and knees, with your knees about hip-width apart.**

2. **Inhale, then exhale and sit back with your buttocks onto your heels, bringing your torso down to rest on your thighs.**

   If it is uncomfortable for your knees or legs to sit back on your heels, put a folded blanket between your thighs and calves. You can also place a pillow or blanket under your knees for support. Or you can widen your knees to allow more freedom of movement.

3. **Lay your arms along your sides, on the floor beside your legs with your palms up, and let your shoulders and breathing relax.**

4. **Close your eyes.**

   Enjoy this as long as you want or need to.

For a modification, extend your arms in front of you, palms down, to add an additional stretch to your back, chest, and shoulders.

Knees to Chest

This is just like the Knee to Chest stretch in the section, "Warming up," and you can refer to Figure 8-3, but this time you bring both knees to your chest, hold them there, and relax your back and hips.

Mountain Posture

The standing asana called Tadasana is a nice way to rest between active postures, too. See the Cheat Sheet along with the steps for Mountain Posture, earlier in this chapter.

Incorporating relaxation and meditation

After you go through your asanas for the day, taking a few minutes to relax your body is always a pleasure, and is also a good time to meditate.

Corpse — Shavasana

Shown in Figure 8-17, Corpse is not only a posture for ending a session, but a fine way to start one if you need a little meditation and rest before beginning. Be sure to breathe and feel yourself melt into the floor. You can start or finish your session with Corpse.

1. **Lie flat on your back on a comfortable carpet or mat.**

2. **Place your arms at your sides, palms up, relaxing your shoulders down into the floor.**

3. **Let your legs roll outward to relax the hips.**

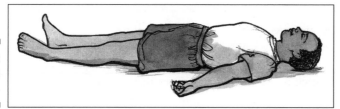

Figure 8-17:
Corpse
Posture.

4. **Close your eyes and practice good deep breathing for a few minutes.**

Try to stay focusedly unfocused (that's a term I just made up) on the moment, without letting thoughts, incidents, stress, or frustration from the day interrupt your flow or possess your mind.

Easy — Sukhasana

Easy, shown in Figure 8-18, sounds easy enough, but if your hips or back are tight, it may be far from it. Easy is basically the classic cross-legged position that is the first step toward getting into the classic (and more advanced) Lotus position. You can modify it by sitting on a folded blanket or block to allow your knees, hips, and legs more freedom. Either way, you stretch your hips and back, and it can be a good way to prepare for other postures as well as to meditate or rest. Try Easy during your warm-up, stretching, or relaxation sections.

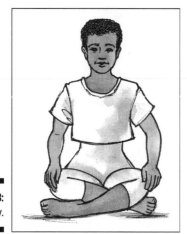

Figure 8-18:
Easy.

1. **Sit on the floor with your legs comfortably extended in front of you.**

2. **Bring your right leg in toward you, then fold the left leg back toward it so the legs are shin-to-calf or ankle-to-ankle.**

3. **Rest your hands on your knees, sit tall, chest lifted, and breathe easily.**

   Imagine someone has a string tied to the crown of your head and is pulling upward. You want to feel tall and light, not sinking and heavy.

4. **Now try sitting with the left leg pulled in first. Notice which side (meaning which hip) is tighter and more difficult to sit with tucked in closer.**

   Remember which is your tight side and be sure to try to sit that way more often to help loosen it up.

What to avoid:

- ✔ Sinking down into a curved back
- ✔ Letting your abdominals pouch and relax
- ✔ Jutting your chin out in front of you

Bringing on the calm with "ohmmmm"

Now I want to introduce the "ohmmmm" that you hear so much about. If you're self-conscious, find a private room and close the door. Or pick a time when no one else is home. Pick a comfortable posture. Good postures for trying an ohmmmm are the Corpse, Easy, or even the Mountain Posture.

First, just say the word, like "oh" with a drawn-out "ooooh" and a good belly breath so it doesn't warble like a bird. Your lips need to be slightly open. Then just close your lips, keep the breath going, and push the sound into your nose. It becomes a slightly nasal "mmmmm" vibration that moves through your entire body.

Try to hold the entire syllable from start to finish for 30 seconds or more. Let yourself feel what the vibration does for your body.

After you repeat "ohmmmm" several times, just hold whatever posture you're in and feel. While you feel your energy rejuvenate, now is a good time to meditate and bring calm to your mind and soul.

Chapter 9

Lining Up Your Yoga Sequence

· ·

In This Chapter

▶ Trying some super sequences

▶ Doing some mini-vinis

· ·

*W*ith all the Yoga postures to choose from, you can certainly go in many directions with your Yoga practice. But whichever way you choose, be sure you go slowly, pace yourself, let your body feel what you're asking of it, and let your mind open and take part.

In this section, I show you a simple *vinyasa* (or flowing sequence of postures) called a Sun Salutation. Of course, if you've taken a Yoga class already or take one after reading this book, the Sun Salutation may be different. The sequence isn't set in stone — there are many variations on this theme.

I also lay out a list of two other sets you can try. One focuses on strength and the other focuses on stretching. I also include three mini-workouts for when you want to work specific areas or when you have a time crunch. Feel free to create any short sampler of your own as you experiment with your practice.

Just be sure to wait at least 1 to 2 hours after a full meal, or as much as 3 to 4 hours, before performing your Yoga session.

Nearly all the postures mentioned in this chapter are described in Chapter 8, so check there for specific instructions.

Warming Up — The All-Important Step

Always warm up before you start a Yoga routine (or any exercise for that matter). You can use the Sun Salutation as a warm-up; just don't push the stretches the first couple of times through.

Don't forget compensation or rest postures. They're yours to use at any time, for any reason. Use them liberally as you develop your practice/routine.

Try to balance your postures, moving from forward bending to extending, and from strength to rest. Also, the order in which I present the postures in Chapter 8 — warm-ups, standing, forward-bending, balance, seated, and relaxation — is a typical order in any session. For example, perform your standing postures before you then come down to sit on the floor for more stretches. You're not only warmer and more ready to stretch your muscles, but you're also fully ready to sit down and rest a bit.

Moving to Vinyasas That Suit Any Fancy

These vinyasas are either classic, such as the Sun Salutation, or a series of postures I have put together for you to try. Use them as your own vinyasas, or use them as templates to put together your own sequences. Name them if you want; for example, Therese's Tiring Ten . . . or whatever.

Sometimes deciding on a theme of a sequence — for example, stretching or balance — can help you decide which postures to string together.

Honoring the sun with a salutation

The Sun Salutation is certainly the most classic of all sequences of flowing movements, or vinyasas. Do the postures in the order I present them, rolling through them as smoothly as possible, rather than jerking. I include instruction only when the movement isn't included in Chapter 8, but you can check out Figure 9-1 for a guide to the various postures. Generally, what I provide are tips on moving from one posture to another.

1. **Mountain Posture (Tadasana): Start with your arms at your sides, then bring your hands slowly in front of you to a Namaste Mudra, which is the position where your palms are held together in front of your breastbone.**

2. **Standing Backward Bend: From Namaste, extend your hands up and overhead, extending your body slightly into a backward arch, but only as far as is comfortable. Look up at the ceiling without crunching the back of your neck.**

3. **Standing Forward Bend: Exhale and lower your arms to the floor as you fold forward from the hips.**

4. **Low Lunge, Right: Inhale and bend your right knee while stepping back with your left foot as far as possible. Keep your hands on the floor.**

   This looks something like a Warrior posture but with your torso leaning forward over your right leg from the hips rather then held upright. If you do any traditional exercise, you may hear this called a "runner's lunge."

5. **Plank: Exhale and step back with your right foot, placing it softly on the floor behind you, beside your left foot.**

   Be sure to modify this if you need to, as explained in Chapter 8.

6. **Caterpillar: Lower your chest, chin, and nose, but keep your buttocks up, as the instructions in Chapter 8 indicate.**

7. **Cobra: Inhale and lengthen your chest down onto the ground and lower your buttocks. Then arch up into the Cobra.**

   After this step is a good time to insert a restful Child's Posture if you need to.

8. **Downward Facing Dog: Curl your toes under you as you exhale and push your hips back and up into the Down Dog, modifying the position by bending your knees as best suits your body.**

   You may want to rest with a Child's Posture after this move also.

9. **Low Lunge, Left: Inhale and step forward with your left foot to return to the Low Lunge (see Step 4 for instructions and tips).**

10. **Standing Forward Bend: Exhale and bring your right foot forward and next to your left foot, bending your knees to ease your hamstrings and back.**

11. **Standing Backward Bend: As you inhale, lift your torso upright, bringing your arms overhead, and bend backward slightly from the hips. Look upward at the ceiling.**

12. **Mountain Posture with Namaste: Exhale and return to a standing tall position, using your abdominal muscles. Bring your hands calmly forward in front of your breastbone.**

13. **Repeat the entire routine 2–6 times (even more as you get stronger), being sure to alternate the leg that comes forward first and the leg that comes forward second in the two Low Lunges.**

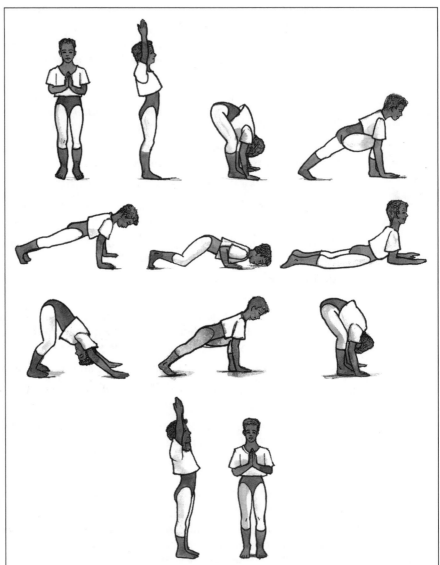

Figure 9-1:
Sun
Salutation.

Centering with the Strength Sequence

Repeat this sequence several times, trying some of the less intense or most intense modifications I explain in Chapter 8, which also sets out all the instructions for each posture in this vinyasa. Remember, as a vinyasa, you want to feel the flow!

Be sure to warm up with some basic postures before starting this sequence. I list warm-up postures in Chapter 8.

1. **Downward Facing Dog.**

   You may want to start from standing then lower into this posture.

2. **Plank.**

   Try a full or modified position.

3. **Caterpillar.**

   A great way to insert a bit of a rest.

4. **Downward Facing Dog.**

   Pull your hips back up.

   You can repeat Steps 2–4 several times if you'd like before moving onto Step 5.

5. **Warrior.**

   Settle into Warrior for some mindful breathwork.

   For extra strength work, try The Tree for balance after the Warrior.

6. **Downward Facing Dog.**

   You may find this posture to be a popular and important transition to the next posture.

7. **Child's Posture.**

   This pose is the big "aaaahh" at the end!

Flexing with the Stretch Sequence

Of course, every Yoga asana works on your flexibility, but this one focuses even more strongly on it.

Be sure to warm up with some basic postures before starting this sequence. Also, be sure to do this sequence at least two times, so you can do each side.

1. **Mountain Posture.**

   Always a great way to start and balance your mind and body.

2. **Standing Forward Bend.**

   Works the backs of your legs and allows you to breathe fully.

3. **Warrior.**

   Place one foot behind you and lift your torso to get into this posture.

4. **Low Lunge.**

   The same "runner's lunge" as in the Sun Salutation.

   Add an extra hamstring stretch here by placing your back knee on the ground and reaching your hips backward until you feel a stretch behind your forward leg. Bend and straighten the leg gently several times. Return to a Low Lunge, if you do this option, before moving on.

5. **Triangle.**

   Follow the foot placement directions in Chapter 8 carefully on this one.

6. **Mountain Posture.**

   If it's good enough to start, it's good enough to finish.

Quickening the Sequence with a Couple of Mini-Vinis

Who's to say you can't put together two to four postures and get a great five-minute Yoga session? Do these mini-vinis (short for vinyasas, of course) as many times through as you have time.

Do a few warm-up movements before you start this sequence. Instructions for warm-ups and these postures are in Chapter 8.

Stretching out that back

Relieving your tight back is never a bad thing, now is it?

1. **Seated Spinal Twist.**

2. **Cobra.**

3. **Seated Forward Bend.**

Un-hamstringing your hamstrings

Loosening up the muscles in the back of your thighs can help your whole body feel better. Even your back!

1. **Lying Hamstring Stretch.**

2. **Standing Forward Bend.**

3. **Downward Facing Dog.**

Opening up your chest

Freeing your chest helps you breathe more freely and deeply. And, speaking of breathing: Don't forget to focus on it during all of these sequences.

1. **Bent Knee Twist on Your Back.**

2. **Cobra.**

3. **Downward Facing Dog.**

4. **Triangle.**

Part IV

The Flow of Ancient Chinese Mind-Body Arts

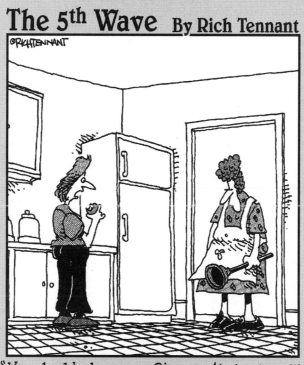

The 5th Wave   By Rich Tennant

"You should do some Qigong. At least you'll unclog your energy channels if not the garbage disposal, the upstairs toilet and the lint trap in the dryer."

In this part . . .

The Chinese have always been a little more in touch with their minds and bodies than we disjointed Westerners. To the Chinese, even the term *mind-body* is kind of laughable — they view the mind and body as one integrated unit in everything they do. It's not surprising then that two of the primary mind-body methods are centuries-old Chinese forms — Tai Chi Chuan and Qigong.

Both of these forms — and their many schools and styles — are all about affecting and feeling your energy through movement. The movements themselves are just the process you use to get the omnipotent and omnipresent energy that should flow freely through your body to actually do just that — flow freely. And that free-flowing energy, so they say, can help make you healthier, happier, and more at peace.

So, turn the page and get your energy going with Tai Chi and Qigong.

Chapter 10

Slowing Down with Tai Chi Chuan

- -

In This Chapter

▶ Checking out the benefits of Tai Chi Chuan

▶ Recognizing the styles

▶ Training yourself on the principles

▶ Setting up a sampler of forms

- -

*T*o Westerners who traditionally think of exercise as working up a sweat, increasing the heart rate, and maybe even hurting a little, it seems like some kind of a joke that something that looks like adults playing freeze tag could actually be legitimate exercise. But it is, oh my, it really is. Tai Chi Chuan just feels so unusual at first because the basic credo is utterly contradictory to most exercise that we in the Western world call traditional.

Tai Chi Chuan's credo is this: Go slow. Go slower still. Go as slowly as you can. If you think you are going as slow as you can, you aren't. So try to go slower. Tai Chi Chuan is certainly the complete opposite of hamsters-on-a-wheel step aerobics, hiking up a hill as fast as possible, or training to go as quickly as you can on the treadmill to burn more calories.

Always think sloooow, slooooower, sloooooowest. You are the tortoise, not the hare. Remember that fable? The tortoise wins the race.

It is the slowness of Tai Chi Chuan movements, in part, that force you to get in touch with your body, listen to your mind, and integrate them both until you're moving as one unified mass. Doing Tai Chi Chuan, you can't let your brain plan tomorrow's dinner while your body goes through the motions — Tai Chi Chuan demands your whole mind-body attention.

You may feel a bit restless at first — it takes patience to move as slowly as Tai Chi Chuan forms require. But with practice and time, that feeling diminishes as you allow yourself to focus, to be calm, and to find the inner peace that enables you to move and breathe joyfully — as mind and body together should.

Practicing Something Mindful, or Martial?

If this is mind-body stuff, why am I talking about *martial* arts, which is fighting and kicking and spinning and rolling and whacking an opponent off the face of the earth — or at least against the wall?

The simple reason is that Tai Chi, the mindful form, comes from the same family, called *Wushu*, as combative martial arts. Wushu is traditionally a self-defense activity carried out with or without weapons, and is actually older than Tai Chi. If you look closely at the forms in this book (for example, the circling, torso-turning, hand pushing, and leg-lifting), you find that if you speed up the movement — and if you had an enemy facing you about to knock out your teeth — you could use the same form to twist off an arm or knock someone off their feet.

Tai Chi actually is a martial art with all the turning, twisting, punching, and grabbing — just a slow, meditative version, which you can use to discover calm and focus before you decide to move faster.

Tai Chi, or Tai Chi Chuan, or Tai Chi Chih, or . . .

You may probably see all three names somewhere, at some point. You may also see this practice written as Taiji *(tie-jee)* or Taiji Quan *(tie-jee chewon)*, which is more accurately Chinese, but isn't so commonly seen in the West. You can see the Westernization of Taiji Quan to Tai Chi Chuan. Same pronounciation, just more comfortable for our eyes because of the way it uses Latin letters. So let's start with that Westernized name as our basis.

Tai Chi, therefore, is just the shorthand I use for Tai Chi Chuan, just as if your name were Susan Marie, but everybody calls you Susan. Same thing. But do recognize the full name.

The name "Tai Chi" can be translated from the Chinese into English to mean many things, from something as simple as "The Grand Ultimate" or "The High Peak" to something more estoeric as "Undifferentiated Unity." Either way, it's the really really big important unified thing. Chuan simply means "fist." That's the martial part rearing its head. So it's kind of loosely translated as, "The Grand Ultimate Fighting."

Tai Chi Chih, on the other hand, is a contemporary method that uses the early classical form of Tai Chi Chuan for some of its components. For a description of this form, see Chapter 17, and refer to the Appendix for resources on both.

Getting *exercise* is not really a goal of Tai Chi Chuan. Fitness just happens as you train your body and your breathing to do the forms of Tai Chi Chuan, which can consist of a few minutes of linked postures or a half-hour or more of very complicated sequences. All incorporate the martial-like moves in slow mo'. I include excerpts from the simplest and most common form, called the Yang 24-movement Short Form. But there are many schools, styles, and forms. Refer to the following sections for an introduction to all of these before I describe the movements.

Going Slow and Sure, Receiving Benefits for Sure

The traditional Western wisdom is that you have to move vigorously and sweat in order to get fit and healthy. Although Tai Chi is far from a Western fitness method, it delivers both mental and physical payoffs, and some of the better researched ones at that.

Getting in the conventional perks

In the following list, I summarize the concrete benefits that sports medicine experts harp on and how Tai Chi helps you realize these gains. Refer to Chapter 6 for more details about health benefits:

- **Aerobic fitness:** You can do Tai Chi very, very slowly, or just slowly (a little more up-tempo) as you become more advanced. Either way, you are moving enough to raise your heart rate just a bit to get your heart and lungs more fit and healthy. You are also complying with research that seems to indicate low-intensity movement can do a lot for your aerobic health over the long haul.

- **Gaining strength:** Depending on your abilities, you can either do Tai Chi with fairly straight knees — just softly bend them a little — or you can do it squatted quite low to the ground to fully challenge all the muscles in your back, hips, buttocks, and legs. You also may find that holding your arms up against the force of gravity and moving them slowly but continuously can be more of an upper body workout than you ever dreamed.

✔ **Gaining more flexibility:** If you're not especially flexible, don't make really large or low movements with your arms or legs. As you progress, you may, for example, lift your legs higher in kicks and squat lower and wider during moving forms, which helps you achieve more flexibility.

✔ **Improving balance:** Tai Chi has also been shown to greatly improve balance through *proprioception* of the nerves and muscles in your lower leg. Very loosely translated, proprioception is sort of like "tickling" your nerves and muscles a little to create better muscle sense of your position in space. With better balance, you won't wobble as much or turn your ankle as often. That can be a boon to performance for athletes, or a life-saver for older people who fall and can break hips and legs.

Realizing the less-than-conventional-but-still-good benefits

The less-than-conventional benefits, the ones most sports medicine experts barely acknowledge, cover the same realm as all the other mind-body methods and workouts in this book, although some methods focus on some aspects more than others. Tai Chi may be one of the more well-rounded methods when it comes to mind-body benefits, although in contrast to Hatha Yoga you gain less strength and flexibility overall. Refer to Table 2-1 in Chapter 2 for a comparison of benefits.

I enumerate the less-traditional benefits you can gain from Tai Chi in this list:

✔ **Relaxation:** Who doesn't need a little more relaxation? You can't do Tai Chi and stay stressed out. If you move slowly and breathe, as required, your stress dissipates, leaving you more relaxed and refreshed. Over time, you find out how to incorporate this stress-release in daily life, for example, while stuck in a rush-hour traffic jam or standing in a long line at the bank behind someone who has 20 million checks to deposit and forgot to sign them first. You train yourself to breathe and relax, letting every moment become a "Tai Chi moment."

✔ **Body awareness:** Have you ever fallen over a step you simply didn't pay attention to? Bump into someone as you tried to squeezed past but didn't have enough room? Had a pain in your foot that you couldn't for the life of you figure out why it started? Many of us meander through life never fully aware of our bodies. It's as if our physical being is completely separated from our mind. We either think, or we move. But we don't think about our movement, or move while thinking, or even do thinking movement. As a result, it's as if a gate of sorts has been slammed shut between our head and the rest of us.

When practicing Tai Chi, you have to think about, and get to know, your body. You find out what muscles are weak, where you're tight, what feels strong, which joints feel loose, how your left and right sides differ (everybody is somewhat unbalanced), and how your ankle bone is connected to your shin bone, and your shin bone's connected to your thigh bone, and so on and so on. You realize how all the parts work and are interconnected. You become aware of all the parts of your body and become more aware of your complete self every day, all day.

✔ **Energy:** Who doesn't want more energy? If you practice Tai Chi regularly and diligently, the theory is that you can unblock the energy superhighways that run up and down and all around your body. After they're flowing smoothly, the energy pulsing all around you gives you more vitality, more verve, and more health, which can translate into getting sick less frequently and less severely. For an introduction to the channels of energy in your body, refer to Chapter 4. For more details, just read on and be sure to take a look at the Qigong information in Chapter 11.

If you want more details about the breadth of benefits that all mind-body methods can impart, skip back to Chapter 6. I give you a peek into what both scientists and practitioners are finding there. Indeedy, science is beginning to look twice, even thrice, at mind-body practices and all the gains you can achieve for body and soul.

Choosing a Style

Saying you practice or want to practice Tai Chi is a bit like saying you want ice cream. What kind?

As a beginner, you may not have to choose the style of Tai Chi you practice, often because if you decide to turn to local schools or teachers, the selections may be like choosing between being offered chocolate or, well, chocolate. One, you take what's offered and, two, you don't know enough to decide what style you may like best anyway. However, the most common style taught in the United States is the Yang form, which is what I offer in the movement sampler later in this chapter.

Still, you want to be aware of what's out there so that you're not confused when a fellow practitioner talks about the Yang form, or the short form, or the Chen school, or whatever.

Bursting with Chen

The Chen style is to Tai Chi what Shakespeare is to contemporary theater. Much, if not all, of what came afterward stemmed from the Chen style (just as much of contemporary theater has a basis in Shakespeare), although it may not be as commonly practiced these days, it remains in about the second or third rung of popularity. Developer Chen Wangting lived around 1600. He was a soldier and a farmer who was also a martial arts practitioner. For decades, the forms he created were handed down from generation to generation. But its style stayed solely in his family until the early 1900s, when a member long down the line began to showcase the Chen moves.

Some parts of Chen style are more explosive than other, more typical Tai Chi disciplines. It bursts from the slow flowing movements typical of what most people think of as Tai Chi into broad, big, jarring movements. Its stances are lower to the ground and involve the whole body.

Flowing with Yang

Yang Luchan was a student of the Chen family in the 1800s. Yang became an exceptionally well-known and respected Tai Chi practitioner and teacher. But it was his son (Yang Jianhou) and grandson (Yang Chengfu) who fully developed the style and its name.

Yang style has an even tempo with larger, more circular movements than the Chen style. The forms incorporate very large movements known for their seamless flowing from one to the other. They're also simpler than other forms. The stances are more middle-height, not too low or high, although they can be taken in either direction based on need and ability.

Hundreds and hundreds of forms to try . . . Oh my!

If you ever immerse yourself more deeply into Tai Chi, you may be amazed at the number of forms there are. The traditional Yang style is a "long form" that has 108 movements. A simplified version (their term, not mine!) has 88. That's simple? Most commonly, you may experience the 24-form style. No worries! This style can keep you busy your entire life of Tai Chi and is what our sampler forms are drawn from. The short form was developed in 1959 by the Chinese government's National Physical Culture and Sports Commission. Its goal: to make Tai Chi more accessible to the masses in an effort to preserve that piece of cultural heritage. After you know the Yang form, it may take you 4 to 5 minutes to get through it once.

If you take Tai Chi in the Western world, you are most likely to experience what is called the "Yang 24-movement Short Form." This is the shortened version of the original 108 movements so it is more accessible to the masses.

Moving rapidly with Wu

Every student has to make his mark, it seems. Wu Yuxiang was a student of Yang, the father, in the 1800s, and worked hard to reach perfection as well as to develop his own version.

Wu style has taller stances, smaller circular forms than the Chen and Yang styles, and has you lean forward slightly, as if reaching from the waist. Its movements follow each other rapidly. This is also about the second or third most popular style today.

Discovering other styles under the Sun

Sun style is a combination of the styles of many teachers. You may see something called Hao, or another style called Wu that came a few decades later than the Wu style I talk about in the preceding section. And, frankly, as with Yoga and many other mind-body methods, every teacher may have a touch of his or her own style that you may take to or not. Nothing is truly wrong. It may just be a different road leading to higher awareness.

Praising the Principles

To properly guide yourself through Tai Chi, take heed of certain principles. Those principles go along with the all the basic stuff that is the foundation of all mind-body work, whether it is called an exercise, a movement, a posture, or a form. In this section, I adapted principles from several sources and teachers (including Tai Chi instructors Manny Fuentes and David-Dorian Ross) and added to them to give you an introduction of the concepts. Enjoy!

Slowing down

Going slowly is the main principle of Tai Chi. As you do Tai Chi movements, pretend you're the tortoise in his race against the hare. If you get nothing else when it comes to Tai Chi, get this: Rushing gets you nowhere, certainly not to mindful balance. Don't just shove your body into different funny-looking poses. When you go slowly, you're able to pay attention to detail, think about what your body is doing, and concentrate on what comes next. Not to mention that you can experience a mindful calm.

Taking it easy

We're used to forcing things. Jar doesn't open? Turn harder. Don't get a job? Call more often. Can't get a board to fit in a space? Shove with more force. Forget the concept of force in Tai Chi. Take it easy. Relax. Look at your hands. Relax your fingers. Think about your shoulders. Shake 'em out! Extra tension in your body means expending extra energy, which you want to avoid in Tai Chi. Save your energy for when you really need it in your forms.

Thinking in curves

From a martial arts perspective, the purpose of Tai Chi's circular motion is to disguise from an opponent where a move stops and starts. That makes it easier to throw an opponent off and win a fight. From a mindful perspective, a rounded or curved joint or limb promotes better energy flow throughout your body. Avoid locking your joints; keep them soft and round or bent.

Being simple

Go with what feels natural to your body. If going from one form to another feels twisted or unnatural, it probably is. Stop! Don't think. Shake out your mind. Then try again, thinking only of the end position of the movement. Just let your body move into the posture naturally — generally you are right!

Sinking lower

The bent-knee stance of Tai Chi is pretty recognizable. Don't be afraid to push yourself just a little. Sink. A little lower. How about a little lower? Bend your knees naturally. The movement flows better because a bent joint lets your body move more easily than a locked joint. And you get a better workout, too!

As you first do Tai Chi, your knees may be nearly straight. As you progress, or if you start out in a fairly fit and flexible condition, you bend your knees more. An advanced Tai Chi practitioner is often quite low to the ground!

Don't bend your knees to the point of being uncomfortable. Mind-body fitness is not about pain. Find a level that isn't too hard, but still challenges you.

Going with the flow

In some mind-body methods, you do a little jerky transition between moves, but Tai Chi is all about continuity and flow, without a break in time or space. Your legs, feet and arms reach the final position at the same time no matter how far each has to travel. But they don't stop there. There are no periods at the end of Tai Chi sentences. When you come to what seems like an end, you only move through it, and flow on to the next place.

Staying balanced

All Tai Chi forms and sequences are a combination of opposites — forward and back, weight-bearing or non-weight-bearing, high and low, reach and pull back. These opposites, or balancing moves, highlight the ancient Chinese philosophy of yin and yang. *Yin* movements typically are higher, lighter, non-weight-bearing, pulled back, and have more emotional energy. *Yang* movements are lower, weight-bearing, attacking or reaching out, heavier, and have a more muscular energy. In Chinese philosophy, yin represents the feminine nature of the universe, and yang represents the masculine. Tai Chi tries to keep you balanced between the yin and yang of movement, creating a flowing and rhythmical dance between the two.

Moving the whole package

When you're doing Tai Chi, you don't move one part of your body, stop to see whether it looks okay, then move another part. Your whole body is one package and moves at the same time, like a snake rhythmically slithering. Your hands and arms don't move independently while your body just hangs out. Rather, your upper limbs merely complete the movement that originates in your feet and legs, and flows up through your torso.

Remember the wet towel you used to twist up and snap at your little brother? You snap your arm and wrist, and the movement rolls out along the towel, snaking all the way to the end where it finally releases its energy. That's something like what happens in your body in a slower sense. The movement starts at one place (your feet grounded into the floor) and reverberates up your legs, through your body, and out into your arms and hands.

Staying rooted

When your feet are on the ground, feel them truly on the ground with your weight centered between the ball and the heel, and to each side of your foot. You want to avoid sitting back on your heels or leaning forward on the balls of your feet, both very insecure positions, but not uncommon ones. You also want to avoid standing or walking with your weight rolled outward or inward on the foot.

Standing firmly grounded not only promotes better posture, but it also allows you to firmly gather in the earth's energy, or chi, through an acupoint in the bottom of your foot. Refer to Figure 11-1 and the rest of Chapter 11 for more information about chi.

Trying a Basic Menu of Forms

On to the nuts and bolts. Here comes the fun! This section is where I lead you through a few Tai Chi movements. I selected these forms and honed the instructions with the input of Tai Chi Chuan instructors Manny Fuentes and David-Dorian Ross. The forms, below, are excerpted from the Yang 24-Movement Short Form, also called the Yang Simplified Form, as a way for you to try some simple, introductory movements from the Yang style that is the most common today. You can actually work for months and months just on these forms and be more than fulfilled. I also try to show you how to link movements so that you can flow from one to another. Refer to the appendix for books and videos that teach the entire short form, if you're interested.

Oh, and to confuse you even more, take note: Tai Chi movements are called *forms.* Several forms strung together are called a *sequence,* if you like. A sequence is a chain of many links; so in this case each link is a form. Every mind-body method uses different terms for directing the body to move. Pilates is *exercises* and its sequence is simply a class, for example. Yoga is *postures,* and its linking together is a practice. Every method has its lingo, and some teachers may use one term while others may use it differently. Some even take offense to the name "exercise." So watch your lingo. Carefully.

When all else fails, call what you do *movements.* The word is so neutral that not only will no one be insulted, but you also won't sound silly or like too much of a newbie.

Ebbing and flowing forms

In this section I boil down the movement to its essence before you get started. Here are the basics in one little nutshell:

> ✔ Your weight shifts back and forth
>
> ✔ Your arms go from reached out to pulled in
>
> ✔ Your legs continually move from open to closed stances

If you ever get stuck in a movement, just move in the opposite direction to get yourself right again. Tai Chi movements are like the ocean: the tide doesn't flow in, then flow in again. It flows in, then flows out, flows in, flows out. That's Tai Chi!

Warming Up

Especially before a short Tai Chi session, you may not need to do warm-up movements. But, if you're a newcomer to exercise, you may feel better if you take a few minutes to do 2 to 3 warm-ups before starting the forms.

Beyond just warming up your muscles and joints, a warm-up session can give you a few minutes to quiet yourself and your mind. You prepare yourself to practice your forms, external *and* internal, with more focus. You can use this time to center your energy, forget any upset, or release any tension.

Repeat each warm-up move for 30 to 60 seconds.

Flop Twists

I started doing this warm-up movement even before a run to loosen up my back. Try these easy twisting motions when you start as a way to shake out your muscles and to make sure your feet are rooted.

1. **Stand with your feet parallel and about shoulder-width apart, with your knees slightly bent. Your arms are hanging at your side.**

2. **Swing your body easily, without any force, from side-to-side, letting your arms flop with your body. Your arms may even kind of whack you on each side or as high as your chest as they swing about like cooked spaghetti. Be sure you continue to breathe throughout.**

3. **Continue to look straight ahead as your body swings.**

If you have a bad back, or have had any back injuries, consult with your physician before trying this warm-up. If you get the go-ahead to practice, keep the swings smaller and more controlled.

Flop Arms

In this warm-up, you may feel as if you're paddling along on an air mattress belly-down or legs-down through the middle of an inner tube — and getting nowhere fast!

1. Stand with your feet parallel and about shoulder-width apart, with your knees slightly bent. Your arms hang at your sides.

2. Raise your arms up to about shoulder-height in front of you, keeping the curve described in the "Praising the Tai Chi Principles" section.

3. Let your arms swing back with a big push, as if you're paddling yourself through water. They only go as far as feels natural.

4. Swing your arms to the front in a passive return from the momentum of your back swing, again let the arms only return as far as they move naturally. Continue to breathe fully and naturally.

I Dunno Shoulders

The movements in this warm-up may make you feel as if you're repeatedly saying, "I dunno." But you do know what you're doing — you're warming up your shoulders.

1. Stand with your feet parallel and about shoulder-width apart, with your knees slightly bent. Let your arms hang loosely from your shoulders. Your arms play no part in this warm-up.

2. Inhale and lift one shoulder as high toward your ear as you can, then let it drop with a full exhalation.

3. Inhale and lift the opposite shoulder as high toward your ear as you can, then let it drop down with a big exhalation.

4. Repeat the individual shoulders 8–10 times each, then start the I Dunno pattern. (See Step 5.)

5. Lift both shoulders at the same time as you inhale, hold your shoulders up and tense them, then drop and feel utter relaxation with a full exhalation.

Circling Shoulders

Because you circle your shoulders and use that joint a lot in Tai Chi, warming up that motion can be helpful, too.

1. Stand with your feet parallel and about shoulder-width apart, with your knees slightly bent. Let your arms hang loosely from your shoulders. Do one I Dunno shoulder lift (both shoulders) and hold it for a split second. Inhale with this movement.

2. With both shoulders still lifted toward your ears, rotate both shoulders backward, then start to pull them downward, feeling the stretch across your chest. Begin to exhale.

3. Then drop your shoulders all the way down as if you were holding heavy buckets full of wet sand in each hand.

4. Finish by pulling your shoulders forward as if you were cold and trying to cower a bit. Finish your exhale, inhale once, exhale again, then start the whole pattern again.

5. Repeat 10–12 times, focusing on opening your chest and releasing any tension in your shoulders. Use the breathwork to help you.

Hula Hoop Hips

You may want to make sure you're the only one in the room when you try this hip-loosening exercise!

1. Stand with feet a little wider than shoulder-width apart with your hands on your hips.

2. Bend your knees a little and swing your hips slowly in a full circle as if you were trying to keep a hula hoop up (only you'd be going faster if you really were).

3. Repeat about 10–15 times in each direction. Make sure you keep the breath moving in and out throughout.

Drawing Circles

Feel as if you're trying to draw a big circle in front of you in the air with your big toe.

1. Stand on one foot, holding onto the wall or a chair as needed for balance.

2. Draw big imaginary circles in the air with the toes of the foot you're not standing on 8–10 times in each direction.

3. Change feet and repeat. Be sure not to hold your breath!

Footing the basics

Although most Chinese Tai Chi instructors just say, "Follow me," and off you go, I describe a few basic foot positions that you use over and over. And over and over. They're the foundations of the forms that follow. Having these basics described and broken-down can make life easier when you try to do the follow-the-leader routine.

You can call these foot positions *steps* or *stances* according to what tickles your fancy.

A Centering Step by any other name . . .

As with all the mind-body methods, different schools, styles, and instructors call different moves by different names. Maybe someone just translated a word or phrase differently; maybe someone felt his or her name better described a movement than another one did. In both the Tai Chi and Qigong chapters in this part, this is particularly true. I try throughout to give you the more common names. But keep an open mind and visualize — the names are all just designed to conjure up an image of what the movement looks like.

Bow Stance (Also Called Bow and Arrow Step, or Arched Step)

Practice the Bow 'til you're blue in the face. Getting this stance down is crucial because it's the foundation of many Tai Chi movements. In this stance, you bend your front leg like a primed bow, and keep your back leg straight like an arrow ready for flight.

Figure 10-1 illustrates all three foot positions: Bow Stance, Centering Step, and Empty Step.

Figure 10-1:
What are those feet doing? The Bow Stance, Centering Step, and Empty Step, that's what!

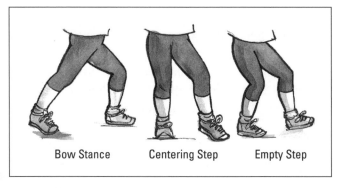

Bow Stance   Centering Step   Empty Step

1. **Start standing with both feet parallel and about hip-width apart. Bend your knees slightly keeping your weight centered over your feet and your hips tucked under slightly.**

   This feet-parallel stance is a typical stance for starting and closing forms, as well as a stance for meditation. I discuss this concept in Chapter 11.

2. **Turn your right foot out slightly (about 45 degrees) by pivoting on your heel to point your toes outward.**

This allows you to keep your hips dropped and your spine aligned and not forced into a sway-back position. If you need to, shift your weight onto your left foot slightly, before you put the weight back onto your right foot to go into the step-out, next.

3. **Nearly at the same time as you're turning your heel, begin bending your right knee slightly and shifting your weight onto your right foot. At the same time, raise your left knee, lifting your left toe off the ground, and step out to the front leading with your heel. Land first (and softly!) onto the floor with your heel, rolling the rest of your foot down flat. Imagine that you're trying to sneak up on somebody and you want to be really, really quiet!**

4. **As your left foot lands, your right leg nearly straightens, pushing about 60–70 percent of your weight onto your front leg, which is bending at the knee. Your stance now looks like a lunge.**

When you get into the position, make sure that your front foot points directly forward. The toes on your right foot should point outward slightly. Plus, you should have some width between your feet as if your heels were placed on opposite corners of a square on the ground.

Centering Step (Also called T-Step)

This transitional step merely shifts your weight. But to do it well is a moment of pure heaven when you feel as if you are floating above the ground, strong in your center, focused in your heart, and totally in control of your body's movement. Developing balance is what gets you to that nanosecond of bliss.

You don't normally just stand around in a Centering Step, but use it to move into other positions. So use this drill to practice your body positioning and balance.

1. **Start standing with both feet parallel and about hip-width apart. Bend your knees slightly (just soften the joint) keeping your weight centered over your feet and your hips tucked under slightly.**

2. **Shift your hips (and your body weight) from a centered position over both feet to a centered position over your right foot, bending your right knee a little more.**

3. **At the same time, lift your left foot and touch the base of your toes onto the ground next to the arch of your right foot.**

4. **Open out your left knee and hip slightly, using the muscles in your buttocks and hips to rotate the knee outward.**

You should be able to stand in this balanced position with no weight on your lifted knee. Try to lift that toe for a moment — you should be able to do this without falling over. Advanced Tai Chi students never touch the ground with that toe or foot when they pass through this position to another one.

Empty Step

This step doesn't really have a name. But teachers who name it often call it Empty Step because your rear foot is *full* (carrying 100 percent of your weight), while your front foot is *empty* (carrying none of your weight). The yin-yang concept of opposites mixing to provide a perfect balance comes into play here.

The Empty step is another transitional step that you don't usually start from a simple standing position. But use these step-by-step instructions to get into a correct position so you can feel and practice it while stationary before putting it into motion.

Empty Step is a lot like the Centering Step (see "Centering Step" in earlier in this section) except the hip of your non-weight-bearing foot is turned in and that toe is in front of the supporting leg, not beside it.

1. **Start standing with both feet parallel and about hip-width apart. Bend your knees slightly, keeping your weight centered over your feet and your hips tucked under slightly. Position your toes as if you are toeing an imaginary straight line on the ground in front of you.**

2. **Step directly forward with your left foot, placing your heel on the other side of the imaginary line.**

3. **Shift your weight backward, bending both knees and lifting just the heel and arch of your left, non-weight-bearing foot off the ground.**

   You should be balanced and rooted on your right leg strongly enough that you can lift the front-left toe off the ground and not fall or be forced to shift your body position.

To help you really feel the weight shift, try rocking this step forward and backward slowly and gently from front foot to rear foot. Just transfer most of your weight onto the front foot, then rock it all backward onto the rear foot, taking a moment to find your balance, then lift your front toe slightly. Be sure to alternate which foot you put forward — one side of your body is always stronger than the other.

Handling your hands

As with feet positioning, many instructors usually don't break apart hand positioning and teach them separately during a sequence or the short form. But, I do exactly that for you since I believe breaking down the movement and seeing it in isolation helps you master a movement or position when you set it in motion. I even offer an illustration, in Figure 10-2, showing the Hold Balloon form and the basic Tai Chi arm position.

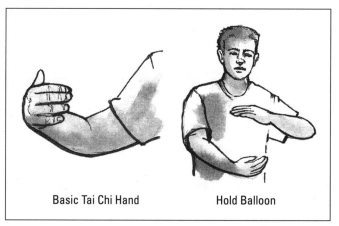

Figure 10-2:
What are those hands doing? Respectively, the Hold Balloon form and the Basic Tai Chi hand.

Basic Tai Chi Hand   Hold Balloon

Basic Tai Chi Hand

The goal for your arms and hands is to keep them curved and soft, but still full of energy and not limp. You do *not* bring your middle finger in a little, as ballet dancers do.

1. **Hold both arms straight out in front of your shoulders, palms facing in, hands and fingers straight.**

2. **Let your fingers and thumbs soften slightly so your palm develops a slight cup.**

3. **At the same time, allow your elbows to soften and widen outward slightly (something they want to do when you soften your hands).**

   You now have one smooth curved line (remember that curves are a key principle of Tai Chi) from your shoulder, around the outside of your elbow and down the back of your wrist and hand to the end of your fingers. Your wrist is soft, but not bent in so much that you have an abrupt change in angle between your forearm and back of your hand.

When the hands go too limp and floppy, the Chinese call it "Too Much Fair Lady Hand." (David-Dorian Ross, who has lived, studied, and competed in China, provided what I assume is that rather loose translation!) At all costs, avoid too much fair lady hand!

Hold Balloon (Also, Holding the Ball, or Embracing the Moon)

The names for this hand position are inspired by what it looks and feels like. I have a soft spot (in my head?) for the name Hold Balloon because it feels lighter and softer to me.

In this position, you feel as if you're holding a balloon in front of your body (well, duh . . .). Your arms and hands look and feel as if they are conforming to the circle of a large inflated balloon.

Start standing in a feet-parallel stance so you don't have to think about it. After you have that down, you can try Hold Balloon with a Centering Step, too.

1. **Bring your left hand palm up and arm across your body at the level of your hips, but don't extend your left hand beyond your right side.**

2. **Bring your right hand palm down and arm across your body at the level of your chest, but don't extend it beyond your left side.**

3. **Soften both elbows and remember to practice Basic Tai Chi Arm! You are now holding a balloon between your arms and hands.**

4. **Try the same position with the opposite hand on top.**

The hand positions and levels change slightly based on the form you are going into or coming out of, as do they also change a bit depending on a teacher's style.

Introducing forms for all folks

The following six forms are part of the Yang Simplified Form. I also include simple opening and closing forms that Tai Chi practitioners believe should be done to properly receive and keep energy, and that are used to open and close the Yang form.

These six key moves can help you understand the basics and help you decide if you want to do more Tai Chi. They also help you center and feel the patterns that come when you start mixing and matching in Chapter 12. In these forms, I have in most cases oriented you to do them in the direction they would face if you were actually doing the Yang Short Form. But you can of course practice them facing whichever way you'd like at first.

Always think about flow. I tell you this over and over. And I won't stop — I'm like a nagging relative. When you practice Tai Chi, what you are practicing is flow, baby, flow.

Grasp the Bird's Tail (Also called Grasping the Sparrow's Tail)

This simple-sounding form actually has four parts and, beautifully enough, covers all of the key movements of Tai Chi in those four! Those four are: Ward Off, Roll Back, Press, and Push, some of which have several parts themselves. I take you through the entire form one side. Be sure to practice it on both sides. For example, you could do it on one side several times, then come into a transitional Centering Step to put yourself into position for the opposite side, where you would do it again several times. You could spend entire sessions doing this one move on both sides over and over! Figure 10-3 shows you all the parts.

Go west, young man! Well, maybe north . . .

Typically, in classical Tai Chi, you find the movement oriented in two ways: by direction (north, south, east, west) or by the face of a clock (12 o'clock, 6 o'clock, and so on). That takes some thinking compared to traditional Western exercise where you just face front, wherever front is, then turn right or turn left. In Tai Chi, the face of a clock is the easiest because your front — wherever that may be — becomes 12 o'clock. (Okay, in most cases. Here we go with another exception. Some call the *rear* true 12 o'clock. Remember, nothing is truly wrong if there is a reason for it and it's consistent.) For you here, then, if your front is 12, then your right is 3, to the rear is 6, and to your left is 9. If you ever hear an instructor say, "Face north," that doesn't necessarily mean true polar north. North may just be a representation of wherever the front happens to be.

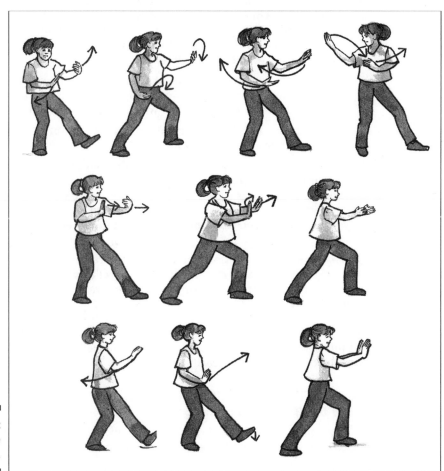

Figure 10-3: Grasp the Bird's Tail.

1. **Start in the Bow Stance (refer to Figure 10-1) with your left foot forward. The foot faces 8 o'clock with 12 o'clock (your front) in front of the open part of the stance.**

2. **Ward Off: Extend your left hand in front of you with the palm cupped and facing you at chest-height. Point your thumb upward so that your elbow is dropped slightly. Your right hand is palm down at your right hip with the elbow bent slightly. (This is where the Bird's Tail gets grasped, so to speak.)**

   If you want to be tricky, you can step into this by starting from a Centering Step with Hold Balloon hands. Inhale, then exhale and start the movement. Be sure to continue to breathe through all four parts.

3. **Roll Back: Turn your left palm down and your right palm up simultaneously as you reach forward with your right hand until both palms are on the same plane (8 o'clock direction still) at about chest-height. Your right palm is near your left elbow.**

4. **Turn your waist to the right as you were trying to shine a headlight in the middle of your chest toward about 2 o'clock. At the same time, shift your weight to your right leg, dropping both hands in a low arc in front of you, ending with both hands also facing 2 o'clock, right palm still up and left palm still down.**

5. **Press: Rotate back to the left from your waist. At the same time, round your left arm as it moves outward to 8 o'clock, palm in, and press with your right hand toward your left wrist, barely grazing it.**

6. **Now shift your weight to your left leg until you return to the Bow Stance and press your hands forward.**

7. **Push: Rotate your hands so you can slide your right palm over the top of your left wrist (some teachers reach to forearm). Then, as you shift your weight to your right leg again, separate the hands to about shoulder-width at navel-height, palms facing down. When your weight is on your back foot, you lift your left toe from the floor.**

8. **To finish, rock your weight forward onto your left leg again and, at the same time, raise your palms to where they are facing away from you as if preparing to push a really heavy tall object away from you. Your elbows do not actually flex or extend. The arm movement comes form the shoulders.**

Grasp the Bird's Tail is one of the longest of the forms I present. When you don't think about doing the forms so hard and just let your body move naturally, you flow through them easily.

Parting the Wild Horse's Mane (Also called Parting the Horse's Mane)

This sequence is actually the first movement after the Opening form of the Yang Simplified Form. The hands may seem similar to the first part of Bird's

Tail at first (see the section, "Grasp the Bird's Tail," preceding this section), but pay close attention and you can feel and see the difference. You can also check out Figure 10-4, which illustrates the differences.

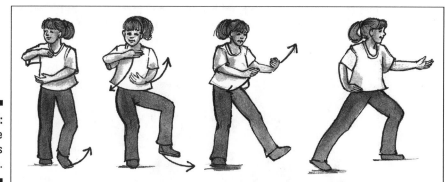

Figure 10-4:
Parting the Wild Horse's Mane.

1. **Start in a Centering Step with your left toe nearly weightless. Your arms are in the Hold Balloon position with your left arm on the bottom and therefore open to your left side that is nearly weightless.**

   Check out the Cheat Sheet in the front of the book for an illustration of the Centering Step, or refer to Figure 10-1.

2. **Inhale, then exhale and step out into a Bow Stance with your left foot. At the same time, sweep outward and upward diagonally with your left hand, and push palm down with your right hand to the inside of your left hand. Your right palm ends facing down at your right hip.**

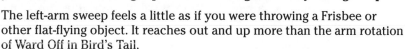

   The left-arm sweep feels a little as if you were throwing a Frisbee or other flat-flying object. It reaches out and up more than the arm rotation of Ward Off in Bird's Tail.

3. **Finish both the forward-stepping and weight-shifting into the Bow stance to face an 8 o'clock position at the *same* time that your left hand reaches the upward position. The fingers are upward and the palm is facing the front of your heart.**

4. **To practice this repeatedly, rock back with your weight onto your left leg at the same time that you float your arms back into a Hold Balloon position. To do that, you can rotate left hand down and sweep the arm to your hip bones, rotating the hand up as you arrive. At the same time, you can rotate your right palm up, sweep it backward, over and back down over the top to "hold" the top of the balloon.**

Think this sounds too easy? Then try repeating it while inhaling on the rock-back and exhaling on the rock-forward, but make the lunge lower. A few minutes of these on either side and you may find yourself mentally challenged to stay focused, as well as physically challenged through your legs and torso to stay low.

Play the Pi'pa (Also called Strum the Lute, or Play the Guitar)

This is a simple move during which you get to try the Empty Step for your feet. As you begin to link the forms in this section, you can use this form as a transition between the others. In the Yang Short Form, it's No. 5 of 24 movements. Imagine you are holding a stringed instrument between your hands to help you with hand placement, as shown in Figure 10-5.

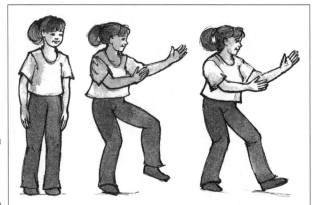

Figure 10-5: Play the Pi'pa.

1. **Start by standing with your feet hip-width apart and arms hanging loose at your sides, in the Basic Stance, facing 9 o'clock.**

2. **Rock your weight onto your right leg as you bend that knee. At the same time, lift your left toe, placing the non-weight-bearing ball of that foot a foot-length forward of its original position to place yourself in an Empty Step.**

3. **At the same time your feet are moving, lift your left arm upward from the shoulder with the palm facing in and the elbow nearly extended, but still curved, as if you were about to shake hands with somebody with your left hand. Your right arm also lifts from the shoulder with that palm also facing in, finishing just below and to your right of your left elbow.**

4. **Repeat on the other side by first stepping back into a basic position with both feet hip-width apart. Then step back out on the other side.**

5. **Finish by placing the front foot back on the floor with the heel down and toe lifted.**

A tall but relaxed posture with your tailbone pulled down can help you stay balanced and not sway.

Repulse the Monkey (Also called Fending Off the Monkey)

You can put together a string of Empty Steps as you Play the Pi'pa, and move backward to Repulse the Monkey — as if there were a Monkey in your living room. (Believe me, I really didn't make up these names!) This form even comes right after the Pi'pa step in the Yang Short Form. So after you get both forms down independently, you can put them together! Figure 10-6 shows you how.

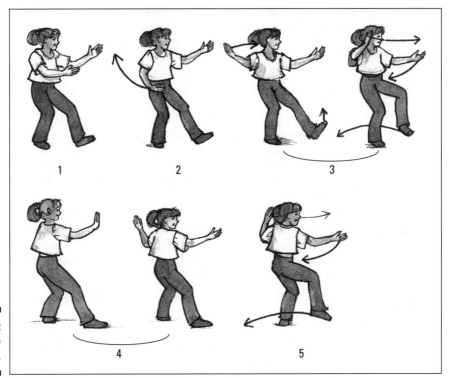

Figure 10-6:
Repulse the
Monkey.

1. **Start in the final position of Play the Pi'pa where your weight is on your right foot to the rear and your hands are forward as if holding the stringed instrument. Your entire body faces 9 o'clock, just as in the finish of Play the Pi'pa.**

2. **Turn your right hand palm up and circle it downward and to the rear in a large arc that moves all the way behind you to 2 o'clock. Turn your waist toward 12 o'clock with the arm circle, as your eyes follow the hand.**

3. **When the hand reaches about shoulder height to the rear, bring the palm straight in to brush past your cheek as if you were pushing something away to your front. Your elbow bends at an acute angle when the hand brushes past your ear. Your waist rotates back toward 9 o'clock with the rear-circling arm movement.**

   Your palm is cupped and sort of grazes near your ear on its path forward as if you were trying to hear something better.

What do I look at?

You can look inward, and you can look outward. Oh, no, there she goes again with these riddles, you say. During all of these moves, you should be almost softening your gaze as if your eyes are open but nobody's home. You want to look inward and focus on your breath and relaxation.

You can even shut your eyes if you want to. If they're open, or just half-open, you can let the gaze follow the fingertips, although it is not really looking at it. The eyeballs are just moving in that direction.

4. **At the moment your right hand moves past your ear, step back with your left foot, touching your toes first, then rolling back onto the entire foot with your weight, to create another Empty Step with your right foot forward. Re-align your new front foot so that your toes face forward.**

5. **Your right hand continues to float forward, turning palm down as your left hand now turns palm up. The two palms float past each other, with your right one continuing its path forward, and your left one now starting its journey to the rear to repeat the entire process starting with Step 2, on the opposite side.**

6. **Repeat as many times as you need to, traveling backward with each step.**

Open Arms Like a Fan (Also called Fan Through the Back, and Unfolding Your Arms Like a Fan)

Think of making a large fanning motion as you complete this step, shown in Figure 10-7. Also imagine an opponent in front of you and one to your left, and you deflect each one with a different arm. Boy, you should be in the movies!

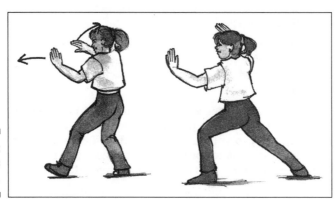

Figure 10-7:
Open Arms
Like a Fan.

1. **Start in a Centering Step facing 12 o'clock with your left toe touching the ground. Your hands are in the Hold Balloon position with your left arm on the bottom.**

   See the Cheat Sheet for these forms.

2. **Step out toward 9 o'clock with your left foot, moving into a Bow Step.**

3. **At the same time, sweep your right arm palm out in a circular motion in front your head, ending with it near your right temple as if protecting your head.**

4. **While your right arm is fanning around palm out protecting your head from an imaginary opponent, your left arm fans upward and outward (moving with your body as it turns to 9 o'clock). Your left palm also rotates outward, and it finishes at about nose-height, also toward 9 o'clock.**

Let your gaze follow your forward-fanning hand, which in the example above is the left.

Separate Hands and Kick (also called Step Up and Kick, and Heel Kick)

Instead of staying well-grounded, with both feet on the floor all this time (well, almost), you get to kick up your legs — one at a time, of course. Wait, though, this "kick" is frankly less of a kick than you think because it's in Tai Chi slow motion. It's more of a lift of the knee, followed by the lower leg lifting up, as Figure 10-8 shows. And that's a lot harder because you can't use momentum!

1. **Start in a turned-out Centering Step (refer to Figure 10-1) with your right toe on the ground and your weight on your left leg, facing 9 o'clock, with your left knee slightly bent.**

2. **Cross your hands at the wrists with palms up, left hand on top of right, about six inches in front of your belly button.**

"At the same time . . . "

How many times have you read that in the Tai Chi instructions I given: "At the same time, do blah-blah . . ." That's what Tai Chi is all about: Flow, baby. And accomplishing flow means the movements ripple as one, like a mountain stream caressing down a meadow. You should work on having all movements arrive at a "finish" position at the same time, even when they are traveling different distances or varied arcs. The catch, however, is that there really is no "finish!" So as soon as they simultaneously reach that so-called finish, they are already — yes, "at the same time" — rippling into the next position as one unit. You should feel like a snake, rhythmically rolling from one place to the other.

When your right leg is kicking, your left wrist is on top. When your left leg is kicking, your right wrist is on top. Opposites again.

3. **Your right knee lifts diagonally to the side without shifting your body in anyway then, keeping your knee firmly stationary in the air, straighten out your lower leg away from you using the knee as a hinge. Kick or push your heel out (imagine your opponent standing there!).**

4. **At the same time as the leg movement, your arms start to lift upward from the shoulders as the wrists rotate so your palms are facing out. Then your hands "separate," palms out, finishing nose-height at about the 7 o'clock and 11 o'clock corners. The position is a bit like the fan in the previous form. Follow your right hand with your eyes.**

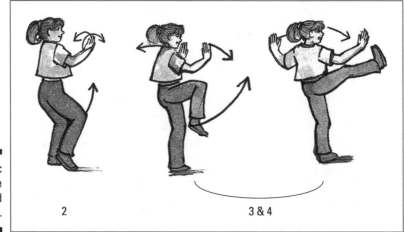

Figure 10-8:
Separate hands and kick.

2

3 & 4

Lift your kicking leg only as high as you can while still maintaining your spinal alignment (no sinking in the ribs or slumping through your back!). You should be able to straighten your lower leg out from that knee without slumping, too. Remember, slumping weakens you and makes you vulnerable to an opponent, who may just knock you off your feet.

Incorporating great beginnings . . . and endings

All the forms start with an opening move — and I don't mean a little Buffalo two-step across your living room! — and finish with a closing move. Basically, these moves help you gather your energy, focus, and breathe before beginning your movement, or finishing and moving on to other things.

Different schools and styles have different approaches to the same opening and closing moves. They vary in knee bend, timing, and stepping, but look very similar. These two are the simplest and are used by most teachers doing the Yang short form.

Open the Door (Or Beginning)

Use this form, shown in Figure 10-9, to bring your mind to the right place for your practice.

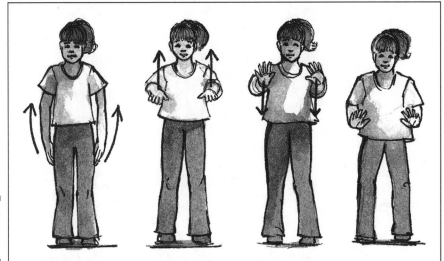

Figure 10-9:
Open the Door.

1. **Start in a narrow stance with your feet together, knees relaxed, arms loose at your side. Take this moment to find your posture and relax in all the right spots.**

2. **Inhale while lifting your arms from the shoulder to about shoulder height (already practicing Tai Chi hands, of course). At the same time, shift your weight slightly and subtly to one foot.**

3. **As soon as the hands reach the top of the move, exhale, step out with your right foot so that your feet are about hip-width apart. Then sink down with your knees and your entire body weight. Let your arms drop slowly and finish at about navel height, wrists cocked slightly so your palms are facing down.**

   Stay here for a moment to breathe and focus, or even repeat this step several times before you begin.

Closing the Door (Or Conclusion)

Enjoy this closing form as a satisfying way to finish your practice. Don't just do the form and run off, though! Stay in the final stance for a few moments and take some deep breaths. Figure 10-10 shows you how.

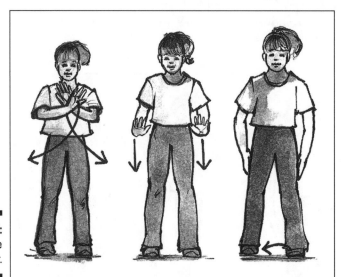

Figure 10-10:
Closing the
Door.

1. **From whatever your last position is before your close: Rotate your body to 12 o'clock. Inhale, and bring your feet about hip-width apart, crossing your wrists, palms in, in front of your chest.**

2. **Exhale, and slowly uncross your wrists, floating your hands to your sides. Palms lead downward until the hands and wrists are extended and at your side, palms facing your thighs.**

Chapter 11

Finding Your Inner Fountain of Energy with Qigong

In This Chapter

▶ Getting the background on Qigong

▶ Mastering standing well

▶ Practicing your microcosmic orbit

*O*kay, so the concept of gaining energy appeals to you, but Qi-who?

First things first — you want to know what this name means and how the heck you pronounce it. *Qi (*pronounced *chee)* is the nonlatinized spelling of the term *chi* or energy (also called "life energy"), and is pronounced the same way. *Gong* (pronounced *gung)* means "work" or "a practice" — something you gain benefits from by dedication to. Combine the two words and you get Qigong, which in the Western Hemisphere, can also be spelled "chi kung" or even "chi gong," which you then pronounce *chee-gung.* You see the concept of chi is right out in front, telling you right away what this is all about.

Put it all together, and you see that *Qigong* is a discipline that focuses on working on the flow of your life energy through a practice of movement.

Feeling the Energy of Qigong

Energy is what Qigong is all about. Working with your energy. Feeling it. Gaining it. Moving it. And letting it help you feel healthier and happier. This is not a medical book, but you should be aware that Qigong, in some forms, can be considered a healing practice, not just an energizing addition to a healthful fitness routine. Some hospitals and practitioners — even a few in the Western world these days — use transference of their own personal Qi to heal disease or injuries, or to keep a person healthy. If you listen, you can hear stories about people who had cancer or other ailments, and who were healed by either consulting with a practitioner or starting a personal Qigong practice (see Chapter 6 for a couple of stories like that). In China, being healed by someone using his or her energy is not uncommon. Sometimes this is done in combination with herbal treatments or other medical care such as acupuncture.

Discussing the practice of using energy for healing is way beyond my scope in this book on mind-body fitness. If you want to delve deeper into that area, you can consult the Appendix for additional resources, perhaps starting with the nonprofit Qigong Institute for research.

Even as a mind-body fitness routine, Qigong can help you dig around inside yourself in a much more spiritual sense than some methods I discuss in this book such as the Modern Classics that focus more on body awareness. The basis of Qigong isn't just to do a movement a particular way, but to use it to learn to listen to your body, to feel the pulsing energy, and to use those feelings to better not only your Qigong practice, but also every other practice and every other part of your life.

The flowing, nearly choreographed and dance-like routines are a more advanced step that can take months and years of practice to accomplish. One that is commonly known, Wild Goose, has an entire series of parts with numerous forms for each part that takes years to grasp, then even more years to fine-tune. Such routines may be low- to moderate-intensity aerobic and full-body workouts in a flowing way you'd never get from a step-aerobics class. But those are awfully difficult to introduce in one chapter. So I have chosen instead a series of stationary or independent movements, rather than an entire routine. Refer to the Appendix for resources to help you dig deeper if you'd like.

Despite only scratching the surface, this chapter on Qigong presents some of the most unfamiliar and slightly esoteric information (to Westerners) I get into in this book. Don't let that scare you off. Take what you want; leave the rest. You may not be comfortable with all this stuff about energy spouting out your hands and up your spine. That's okay. Just use the movements to help you feel your body. Pretty soon, you may find yourself getting in touch with more flow and energy.

Dr. Bingkun Hu, a master Qigong instructor from Berkeley, California, told me once that he thinks the closest comparison to Qigong familiar to the Western world is psychic practices. Somehow that doesn't seem so odd since the basis of psychic ability is listening to your gut feelings. You try to listen to and trust your intuition, don't you? Well, in a loose way, Qigong is like intuition. You have to train yourself to listen and to trust.

Infusing a Chinese medical tenet into Western health care

To the Chinese, ongoing Qigong practice is considered one way to keep disease at bay. The Chinese philosophy is: Prevent disease from occuring rather than try to cure it once it occurs. Slowly, ever so slowly, Western health care is beginning to accept this concept. The U.S. government-funded research body, the National Institutes of Health, has a branch devoted to alternative medicine and health that has begun to fund research into areas like Qigong and meditation. Some health insurance policies now cover such things as acupuncture and massage as well. Coverage of preventive measures such as Qigong may be in the future. Stay tuned as the world changes.

Uncovering Qigong's Benefits

What you gain from a Qigong practice extends way beyond the basic aerobic fitness you can achieve in a traditional fitness class. Fitness is in fact secondary, as it is in the other Chinese mind-body art, Tai Chi Chuan, that I discuss in Chapter 10. Fitness, in the traditional Western sense, turns out to be a pleasant and perhaps surprising outcome of a Qigong practice.

Interestingly, Qigong is one of the methods in this book with the most credible scientific proof behind it. (See Chapter 6 for some of the details.) For analytical Western minds, that fact may be quite astounding because, on the face of it, Qigong seems to be the least scientifically provable discipline of the bunch. But in China, Qigong has long been recognized as both a science and an art, so no one raises an eyebrow about gaining such a range of good things from the simplest of movement forms.

"Use your mind to promote your health and your mental state," says master instructor Dr. Bingkun Hu.

The following sections outline several benefits you could gain from a regular Qigong practice.

Finding the awareness

Your mind discovers how to open up and become more finely tuned-in to what is happening within you and outside of you, as well as how they are connected. That can mean awareness of your health, your body's movement, any tension or stress, particular feelings, or your relationship to the world you move through. That awareness is the first step in allowing you to take control of anything that may need action, such as releasing stress or healing a disease.

Feeling the focus and calm

The meditative, repetitive, and awareness movements, as well as the flowing routines, bring on a sense of calm, peace and mental clarity that then can permeate everything you do in life. Of course, it's not scientifically proven, but you try it and see. You may become more focused in work, in relationships, in school, and in all interactions. You may become more relaxed (not a space cadet, oh no, just calm and clear) and you may be able to deal with what comes at you day-to-day better than you could otherwise.

Gaining higher energy

With more awareness of body and mind, and a more focused calm, also comes a higher energy level. And the energy you gain is vibrant and alive, not like the burst you may get from the likes of caffeine or adrenaline. You carry this energy throughout all you do, long after a Qigong session is over and done.

Feeling the fitness

Yes, yes, you do get exercise and therefore can see many of the healthful gains that come from moderate aerobic activity, such as lower risk of disease and increased strength and flexibility. Okay, okay, the fitness connection to Qigong isn't truly proven by science, but you try it. These gains of course depend on the intensity, level, and type of movements you do. Many of the exercises in this chapter focus on increasing your awareness and getting in touch with your chi and are more stationary. They may bring on only higher relaxation and clearness of thought. No real fitness benefits there.

Practicing the Principles of Qigong

Qigong exercise is a series of linked postures or forms that flow from one into the other like a smooth, very slow dance. The practice also includes simple, stand-alone stances where your mind does all the work, such as standing meditations, self-massage from standing or seated positions, and breathing practices. Qigong, in this case, can hardly even be called exercise in the traditional Western sense.

At least five schools, including Daoist, Buddhist, Confucian, medial and martial, take a slightly different approach to the method. Just like Tai Chi, some Qigong styles are a martial art that can also be combative! But, not to worry, you won't be kicking out anybody's teeth any time soon.

In this section, I start your journey by exploring the common tenets of Qigong forms.

Breathing bonanza

Where some mind-body methods in this book instruct you to continue to breathe, in Qigong, breathing is what the entire practice is really all about. "Qigong is breathing. Breathing is Qigong," says Dr. Bingkun Hu, a master instructor in Berkeley, California. That doesn't mean that you just sit and breathe (although you can). Using movement is the best way to train your breathing to be full and conscious. With the movement of full breath follows the stabilization of your energy in your body's energy channels (see the next section in this chapter). After your energy is stable and balanced, you can move your energy better.

Meeting your Microcosmic Orbit

Microcosmic Orbit certainly sounds like a term out of *The Jetsons.* But do take it more seriously than a cartoon. This is a path used to create a rushing flow of chi through two of the largest of your energy channels, the one up the front and the one down the back. If you look at yourself from the side, imagine an oval with one side of the oval kind of running up the front from below the Dan Tien to the crown of your head (Bai Hui), then the other side of the oval running back down your back. The oval finishes the path again at the bottom where they connect at the Dan Tien. When you do microcosmic orbit meditations, you're working to free the flow along these super highways. The exercises in this section help your energy channels flowing smoothly. Be sure to keep breathing during all of them to help your energy move.

Historically speaking

More people have at least heard of Tai Chi, but what most don't realize is Qigong is actually an older form of exercise than Tai Chi. Traces of Qigong have been found in historical pictograms that date back to hundreds of years B.C. Over the centuries, some Qigong practices were influenced by Daoist masters and even Buddhist monks, creating hundreds and thousands of different styles. Just like other mind-body methods, nothing is truly wrong; it may just stem from a different teacher. The ultimate goal in all cases is to balance the body's energy to achieve greater health and happiness. The forms in this chapter stem mostly from Daoist and Buddhist schools.

So why, if Qigong is so ancient, have so few people heard of it, and are even fewer doing it? Because for a very long time, Qigong was a very secretive practice, passed down in families (even royal ones) from generation to generation, and kept mostly behind closed doors. Although more research and practice was done in the mid-1900s, it wasn't really until the 1970s that interest blossomed. The Chinese government watched the growth, and finally granted its support and approval in 1985. As a part of that government approval, researchers now present results from hundreds of scientific papers at annual Qigong conferences.

Your energy isn't really just sloshing around under your skin. Qigong practitioners see it moving through different *meridians* — like a little network of energy highways running throughout your whole body, with certain gathering centers (highway interchanges) and points of access (on- and off-ramps) where energy more readily flows in, out, and around. Figure 11-1 shows these energy channels, with their names. The points (sometimes called *acupoints* because they are also used as gateways in acupuncture) are the chi on- and off- ramps. Every spiritual school has different numbers and locations of on- and off- ramps, but the ramps all serve the same purpose.

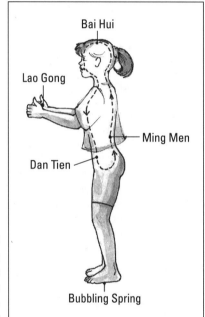

Figure 11-1:
The
Microcosmic
Orbit.

In Qigong, you work one major center (the Dan Tien, located in your abdomen) with several major on and off ramps. Depending on your teacher, he or she may use different names or even vary the location slightly.

Dan Tien

Before I knew a Qigong teacher who was actually able to answer my probing questions, I took some classes from an Asian man who could speak very little English. He'd say something about a "dawn ten" and sort of point to his belly. I just figured I couldn't understand what he was saying and kept moving.

How wrong I was about misunderstanding. The *Dan Tien* (pronounced *dawn tyen* and meaning literally "elixir field") is akin to NASA's Mission Control for your body's energy, according to Qigong theory. Located between your navel and your pubic bone in the center of your abdomen, the Dan Tien (practice saying this word — you'll hear it often if you read about or do any Qigong) acts as a storehouse for your body's energy, as well as a pump to get your energy gushing to all the right places when you need it. Doing the right practices and the right movements makes sure you don't lose or gain too much from this center. But this pump needs priming. If you let it just sit unused, it dries up. Practices such as Qigong movement, other mind-body methods, and meditation can help prime your pump and keep the chi flowing smoothly.

As a Qigong student, you may find that nurturing what is underneath a very innocent-looking belly becomes a way of life since the "elixir field" holds long life, health, and wisdom. Man, that's nothing to leave out in the rain.

Now that we've settled that, let's expand, because there are actually three parts to the command central:

- ✔ **Lower Dan Tien** is in your lower abdomen and stores sexual energy.

- ✔ **Middle Dan Tien** is in your center about at your heart and relates to the health of your internal organs.

- ✔ **Upper Dan Tien** is what other Eastern practices call the *third eye chakra* — a spot on your forehead between your eyebrows. It is logically associated with the brain.

If someone ever just says "Dan Tien" without qualifying the location, they mean the belly area, or the lower Dan Tien.

Note that you may also see different spellings, such as *dantien* and *dan-tien*.

Ming Men

This was another term my barely English-speaking instructor would use. I strained to hear it each time, rolling it around in my brain, trying to figure out what he meant. Turns out I heard it right. I just didn't know what he meant when he said "ming men" and rubbed his low back. Literally meaning "gate of life," the *Ming Men* (pronounced *meeng men*) acupoint controls your kidneys and is located in your low back. If stimulated properly, Ming Men keeps the kidneys functioning well and can increase your vim and vigor. You can use your fists to rub this area, the same way some people rub their low back when they stand up to stretch and sort of lean backward a little. This rubbing is often done before or after practices, or if you feel your energy waning. Better than a cup of joe!

Bubbling Spring

Also called Bubbling Well or Yong Chuan, these are points in the front part of the instep near the ball of the foot. They allow you to feed your Dan Tien and Ming Men with chi from the earth. If stimulated properly, they can help feed even more vitality up into your Dan Tien by helping to prime your Ming Men. Got that?

Stand up for a minute. Don't move. Just feel how your feet are placed on the floor. Many people subconsciously stand on the outside of their feet or with their weight sort of thrown back on their heels. But planting yourself firmly, as I describe in the Tai Chi chapter (see Chapter 10), allows your Bubbling Spring points to fully access chi from the earth and feed it up to your body's Mission Control.

You can massage the balls of your feet with your hands to stimulate this acupoint, also.

Lao Gong

If you cup your hand as if you were trying to hold water to drink, right in the center of the bottom is the *Lao Gong* acupoint. (Translated, you can call it the Labor Palace.) Pronounced like an "ow" exclamation of pain with an "l" sound in front, the Lao Gong ("gong" rhymes with King Kong) is an energy point that I use often in this book. It can perhaps be felt most easily by someone beginning to experiment with the flow of their chi. Look for this little experiment, Feel Your Chi, later in this section.

Bai Hui

Balanced in the very tippy top of your head, the *Bai Hui* (pronounced *by way*) literally means "hundred meetings" because many energy channels up and down your body converge there and mix before continuing their journey. In other practices, the point is called the Crown Chakra.

Practicing Powerfully Quiet Postures

The essence of Qigong lies in its deep stillness — a stillness that exists even when you're moving. Because this chapter is but an introduction to Qigong, I focus mostly on standing and walking movements, and stand-alone meditations. The longer forms — such as Wild Goose — that string together twists, turns, bends, reaches, and move all around, are quite complicated, although experiencing them is worth the effort to seek out further instruction at some point. Before you can understand and fully gain from those forms, however, you need to be able to get in touch with your chi. For many, that takes non-moving or less complex postures so you don't lose your focus on the chi while trying to untangle your feet and arms.

One of the best ways to start dabbling in Qigong is to incorporate small pieces of it into other parts of your mind-body routine or just scatter it throughout your day. Of course, for many people, Qigong exercise can be an entire program in itself.

The following list offers examples of how you can use it in combination with other routines you may do.

✔ **Warming up mentally or physically:** The gentle movements bringing focus and calm can be a superb way to center yourself as a part of a mental warm-up so you're ready to proceed with the rest of your practice or exercises. With mind-body or even traditional exercise for fitness or performance, it is vital to be mentally johnny-on-the-spot and ready to go. Qigong movements can also be a way to start moving and warming up joints and muscles to prepare them for either more active and intense Qigong routines or other exercises.

✔ **Cooling down after exercise:** Same as above for warming up, but in reverse. When you're done, you need to cool down your muscles and joints. You also need to settle your mind and bring it back to the other duties and tasks you may be moving onto.

✔ **For relaxation:** If you stick to the basic, meditative movements, Qigong can serve as a wonderful way to calm down and prepare for a good night's sleep. Or, if you've had some high-stress in your day, you can use a few minutes to recenter, focus, and bring back the calm you had earlier.

✔ **Preperformance focusing:** Whether before a lecture to a ballroom full of people, prior to an athletic event, or as you get ready for a dozen dinner guests, a little Qigong can let you focus on what you need to do and decrease nerves, anxiety, fear, or tension. Without such ogres leering over your shoulder, your lecture, athletic endeavor, or dinner can come off without a hitch.

Reviewing principles for your postures

I'll keep this simple, simple, simple since thinking too hard is an antiprinciple in Qigong! Just keep the following principles in mind as you practice.

✔ **Be relaxed:** Above all, don't stress about whether you're doing it right. All that Type-A anxiety can put one big kink in your energy hose and do just the opposite of what you're trying to accomplish.

✔ **Be quiet:** Both your mind and body should be quiet. Think too hard, jiggle too much, get your mind caught up with a to-do list, and you curtail any benefits from a Ming Men massage you hoped for. Ever notice how calm yogis and other advanced mind-body practitioners are? Try it. Take a breath. Let your mind quiet.

✔ **Be natural:** Let your body move in the way that feels right. Don't work too hard, contort yourself, or do anything that doesn't feel good or right to your body and mind. Qigong should feel second nature to you. And if a movement doesn't feel second nature the first time, it may feel natural the third or fifth time.

Energizing with basic Qigong

Qigong is a bird of a different species. Whether you can really pick up the essence from a book depends on how you think and learn. Everybody can get an idea of what it's all about and what the movements should look and feel like. But Qigong is about finding that inner energy center and then activating it. Some people may have a great sense of what this means and be able to feel the practice on their own through movements they read about in any book, including this one. Others may crunch through some movements, wonder what it's all about, Alfie, and turn the page.

If you're one of those people who is intrigued but can't seem to quite feel it on your own, taking a class or workshop can work wonders. A good instructor can help you feel the energy and coax you into letting go just a bit. If you're in a group, the energy of the class can help you unkink your energy highway, too. If you need to experience an activity, do seek local resources by looking in your area telephone book, or use the referral system through the Qigong Institute's database. See the Appendix to find it.

Bottom line: Try the following movements on your own and get an idea of how they feel. Be patient. Even with a group or a teacher, it may take you weeks or months to begin to feel the energy flow. It's not a quick fix. This is crockpot cookery, not microwave magic.

Standing Makes Perfect

In Qigong, pulling in your abdomen and aligning your spine isn't something you want to get all wrapped up about. A perfect posture means relaxing everything. That doesn't mean just hanging there above the ground like a puppet on a string. That means actively relaxing so you're not forcing yourself into any one posture, but still using your muscles. Figure 11-2 shows you the proper position.

You know you're standing correctly when these factors are in place:

- ✔ Your head is erect as if someone were pulling on your crown with a string.

- ✔ Your shoulders are relaxed and down.

- ✔ Your chest is slightly concave.

- ✔ Your lower back is straightened slightly by allowing your tailbone to tuck under just a little. Don't crunch down and force any tucks. Just let it sit underneath you.

- ✔ Your arms and hands are hanging at your sides very relaxed and not forced to face any particular way.

- ✔ Your feet are planted firmly on the floor with your weight centered so your Bubbling Spring acupoint (refer to Figure 11-1 to locate this) is fully in touch with the earth's chi.

✔ Your teeth touch lightly but aren't clamped, nor are they hanging open and loose.

✔ Your tongue is lightly touching the top of your palate just behind your front teeth. That touching is thought to connect one meridian in the front to another in the back so the energy can circulate freely.

Okay, now that you're standing pretty, you're ready to move your chi.

Standing Like a Tree

Sometimes standing meditations — that's what Standing Like a Tree is — can be difficult for beginners because you can get fidgety and start thinking about the laundry or what the kids are up to. But meditations standing stock-still are powerful and worth trying at the beginning or end of a routine, or even for just a minute or two here or there during your day. Figure 11-3 shows you the proper form, with three different hand positions. You can add various hand, arm, and feet positions to your standing meditation. I introduce three later in this section.

If you're really uncomfortable standing, try sitting at first. The Chinese believe that you're more likely to stay quietly alert while standing because you can't actually fall asleep on your feet. (If you did, you'd fall over and that's not much of a tree.)

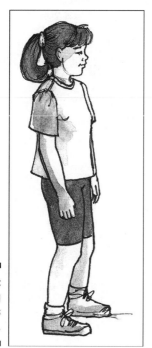

Figure 11-2:
Standing
Makes
Perfect.

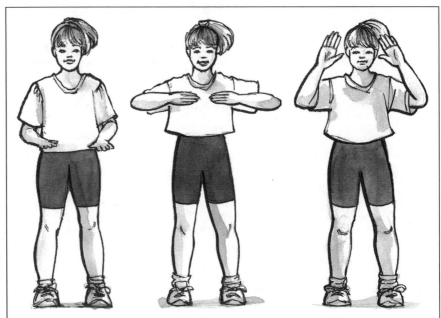

Figure 11-3:
Standing
Like a Tree.

It does seem odd in our fast-paced society to just stand there. Qigong doesn't ask you to actually do anything while there. You just feel your body and become aware of the chi and its movement . . . or not. Also, try to become aware of any tension you may hold and let your breath go to that spot and help release it. If an odd thought bounces through your mind, acknowledge it, then let it go.

Your eyes are open but relaxed, practicing the inward focus. Refer to Chapter 4 on movement basics and Chapter 10 about Tai Chi for more information about an inward focus. If you like music, try playing something soft without vocals.

Start with just 5 minutes, gradually building your time to 20–30 minutes. You can hold one hand position for the entire time, or change positions every few minutes. Experiment with the different hand positions as you "stand like a tree" to see which ones feels best to you.

Hang Hands at Side

This is of course the simplest since your arms just hang at your side as I instructed in Standing Makes Perfect (earlier in this section). Just assume the basic standing posture with your arms at your side. That's it. Stay there, and follow the directions above for your meditation.

Place Palms on Table Top

Hands are held in front of your hips with the palms facing down and the elbows slightly bent. Fingers are facing forward. You feel as if you have your palms resting on a hip-high table in front of you. (See Figure 11-3.)

Embrace the Tree

Hold your arms out in front of you with the elbows soft and rounded. A slight curve goes from your shoulder down to your fingertips. Imagine you're hugging a tree very gently.

Hold Arms Chest High

Lift your elbows (not your shoulders!) in front of yourself so that your hands are at chest-height. Your palms face down and your fingers are facing in but remain a few inches apart. (See Figure 11-3.)

Frame your Face

This is the most advanced position because it takes the most endurance to hold your arms here. From the chest-high hand position, lift your hands up so your fingers are just below eyebrow-height. It looks a little as if you were holding very large binoculars except your palms are turned slightly more outward and your fingers are softly extended. (See Figure 11-3.)

Feeling your Chi

Try this sitting or standing. If you're sitting, make sure that your feet are flat on the floor so your Bubbling Spring is fully in contact with the floor. It doesn't matter what kind of shoes, if any, you have on.

This isn't really a formal Qigong movement, but gives you a moment to try to feel your chi's movement and warmth in the acupoint in your hands — the Lao Gong (or Labor Palace).

Feel your chi with this simple Qigong movement:

1. **Let your palms face each other, playing with the distance between them from 6 inches to a foot or two.**

2. **Allow the energy emitting from each palm to connect and circulate through your body.**

   Choose something to visualize between your palms such as a glowing ball that you're holding, a light beam moving between your palms, an electrical current blazing between the two, or something else that helps you.

3. **Feel a warmth in your palms moving back and forth between them.**

4. **Try stretching your palms open and closed to prime your hands' energy pump.**

5. **Try slowly circling your palms as if you were rolling a large piece of dough into a ball between your palms.**

You may be surprised with the warmth that begins to emanate from your palms. Remember that feeling and use it in other movements.

Try this little experiment for a short time in different places. For example, if you get stuck in a grocery line or at a long stoplight, no one will know what you're up to if you just start moving your hands around a bit.

Rocking

This move, which massages your Bubbling Spring acupoint (see the section, "Finding energy channels, centers, and points" earlier in this chapter), can even help athletic performance because it can draw chi into your body. But aside from performance, you stimulate your Ming Men and increase vim and vigor. Figure 11-4 shows you how.

Massage your Bubbling Spring acupoint with these steps:

1. **Stand with your left foot pointing straight ahead and your right foot turned out to about 45 degrees.**

2. **Position your right foot so its arch is even with your left heel.**

3. **Place your hands on your thighs and slide them down toward your knees so you're forced to lean over just a little from your waist.**

Keep your shoulders back and your back flat so you have a straight line down your back to your tailbone. Don't rest your hands right on your knees — you don't want to put strain on the joints.

4. **Rock forward slightly so your right heel comes off the ground. Inhale.**

5. **Rock backward, lifting your left toe off the ground. Exhale.**

6. **Continue this slow rock with the alternating toe and heel lift for a few minutes. Then switch sides.**

If it is uncomfortable to bend your knees so low, you can place one or both hands at your hip joint.

Big Guy (Or Whole Body Breathing)

This is a name that Dr. Bingkun Hu, a Berkeley, California, master instructor, devised for a common Qigong movement because, well, it looks like a really Big Guy kind of puffing out his chest. Use this to prepare your chi for the microcosmic orbit.

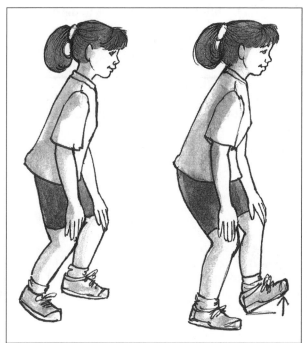

Figure 11-4:
Rocking.

1. **Stand centered on both feet with your arms hanging at your sides.**

2. **Inhale and, at the same time, let your elbows float upward a little. Keep your arms rounded as if a helium balloon were tied to each elbow but your forearm remains heavy. Lift the arms slightly in front of your body.**

3. **Exhale, and release the arms back down toward your body slowly, allowing your knees to bend slightly and your body to sink.**

4. **Repeat for several minutes. Your spine and whole body should relax through the movement so it feels nearly effortless. The movement feels like a circling motion, rolling forward and backward.**

If you ever begin to feel dizzy, lightheaded, or uneasy in any way during any of these breathing movements, stop immediately.

Row the Boat

This is another preparation for the microcosmic orbit. Imagine you're rowing a boat to get the feel for the way this moves. Think about lifting your energy up through your body, then pushing it back down again. Let your spine move freely in this move for added flexibility as well as to massage your Ming Men and Dan Tien acupoints.

1. Stand centered on both feet with your arms hanging at your sides.

2. Inhale, and draw your hands up your sides so the V between the thumb and your first finger is sliding up your side toward your armpits. Let your back arch slightly as the hands move upward.

3. When your hands reach to just below your armpits, circle them to the front away from your body. Exhale as they move downward and away from your body. Let your back round when the hands circle and drop to the front.

4. Repeat the circling motion for several minutes, remembering to keep your breath moving fully.

Dog Paddling

One hand of this movement looks as if it is doing the dog paddle, while the other sort of scoops up along your body then pushes back down. This is actually part of a series of movements in a Daoist practice — one of the schools of Qigong — that is translated roughly as "Live 100 Years Like A Turtle." Although Dog Paddling is a flowing and rhythmical movement, you need some breakdown to understand the pieces. Don't think too hard while you're mastering it. Let's do the Turtle!

Before I go through the exact movement, I want you to get the feel for the scoop and paddle of the hands, and the sway of the body. Simply standing in one place, lift the right hand palm up as if you were scooping water up to your mouth to drink. As soon as you have the drink of water, so to speak, turn the palm down and run it down the front of your body. Now, just with your left hand, keeping the palm down, lift the hand up along your side in the start of a forward-moving circle and then push it back down to your front as if you were dog paddling. Got those separately? In the movement, we put them together.

1. Stand centered over both feet, arms hanging relaxed at your sides.

2. Inhale, and turn the right palm up with the pinkie turned inward and upward. Scoop your cupped hand, with pinkie inward, along the middle front of your chest. You think of lifting the chi along with the hand.

3. When your cupped hand reaches about your chin level, rotate the wrist and push downward leading with your thumb, exhaling, and thinking of pushing the chi down. At the same time the hand reaches the chin, rotate the left hand and lift the left hand upward just as you did in Step 2.

4. Keep the alternating motion going: Right hand scoops up when the left hand paddles down. Right hand pushes down when the left hand lifts upward in preparation to paddle.

5. **Now that you have the arms, add the body: When the right hand scoops up, shift your weight slightly to the left and rotate the left side of the body inward a little. When you push the right hand down, the weight shifts back to the right and the right side of the body turns inward slightly.**

   The lower body resembles a small figure 8 movement.

6. **Repeat this swaying and breathing motion for several minutes. Then change to the other side.**

Small Heavenly Circulation (Also called Microcosmic Orbit)

This is the smallest of movements for such an important one. At first, as you figure out how to move your chi in its orbit, you let your hands and arms take part. Then, you stop that movement and try to feel the chi circulating without the aid of your hands and arms. It may take months to truly learn to control and feel the orbit of your chi without your arms. When you first experiment with this, you may want to try only Steps 1–4, then add 5 when you're comfortable. Wait until you feel at ease with this to move to Step 6 for any length of time.

1. **Stand centered over both feet with your hands relaxed at your sides.**

2. **Inhale through your nose, feeling the breath and energy move from the base of the spine up your back to the Bai Hui acupoint in the crown of your head. Let your hands and arms move freely upward as if tracing the circular path on the outside of your body that you are trying to achieve on the inside.**

3. **Exhale, and feel the breath and the energy move from your crown back down the front of your body to your perineum at the base of your torso between your thighs. Let your hands and arms now mimic that path down the front as they continue their soft circle to the front.**

4. **Do 9 full cycles as your Orbit "warm-up."**

5. **After you have your chi moving, forget the pattern of the breath and just feel it and imagine it circling in your body on its own.**

6. **After you have the chi circling, drop your hands and let your body and mind take over the job, continuing the circling mentally.**

Some people may not move their bodies at all when they do this. Others may sway, rise, and sink as if possessed. Just let your body move as it's comfortable. Don't force it one way or the other.

Qigong Walking

Don't be misled by the term "walking." This forward-moving motion is more meditation than transportation, and certainly isn't what's known as fitness walking. Each step becomes a moment of quiet, stable meditation. Try to practice this somewhere outdoors where you have trees, plants, animals, and green around you if at all possible, and it's best to do it after a few moments of standing meditation.

When you first do this exercise, you may have to focus harder on the actual movement than meditation. But once you get the details and stability down, think about the peace and your energy flow. This is also great balance training — good for anyone prone to sprained ankles or seniors who may be prone to falls. Figure 11-5 illustrates the steps.

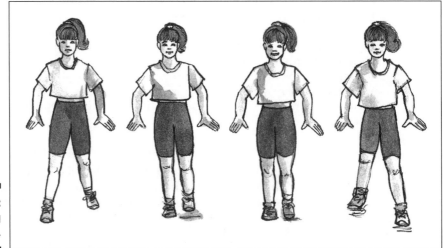

Figure 11-5:
Qigong
Walking.

1. **Place your hands in the Table Top position as described in Standing Like a Tree, then float your hands to your sides as if you were propping yourself up between bars to let your legs swing freely. Your fingers should face front and your entire hand should feel light.**

   In Table Top hands position, you hold your hands in front of your hips with the palms facing down and your elbows slightly bent. Fingers are facing forward. You feel as if you have your palms resting on a hip-high table in front of you.

2. **Step out with your right foot, softly planting your heel first so your left foot is still full (bearing weight) and your right foot is empty (non- weight-bearing). (See Chapter 10 on Tai Chi to get the full scoop on the concepts of empty or non-weight-bearing, and full or weight-bearing.)**

3. **Slowly roll through your right foot as you transfer your weight onto that foot to make it "full" while the left foot now becomes "empty."**

4. **As a transition between steps, pull the rear foot forward (in this case the left foot) and touch the ball of the foot and toe beside your right foot. Keep it empty.**

5. **Now move the left foot forward, repeating the directions in Steps 2–4 on the opposite side.**

   You can continue this walking meditation for several minutes, lengthening it as you become more comfortable.

Your next challenge: After the forward motion is comfortable, try the movement moving backward, leading with the ball of your foot, instead of the heel, to the back. This is quite a bit more difficult, so don't jump into it!

Aspects of the movement to concentrate on:

✔ Staying strong and stable like an oak tree; not wobbling.

✔ Moving slowly. This is not something to rush.

✔ Avoiding a big thunkety-clunk when you put your heel or toes down.

✔ Relaxing your muscles in your leg when it becomes "empty."

✔ Breathing! You'll be surprised how easy this is to forget.

Wake Up to the Sun

Find some space in your home to do this walking meditation, perhaps a hallway or even a driveway or backyard. You've heard of airing your dirty laundry? Well, this is said to be a way to disperse dirty chi and gather up more powerful yang energy. In the reach upward, you're opening up your chest and closing the meridian in your back. Turn to Chapter 4 for more information about meridians. In the following position, shown in Figure 11-6, you close your chest and open your back. The breath and movement may take some coordination. If you don't think too hard, the rhythm should come naturally. Analyze it, and you may end up tied up in knots.

1. **Stand centered over both feet with your arms relaxed at your sides. Inhale.**

2. **Take one quick exhale, and at the same time kick your lower right leg out quickly, heel first, as you fall forward onto that foot into a small lunge about 2–4 feet in front of you (depending on your leg length) with your arms at your side. Take two quick inhalations through your nose as you settle into the lunge.**

   Much of your weight is forward on your right foot and your right knee is bent. Your rear foot is slightly turned out, much like in Tai Chi's Bow Stance. Chapter 10 has details about the Bow Stance.

3. **Now, exhale long and very drawn-out, letting the exhalation create a sound like "aaaahhhhh" through your open mouth as the air moves across your vocal cords. Keep the sound and exhale moving as you**

sink down into the lunge while your palms move upward and push to the sky. Elbows stay a little bent and in front of your head, and you look up toward your hands. Don't rush this move, and stop before your arms are completely straight.

4. When the breath is complete, inhale long and slow, and pull your back foot in so the toe touches the floor next to your front foot. That heel is lifted. You're canted slightly forward at the hips and your hands have moved with the foot in one motion from the lifted position to your belly. There, the thumbs and first fingers are touching to create a circle at your Dan Tien, and your arms are curved as in a lower Embrace the Tree position. (See information earlier in this chapter on the Dan Tien and on the Embrace the Tree hand position.) Relax for a moment.

5. Repeat the stepping movement forward, alternating legs. You can do 18 forward, 9 on each side, or more if you're comfortable enough.

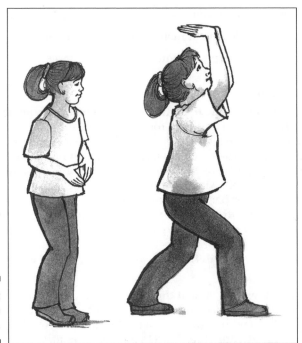

Figure 11-6:
Wake Up to
the Sun.

Chapter 12

Mixing and Matching Chinese Mind-Body Arts

The beauty of both Tai Chi and Qigong exercise is that you can build a routine using just one discipline, you can combine both forms, or even practice just one form or movement from either one repetitively for a few minutes for superb benefits.

In this chapter, I show you a couple of sets of Tai Chi lineups, then a couple of sets of Qigong lineups. Then I put them both together in a couple of sets so you see how broad the possibilities are! As always, when mixing and matching mind-body exercises, feel free to pluck out and put together a series that suits you, your body, your mood, your ability, and your tastes. Just use these as templates. If it feels good, just do it and enjoy. Then add more as it feels right.

These short lineups are just experiments, like stepping stones to help you navigate the waters of Chinese mind-body arts. So, like stepping stones that may not carry you all the way across a river, these little bitty forms may not help you derive all the benefits of a longer practice. But you can certainly start to get a feel.

Fitting Forms to Your Tai Chi Mood

The forms I explain in Chapter 10 are all pieces of the 24-form Yang Short Form. But that's not to say you can't put them together in different patterns for the length of form you want. Call it Jane's 3-Form Really Very Short Form, if you will. Or Jonathan's 5-Form Still Pretty Short Form.

Tips for lickety-split form linking

The way I present these mini-combinations to follow may have each form ending in a way that allows you smoothly to step into the next form if you follow the form instructions in Chapter 10. Note that the instructions there to each form are in isolation and don't include repeats on each side, or transitions that move you into the next form in the Yang Short Form. No problem, no worries! You can find answers in a couple of the basic steps.

Use these tips to help you link your forms together like a pro:

- ✔ **Add transition steps:** All you have to do is remember your transition steps — the Centering Step, the Bow Stance, and the Empty Step — particularly the Centering Step. I broke them down in Chapter 10. Between each move just gather yourself and your limbs back close to your body and to the center, softly and controlled of course, then step or reach back out into the next form.

- ✔ **Use the concept of "empty" and "full":** The concept of weight-bearing and nonweight-bearing applies to these shorter forms, too. If for example your weight is on your right foot ("full") at the end of one form, then transfer the weight to your left foot (making your right now "empty") so you can step back into the next form on the opposite side.

- ✔ **Avoid movement stuttering:** Avoid stuttering between forms. That is, try not to stop and start a lot. If you have to hold for a second to think about what comes next, that's okay at first, but aim for total smoothness eventually. Try linking only two forms at a time, and become fluid in moving between them before you move on.

Shortie Form #1

Tai Chi instructor and performance champion David-Dorian Ross put together this line-up for you to try. Do it in parts — for example, do Steps 1 and 2, then Steps 3 and 4, then Steps 1–4, then Steps 5 and 6, then Steps 5–7, then all 7 steps.

I explain all these forms with detailed instructions in Chapter 10.

1. **Open the Door:** Always a good place to start to connect yourself with your energy.

2. **Part the Wild Horse's Mane.**

   Bring your rear foot into a full position closer under you to get into an empty step for the next form.

3. Play the Pi'pa.

4. Repulse the Monkey: Move backward once or more on each side as you better learn these steps.

5. Grasp the Bird's Tail: Get the movements of this one down before you incorporate it into a sequence like this.

6. Separate Hands and Kick.

7. Close the Door.

Short-Short Form #2

Instructor and exercise physiologist Manny Fuentes offered this line-up for you. Notice some similarities to Shortie Form #1. With so few forms to choose from in an introductory menu as I offer in this book, you end up repeating them but in a different order. Plus, some naturally link together better than others.

1. Open the Door.

2. Grasp the Bird's Tail: Pivot 180 degrees to repeat on the opposite side before moving on.

3. Separate Hands and Kick: Kick right first, then left.

4. Return to the all-encompassing Centering Step to set yourself up for the next form.

5. Open Arms Like a Fan: Move to the left, then to the right.

6. Close the Door.

Still Short Form #3

One more for you to try in your Tai Chi adventure! I put this together for you since three's a charm!

1. Centering Step: Keep your right foot "empty" or nonweight-bearing.

2. Play the Pi'pa: Step forward with your left foot, then step forward with your right foot, transferring the weight and changing your arms with each step. To transition your arms, you can simply drop them as you move, then lift them back up into the Play the Pi'pa position as you sink your weight to the correct foot.

3. Separate Hands and Kick: On each side, start with a left kick by placing your weight back onto your right foot and pivoting to face to the right side so your left foot does not have any weight on it.

4. **Repulse the Monkey: After the kicks, turn back to your left and place your weight on your right foot in a Play the Pi'pa step as transition. Start with your left foot stepping backward. Step back once each side, or more as you prefer.**

Return to a Centering Step, facing to your right with your weight on your right foot.

5. **Part the Wild Horse's Mane: Do this 3 times.**

6. **Close the Door.**

Freeing Your Chi with Meditative Qigong Moves

A great part of Qigong is letting the meditative powers encompass much of what you do, all day long, and in other exercise forms. But 5–15 minutes at a time all by itself can let you focus so you can better apply your energy to other movements. Using the Qigong movements, for example in these sample combos, can help you unkink the energy channels to free your energy, or chi. (Refer to Chapter 4 for overall details about the energy channels, and to Chapter 11 for details about the Qigong-specific name and insights.)

Prepping and pacing for Qigong

Certainly Qigong can help you calm down, but you should probably still avoid starting your practice if you are particularly angry or stressed. If you don't feel emotionally ready, try doing some Whole Body Breathing ("Big Guy," see Chapter 11) to help center yourself. Once your breathing is okay, everything is okay.

Don't think too hard during a Qigong session. Just let the process happen.

Turn to Chapter 11 for the details on the moves in the following samples.

Stationary Exercise Practice #1

This short lineup works specifically on prepping and using your microcosmic orbit, a basic tenet of Qigong exercise. You stay stationary, preferably standing.

1. **Row the Boat.**

2. **Dog Paddling.**

3. **Small Heavenly Circulation.**

Moving Exercise Practice #2

This starts out stationary so you can focus, then directs you into a walking meditation.

1. **Standing Like a Tree.**
2. **Qigong Walking.**

Morning Exercise Practice #3

Of course you really can do this anytime. But in the morning is the best time. The Big Guy breathing helps loosen your spine and breath for the movement to come.

1. **Big Guy.**
2. **Wake Up to The Sun.**

Tai plus Qi: Doing Them Together

Some students and teachers like to keep Tai Chi and Qigong separate, partly because each practice can take so much time and focus. Others feel that starting with some Qigong meditation helps balance you for subsequent Tai Chi moves. While others recommend concluding with Qigong exercises to regain the energy you may have lost doing Tai Chi. Notice that you don't necessarily start each series with Tai Chi's Open the Door or end with Closing the Door — you may start or end the entire combination with some Qigong movements.

Chapter 10 explains the Tai Chi forms and gives detailed instructions, while Chapter 11 shows you the Qigong movements, also with detailed instruction.

Qi-Tai-Gong #1

Start with some Qigong to prepare for Tai Chi, before concluding with more Qigong.

1. **Stand Like a Tree** (Qigong), **using several hand positions.**
2. **Part the Wild Horse's Mane** (Tai Chi) **several times, moving with your left foot out to 9 o'clock, then several times with your right foot out to 3 o'clock.**

3. **Move into a Centering Step** (Tai Chi) **between sides and change which arm is on top of a transitional Hold Balloon hand position to move to the right.**

4. **Play the Pi'pa** (Tai Chi).

5. **Repulse the Monkey** (Tai Chi): **Move backward once on each side.**

6. **Close the Door** (Tai Chi).

7. **Qigong Walking** (Qigong — you're not surprised, are you?).

Qi-Tai-Gong #2

This series can help prep the circulation of your energy with both Qigong and Tai Chi movement — like priming the pump — before you try a full meditation.

1. **Big Guy** (Qigong).

2. **Row the Boat** (Qigong).

3. **Open the Door** (Tai Chi).

4. **Grasp the Bird's Tail** (Tai Chi): **Pivot 180 degrees to repeat on the opposite side.**

5. **Separate Hands and Kick** (Tai Chi): **Kick right, then left.**

6. **Return to the all-encompassing Centering Step here to be able to move on.**

7. **Open Arms Like a Fan** (Tai Chi): **Move to the left, then to the right.**

8. **Close the Door** (Tai Chi).

9. **Small Heavenly Circulation** (Qigong).

Part V
Presenting Pilates®

The 5th Wave   By Rich Tennant

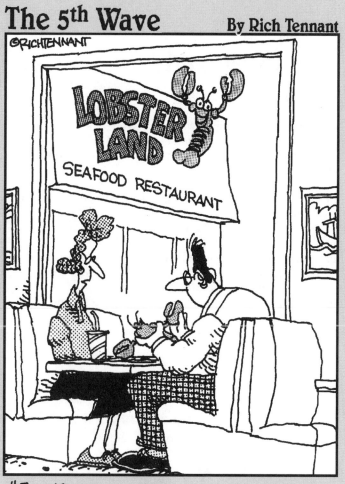

"Is there a way you can explain
Pilates to me without using the
carcass of your lobster?"

In this part . . .

Compared to the meditative aspect of Hatha Yoga, the flowing aspect of Tai Chi Chuan, and the healing aspect of Qigong, Pilates work may seem a bit structured. But it is a substantial and vital element of the mind-body world and one that you can use to complement other routines.

In this part, I tell you a little about where the Pilates work came from because the history is an important part of understanding this method. I help you decide whether this method appeals to you by reviewing its benefits. I also introduce basic movements you can do without equipment with this book as your guide, and show you how those movements can fit together as one workout. Of course, I also touch on some of the classic Pilates work done on Pilates equipment — and describe that equipment — so that you can decide whether you want to explore that avenue.

Chapter 13

Benefitting from the Power of Pilates Movement

In This Chapter

▶ Gaining strength and flexibility with Pilates

▶ Using your power center

▶ Getting on a Reformer, and using other Pilates equipment

*P*ilates may seem like a silly-sounding word for an exercise method. But don't tell Joe that — Joseph H. Pilates (pronounced *puh-lah-tease*), that is, the German immigrant who developed the method early in the twentieth century. The basis of all Pilates-inspired methods — no matter who teaches them or what they're called — comes from his work. Having been a frail and sickly child, Mr. Pilates merely wanted to become a stronger adult and help others become stronger adults, too.

With Pilates, you constantly check in with your body, allowing yourself to focus on what it's doing, thereby allowing your mind and body to become one in movement. *Pilates* is an extremely orderly system of movements that demands a very powerful focus on what you are sensing in your muscles as you use them in exercises both on the floor and on machines, without taking the full step into the inner flow of energy as some Eastern forms do.

Discovering Pilates

In 1926, Mr. Pilates decided to head to the United States, the land of opportunity; and, naturally, he set up a studio in New York City. Because New York City was the home of dancers and performers — always a crowd willing to try something new and trendy — his method quickly became a must for anyone who used their body for their profession. Dancers, movement artists, and actors all flocked to Mr. Pilates to take his classes in muscle conditioning. But it remained the little secret of the performing community . . . until the early 1990s.

As the traditional exercise world tired of high leg kicks and non-stop aerobic dance, it began to search for alternative forms that were softer, less of a strain, yet could accomplish muscle tone and flexibility without bulking up with large muscles. And the little secret called Pilates exercise slowly spread as physical therapists, chiropractors, doctors, fitness instructors, athletes, and today's movie and TV celebrities rediscovered his old method.

Reaping the benefits of Pilates

Pilates movements are a super base for getting in touch with your body and discovering how to use your core's power center (which I talk about in Chapter 4). Your *power center* is your abdominal and torso area — which is your mid-section or *core* of your body — that needs to be strong to move better. Using your power center correctly enables your body to move freely from the torso's strength, rather than to move from throwing around your limbs without a strong core of support.

In most people, a lack of core strength or some muscle imbalance results in injuries, from ankle sprains to low back pulls.

Especially for dancers, many of whom have strongly embraced this exercise system, strength is king. But strength isn't beneficial to any dancer — or anyone else for that matter — if it costs them their limberness or forces a loss in litheness. Can you imagine watching Swan Lake if the prima ballerina has shoulders the likes of Arnold Schwarzenegger? Or can you imagine her partner managing feather-like leaps across the stage if his thighs are so bulky they rub together with every step? Can you imagine enjoying fitting into nice clothes if your thighs were thick with muscles? Would it be possible to play with a child or grandchild if you didn't have the flexibility to sit on the floor with them?

The Pilates method can help a dancer gain strength and flexibility, with a torso and abs of iron, while maintaining long, lean, flexible muscles. Now that probably sounds like a body you'd want, even if you're not a dancer. Long, lean, flexible muscles can not only be attractive, but can also be very useful to getting around in daily life and doing chores and work.

What can you get from using Pilates-inspired movements?

- ✔ A tall, open posture
- ✔ Strong abdominal muscles
- ✔ Long, lean leg and lower-body muscles
- ✔ Balanced muscle development so you aren't prone to injury
- ✔ Physical grace

Pilates by another name: The Art of Contrology

Mr. Pilates didn't originally call his exercise after himself. That didn't happen until after he was in the United States. He actually called it The Art of Contrology — not exactly a name that Hollywood would flock to, huh? His program — consisting of twisting, stretching, pulling, pushing, and rolling movements both on the floor and on various machines — may well have been one of the first true mind-body methods born in the Western World. The entire concept is based on using the mind to control the body and master the muscles. Some exercises may look familiar if you have exercised in the past, but are executed with a different sense of control. Hence, "Contrology."

In Germany, Mr. Pilates taught his unique form of mindful muscle management to fellow internees during World War I to help them maintain their conditioning. Later, as a hospital orderly in the latter part of the war, he taught his methods to bed-bound patients. Pilates has a simple heritage, that's for sure.

Easing into Pilates

Pilates exercises are for anyone who likes slow, controlled, distinct movements. Perhaps stemming from Mr. Pilates' German background, each form has a very structured set of directions. Deviating from them is, in a word, incorrect. Having lived in Germany for a number of years, I can see a mirror of the exactness of that society in the style, which is not necessarily bad, just different than many less structured mind-body methods that have an Eastern heritage and usually tell participants to do whatever feels good.

Of course, other schools and methods that are off-shoots from his original style have developed some of their own instructional patterns, but all of these off-shoots still lead home — to a controlled and exacting style. According to Elizabeth Larkam, founder of the Polestar Education Program for Balanced Body, methods can differ in several ways: Speed and rhythm of movements, choreography or arrangement of movements, assumptions about the way the body moves, instructional style, and what a correct alignment looks like. That's not to say that one school is wrong and another is right — they're just different, which allows the various styles to appeal to different personalities, needs, and experience.

If exacting isn't for you, maybe Pilates movements won't be what you find you like the best. Still, you may be able to draw from some part of this work and apply it to your mind-body practice along with other forms. And don't ignore trying different schools because one type may be your cup of tea even if another isn't.

Because of its emphasis on core strengthening, Pilates can be particularly well-suited for injury rehabilitation, particularly if you're predisposed to low back pain. But, as always, you should consult your physician to make sure the Pilates moves are okay for your particular rehab needs if you have an injury or a history of injuries.

Assembling Your Pilates Stuff

Do you need any equipment to practice Pilates? Yes and no. Oh, aren't I definitive? It depends on which part you choose to do and where you choose to do it. I mostly discuss doing Pilates exercises on a mat, because that requires nothing more than a soft surface. So no stuff. I introduce a few exercises using some other equipment, such as the Reformer. But before you invest in equipment, try the machines in a club somewhere, getting some instruction so you can, one, make sure you like using it before spending a bunch of money and, two, get some training so you don't hurt yourself. The equipment can be large and expensive, although it offers great benefits and toning once you know how to use the pieces.

Just the mats, please

Most people choose a home workout without equipment because it's just easier and doesn't require space-hogging equipment. The Pilates-inspired *mat workout* uses only your floor, or perhaps a mat (which is, of course, why it's called a mat workout). If you see a video or a health club class titled "Pilates Mat Workout," don't be confused! This is the real deal of Pilates workouts. You don't have to have the equipment.

See the exercise section in Chapter 14, where I lay out basic exercises for you to try. I selected these exercises from a huge number of Pilates-inspired exercises, partly in consultation with Moira Stott, co-founder of Stott Conditioning, a company in Toronto, Canada that teaches a contemporary approach to the system of exercise pioneered by Joseph Pilates. Many approaches to this system exist, none of which are inherently good or bad. Some adhere more rigidly to the exacting creations of Joseph Pilates. Some take the basics and add contemporary knowledge about the way the body moves. Some take the basics, add a contemporary approach, and movements influenced by other mind-body methods. I tried to keep these movements more purely Pilates-based with modern touches based on today's knowledge about movement and exercise. You will notice bits of information from or about several methods. I encourage you to explore them!

A Reformer may reform you

If you've heard of Pilates work, you've probably heard about the funny contraption called a Universal Reformer, and its resemblance to some Medieval torture device. No, really, I'm not kidding. With all the straps and springs and things, it looks pretty scary, but it's not really. You're totally in control, applying many of the same basics and movements as you do on the floor. The *Reformer* is a table-like machine with springs at either end and sliding platforms that you lie, sit, kneel, or stand on, to push and pull with your feet and arms against the resistance provided by the springs. An old-time version of modern weight machines. Mr. Pilates was actually very ahead of his time!

Someone inventing the Reformer today probably would dub it something like, "Killer Gut and Butt Flexer," and design it with shiny sidings and sleek colorful cables. Of course, its sales would skyrocket into the millions of dollars. Mr. Pilates obviously didn't have an agent. So a Reformer it was, is, and will stay.

I introduce a handful of exercises you can do on a Reformer — just in case you find the resistance of a Reformer intriguing (and it does feel good) — so try them out if you want. If a Reformer truly strikes your fancy, you may also consider getting some instruction though videos or in a studio before you try it by yourself.

Is that a pink Cadillac? And what a Wunda-ful chair!

In today's exercise world of gleaming metal, slick designs, and high-tech concepts, the other equipment that Mr. Pilates came up with is pretty simple, and it's oh so practical in its simplicity.

Several pieces, other than the Reformer, that you may hear about in connection with Pilates are:

- **Cadillac/Trapeze Table:** The Trapeze Table is a table (duh), with trapeze-like bars hanging from a top "cage" over the top or end, plus ankle loops cuffs, belly straps, and miscellaneous bars and other jungle-gym devices. The exact configuration depends on the manufacturer. You use it for various stretching and toning exercises.

- **Wunda Chair:** This "chair" looks sort of a like an overgrown kitchen step stool made of wood and with a padded top (that's because you sometimes sit on it and you don't want your tush to complain). You do many of the same movements on it that you do on the mat, but it requires more strength and balance.

✔ **Barrel:** Actually, more like half barrels cut lengthwise so the opening is long (in contrast to those half barrels cut through the middle and in which you plant flowers). The flat, cut part lets it sit securely on the ground. You do various movements over the curved top, for example, and the curves intensify back and side stretches.

✔ **Spring Circle:** You have to wonder where Mr. Pilates got his ideas. You have the barrel, now you have circles made of metal that look something like the metal bands that keep the barrel together! These bands are about a foot or so in diameter and kind of springy, so you can push in on both sides with the floor, your arms, hands, legs or feet, or any combination. That pushing creates a muscle-toning resistance.

In the last decade, the concepts and equipment of Joseph Pilates have inspired contemporary methods based on his teachings, some of which have altered and expanded the equipment used. Check out some of the Pilates-oriented Web sites in the Appendix to find a wide range of equipment.

If it looks like Pilates movement, and feels like Pilates movement, why isn't it called Pilates?

Oh boy, here is a tempest in a teapot. I'll make this summary quick since lawyers are involved. Basically, Joseph Pilates and his wife Clara ran The Pilates Studio in New York until Mr. Pilates died in 1967. Before his death, he had turned over the reins to one student, Romana Kryzanowska. In 1992, teacher Sean Gallagher bought the trademarks, which had been granted to an intermediate owner in the 1980s, and began additional promotion of the movement style. Mr. Gallagher subsequently began sending out cease-and-desist letters to many teachers, companies, classes, and studios that were using the Pilates name without his permission.

Funny thing is, many people who were running these other companies and studios had their original training in New York under Romana (as she is called), but eventually branched out on their own with their own interpretation of the method, which is, of course, the entrepreneurial way.

Several lawsuits began to surface around 1994, with various clubs and programs suing Gallagher, and vice-versa. When this book was going to press, the largest lawsuit — a class-action lawsuit that began in 1996 — was still scheduled for trial. This suit claims that the name Pilates has gradually become a generic name for this type of exercise and should not be allowed a trademark. In one survey by a professional association of fitness teachers, instructors said there was no other way to describe the method of exercise as precisely. If you're interested in the legal hoopla, go to www.pilates-cancel.com.

So, if you come across classes or videos called "The Method," "Stott Conditioning," "Balanced Body," "Dance Conditioning," "Body Conditioning," "Synergy," "Long, Lean and Strong," "Body Lines," or other descriptive titles, don't be fooled. If you dig into a description, you are likely to find a phrase like "based on the work of Joseph Pilates," or some other phrase that doesn't set up the teachers or owners for a lawsuit.

Chapter 14

Performing Pilates-Inspired Exercise

*O*ne of the discoveries you make about Pilates as you try these exercises is that you can't cheat. Oh, I suppose you can, but it's not easy. And that's the beauty. You find out how to truly isolate small movements and really use the muscles needed. With traditional exercise, it's a piece of cake to kick a leg lower, yank on your head with your arms to lift into an abdominal crunch instead of using your ab strength, or throw your entire body into a weight-lifting movement. And that may be okay at that moment because you're still getting a workout. But you can't do that here. It's just you and the mat (or other apparatus). And if your spine isn't aligned or your feet aren't positioned properly, you often can't do the exercise at all.

The other beauty of Pilates movement is that it emphasizes quality over quantity. Mr. Pilates never wanted anyone to bust a gut through countless repetitions. In fact, through deep focus of your mind on your body's movement in each exercise, you may find that you use your muscles more and actually need fewer repetitions.

Understanding Key Concepts for All Pilates Moves

No matter what Pilates exercise you attempt, if Joe (that's what you may hear some teachers call Mr. Pilates) were standing nearby, he'd talk about the basic concepts in the following list. He'd likely even hound you a bit if you weren't doing movements correctly. Looking down this list, you can see that these tenets actually can, and actually *should*, apply to almost any fitness routine. Unfortunately, most people don't think about them.

✔ **Stay in focus and in control:** One of the very clear principles of any mind-body workout is the necessity to use your mind to focus deeply on what you do as well as to control your movements. Pilates movement is no different. You need to turn your mind inward and be aware of exactly what each limb and each muscle are doing.

✔ **Keep calm and centered:** Despite the fact that you're focusing on each muscle and each movement, you need to be calm and not grip tense muscles in your attempt to do the movements. You stay actively centered in the moment of each exercise, and use proper spinal stabilization to accomplish each movement.

Another of Pilates' original recommendations was to tuck the pelvis under to flatten the spine. (Aerobics instructors also recommended this posture as late as the 1980s.) Many contemporary methods advance the concept of a strong center to include a spine that is aligned but maintains its natural curves. See Chapter 4 for more information about body alignment to achieve a neutral spine and other movement basics common to mind-body methods.

✔ **Move fluidly:** In contrast to traditional exercise, all movements flow from one to the other, without clunky breaks. Jerking, bouncing, and static movements are not a part of the concept because these movements aren't those you commonly do during the course of a day. Your movement is linked, like a steady stride. Movements are done continuously and in a steady tempo, with some sequences sped up if you want them to become much harder or more aerobic.

✔ **Be exact:** Close isn't good enough. You're either right or you're wrong, according to this philosophy, which can differ a bit from the more free-form philosophy of other methods. Doing one or two very precise moves is much better, according to the Pilates system, than doing a whole string of almost-right moves.

✔ **Lengthen your body:** Continually keep all your muscles activated and energized — do not just lie or sit there, letting your spine and muscles just hang. Even when you're just lying or standing, your entire body lengthens upward through the spine and head, outward through each limb, and downward out your feet. Don't just mindlessly flip an arm around without an active and energized lengthening through the whole body. Imagine you are a tiger ready to pounce, not a polar bear hibernating.

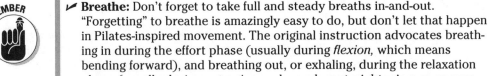

✔ **Breathe:** Don't forget to take full and steady breaths in-and-out. "Forgetting" to breathe is amazingly easy to do, but don't let that happen in Pilates-inspired movement. The original instruction advocates breathing in during the effort phase (usually during *flexion,* which means bending forward), and breathing out, or exhaling, during the relaxation phase (usually during *extension* such as when straightening up or even bending backward).

Some modern approaches encourage just the opposite — breathing out during effort or flexion (like when you roll up in a sit-up) and breathing in during extension or straightening (like when you lay back from the sit-up).

✔ **Maintain proper posture, head-to-toe:** Open your chest, pull down your shoulder blades, tighten your abdominal muscles, align your spine properly, lengthen your neck, and place your head squarely on top of your shoulders. Establish this posture at all times so that when you move your legs or your arms, the rest of your body doesn't get thrown out of whack. Imagine a ballet dancer on stage: Their legs and arms seem to move effortlessly around an oak tree of a torso.

The principles outlined in the previous list can help you master the exercises I present throughout this chapter. Ready to begin the program?

Mastering Preliminary Exercises on the Mat

Mat work isn't an end, but rather a means to an end. The goal of mat work is to help you discover how to move better and stronger in daily life (or on stage or even in other activities), although it offers great toning, strengthening, and flexibility, too.

Actually, you can use the floor or a towel instead of a mat. But some moves require some cushioning for your neck, spine, and pelvic bones. So I recommend having a mat around for when you do need it.

Most modern approaches to the work of Joseph Pilates incorporate a series of first-step movements, which were not part of his original work. But creators of off-shoot methods these days find it helpful to break down some of the basics before proceeding to their other moves. Depending on the method, you may hear them called "fundamentals," "essentials," "principles," or even "beginner." Long story short, they show you how to walk correctly so you can then run correctly.

Getting warmed up with the basics

These first-step or preliminary movements of Pilates are a great opportunity to familiarize yourself with focused movement. They can also help you assess your body's alignment and help you breathe when it is aligned, as well as help you check your progress. And if you have injured your foot or back (or ever do get injured), they can be a nice road back.

Aligning your spine the Pilates way

To Joseph Pilates flattening your abdominals and aligning your spine was a technical art that was not only crucial, but made a lot of sense. Start by lying on your back with your knees bent. Put the heel of your right palm (the meaty part of your palm where it meets your wrist) on your right hip bone, and the heel of your left palm on your left hip bone. Now flatten your fingers toward your pubic bone, as if you were trying to hold your stomach. Note the position of your hands. They *should* be on the same plane or parallel to the ground. If your fingertips are higher, your pelvic girdle is tucked under slightly. If your wrists are higher, you have too much of a sway back. Try to straighten out the plane of your hand.

These may seem childishly easy. But if you focus correctly, you get more of a workout than you imagined.

First, though, try these three starting positions. I use them for every exercise I instruct, including all of the preliminary exercises. These are the exercises that help you first discover alignment and position, and the basic exercises, which are the beginning exercises of the program (see the section, "Basic Exercises on the Mat" later in this chapter). Refer back to these three as you progress to remind you what they are:

Starting position #1: **Lie flat on your back, with your knees bent and your feet flat on the floor (see Figure 14-1).**

Figure 14-1:
Pilates
Starting
position #1.

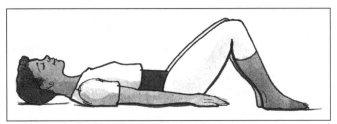

Elongate your arms and rest them at your sides. Properly align your pelvis, find a neutral spine, and tighten your abdominals.

Starting position #2: **Lie flat on your back with your legs extended (see Figure 14-2).**

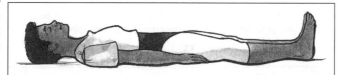

Figure 14-2:
Pilates
Starting
position #2.

Keep your arms elongated and resting at your sides. Check your pelvis. Is it still aligned?

Starting position #3:   **Sit up on your buttocks with your weight just behind your pelvic bones (see Figure 14-3).**

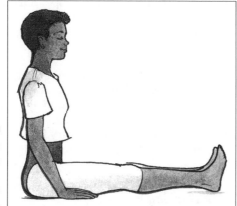

Figure 14-3:
Pilates
starting
position #3

Extend your legs, straighten your back, and open your shoulders, as I discuss earlier in this section when describing good Pilates positioning.

Any exercise that starts with #3 can be done sitting on a folded-up blanket or towel if you have tight hamstrings and have trouble straightening your legs or sitting up tall.

Breathing

"You're going to teach me how to breathe?" you ask. Yes, I am! Because it's likely that you sometimes forget to breathe consciously. But breathing fully is very good for you, and essential for performing Pilates exercises, and any mind-body routine, well. Use these steps to help you breathe more fully:

1. **Use Starting position #1 (refer to Figure 14-1).**

2. **Inhale and exhale slowly but actively.**

When you inhale, feel the back and sides of your ribs expand and press downward and outward. When you exhale, contract the ribs, progressing to an end point where you are contracting your abdominals to press out all the air you can.

You need a sense of fully using your breath, and not just of breathing shallowly in the upper chest.

Using proper body positioning

Most Pilates methods talk about "imprinting" the body into the mat or floor as part of a basic exercise progression so you are fully connected. Basically, *imprinting* refers to lying on your back with your shoulders, upper back, mid-back, low back, and buttocks all touching the floor in proper alignment, as if you were lying back in soft snow and trying to make a complete snow angel; then doing some basic movements while "imprinted" to make sure you can stay stabilized and focused.

Some modern approaches to Pilates movement, on the other hand, take you through the positioning of each body part separately instead of just telling you to make contact with the ground. For the Western brain, that makes a lot of sense, so I follow that procedure here. After I go through the position of one body part, I tack onto it a basic movement you can try to "test" your alignment while you're in that position to check your stabilization.

Proper pelvic placement (Also known as Pelvic Bowl, Pelvic Rolls, or Clocking)

How many times am I going to talk about aligning your pelvis and staying in a neutral spine? Probably not enough since most people walk around curved in all the wrong places (see Figure 14-4). So I'll mention alignment again.

Figure 14-4:
Pelvic
alignment.

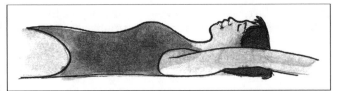

1. **Use Starting position #1 (refer to Figure 14-1).**

2. **To help you find your neutral spine, roll your hips around as if you were trying to swing a hula hoop while lying flat. You feel as if you are using the part of your pelvis that is pressing into the ground to draw a circle on the floor under your buttocks. First, push your low back into the mat and your tailbone toward the ceiling. You've started drawing the circle under your low back.**

3. Now, push the right side of the back of your hip into the mat, trying to keep your knees from flopping around and your torso from twisting, and trying to isolate the movement in your pelvis. The line of the circle you're drawing continues from your low back out to the right.

4. Next, roll down from the right side with your hip and push the tailbone into the mat creating a space under your low back and the mat so you are kind of arching your back. The "line" you're drawing on the floor completes a half-circle, from your low back around the right and to the tailbone!

5. Then roll back up the left side, pressing with your left hip into the ground, using the same stabilization as in Step 3. Your imaginary circle on the floor is ¾ drawn.

6. Finish by returning to the position in Step 2, so you now have a full imaginary circle drawn on the floor beneath you. Repeat the process several times in each direction. Be sure to tighten your abdominals to control the movement.

You may find that one side is harder to control then the other along one curve of the circle. This means you have to work harder with your abdominals and torso to remain stabilized.

7. Finish by finding your neutral spine back in the center position, without being arched up, pressed down, or rocked to one side or the other.

8. Test your pelvic placement: With knees bent, lift one knee toward your chest without disturbing your neutral spinal alignment. Return that foot to the floor. Repeat with the opposite knee. Repeat several times on each side, lifting the knee only as far as you can without knocking your pelvis out of kilter.

Rib cage placement

Use this placement to properly align your rib cage.

1. Use Starting position #1 (refer to Figure 14-1).

2. Breathe while continuing to lengthen and expand your ribs. Feel the spine between your shoulder blades pressing into the mat.

3. Test your rib cage placement: Keep your elbows straight and raise your hands toward the ceiling.

Continue the movement as though you were reaching overhead, but only go as far as you can without feeling the ribcage "pop" up, open, or off the mat behind you.

4. Return your arms to your sides. Repeat this stretching exercise several times.

Shoulder blade placement

Your shoulder blades (or *scapula*) are not attached to the back of the ribs by any bones, so you can move them quite freely — you can elevate them, depress them, and rotate them in various directions. If your shoulder blades don't move so freely, then you may need to work on freeing them.

1. **Use Starting position #1 (refer to Figure 14-1).**

2. **Keep your scapula rotated open and flat on the mat.**

3. **Test your shoulder blade placement: Reach your arms out to each side. Rotate one shoulder forward, as if reaching the top of the shoulder to your toes. Roll it back to the floor. Rotate the opposite shoulder up and forward, then back to the floor. Repeat several times on each side, but make sure your opposite shoulder blade stays anchored to the mat.**

Head and neck placement

Joseph Pilates advocated scrunching your chin down to your chest. But we know today that can be stressful to the neck and spine. Try this instead. See Figure 14-5 for proper head and neck placement.

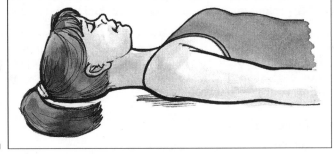

Figure 14-5: Proper head and neck placement.

1. **Use Starting position #1 (refer to Figure 14-1).**

2. **Lengthen the back of your neck toward the mat, as if someone has grabbed the hair on the top of your head and is pulling.**

   Your chin drops slightly. You should feel as if you could hold a tennis ball between your chin and your chest.

3. **Test your head and neck placement: Nod your head (as if you're saying, "Yes, Therese"), but use a very small range of motion so the movement is happening only at the joint where the head sits on the top vertebra of the neck. The chin still doesn't drop to the chest or "scrunch" the neck.**

Basic Exercises on the Mat

This section presents you with a menu of basic exercises, which are sometimes called advanced beginner and sometimes called intermediate exercises. Everybody has a different idea of what a beginner or an intermediate level is. I call them basics since all levels can and should do them.

It's best to master the essentials of alignment and placement before you try these 14 exercises. See the section, "Preliminary Exercises on the Mat," earlier in this chapter.

Joseph Pilates had dozens of different mat exercises, and the contemporary methods that have developed in the last decade have expanded that repertoire. Many variations exist, either to accommodate a less-fit student, a student with a special need, such as someone who is pregnant, or to make sure an advanced student is challenged. Modern-day creators dream up their own variations that evolve from whatever their personal exercise or movement background is, too.

Whatever the method or background, no matter what class you go to, or what video you may watch, you can see certain similarities.

The same concepts that are key to Pilates movements, as I present at the beginning of this chapter, still apply. Never forget your breathing, focus, lengthening, fluidity, and proper alignment, no matter whose program it is.

Your Pilates mantra: Is my spine neutral? Is my body aligned? Am I focusing and centered?

I describe 14 basic exercises for you to try in the following sections.

Ab Preps

These Ab Preps prepare your core for the work to come (see Figure 14-6). The original work of Pilates, as well as other methods today, prescribe that you go straight without stopping in one session from the first exercise to the next one, and then straight through the 14 exercises, which can be pretty hard. So make sure you are comfortable with this basic of the basics first because it takes all the alignment concepts and now has you move a little with them.

1. **Use Starting position No. 1 (refer to Figure 14-1).**

2. **Inhale and lengthen through the back of the neck. (Refer to the section, "Mastering Preliminary Exercises on the Mat," earlier in this chapter).**

3. **Exhale and crunch, or flex, your upper body slightly by sliding your rib cage down toward your hipbones. Reach your arms long along your sides. Inhale.**

4. **Exhale, and slowly lengthen your body back to the mat.**

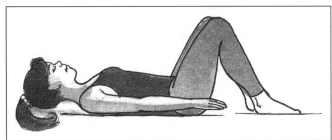

Figure 14-6:
Ab Preps.

Notice I didn't just say "return to the mat." Most people would just collapse and not lengthen or continue to use their muscles actively.

What to avoid:

✔ Tightening your neck

✔ Tucking your pelvis

✔ Clenching with your chest muscles

Hundreds

If any exercise is the "classic" Pilates-inspired movement, this is it. Every teacher, every method, every class does this. You do Hundreds every time you do a Pilates workout. You also learn to love the ab toning you gain from its simplicity (see Figure 14-7).

Again, think and breathe actively as you do Hundreds. Avoid flailing with your arms as they pulse. And only do as many as you can without tension or collapsing your form.

You want to know why it's called Hundreds? Because in advanced sessions, you do a hundred of these.

1. **Use Starting position #1 (refer to Figure 14-1).**

2. **Lift your knees so your thighs are perpendicular to the ground and your lower legs are parallel to the ground with your inner thighs glued together. Remember your neutral "imprinted" spine.**

3. **Lay your arms alongside your body palms down, but lift them slightly off the floor with your fingertips reaching toward your toes so your arm muscles are actively contracting.**

4. **Inhale, then exhale as you lift your upper body off the ground and lift your arms level with your shoulders.**

5. **Alternately inhale for 5 counts (just count to 5 quickly) and exhale for 5 counts (keep the 5-count repeating) while pulsing the arms in small up-and-down movements from the shoulder joint. Emphasize the pulse down.**

6. **Repeat for 10 repetitions of 5 inhales and 5 exhales, which makes 100 repetitions, thus the name "Hundreds." Even though this is called Hundreds, if you don't have the strength to hold your alignment for that many repetitions, stop at any time you are losing your form.**

7. **Finish by lengthening to the ground while exhaling. Avoid just collapsing down, but continue to use your muscles.**

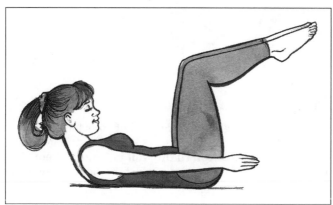

Figure 14-7:
Hundreds.

What to avoid:

✔ Tensing your neck (hold your neck with one hand if that helps)

✔ Letting the abdominals poke or bulge upward or outward more than when you started. That indicates you are losing the muscular hold.

✔ Losing your neutral spine

Leg Circles

Circling your leg can be hard because you need to keep a neutral and strong center while you move your leg in the circles (see Figure 14-8). You need extra focus.

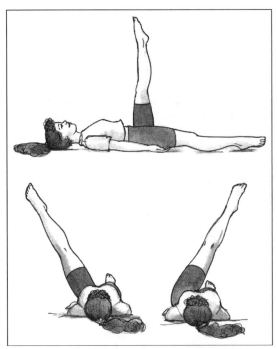

Figure 14-8:
Leg circles.

1. Use Starting position #2 (refer to Figure 14-2).

2. Lift your left leg straight up so the toes of your foot are pointing toward the ceiling while your right leg stays long and strong along the floor, with your toes pointed toward the wall in front of them. Keep your arms at your sides, palms down against the floor for some support.

   If your hamstring is too tight for this, bend your right knee so that your right foot is on the floor.

3. Circle your left leg in one direction as if you have a pencil in your toes and are trying to draw a circle on the ceiling. Keep your knee extended and straight. Repeat 5 times in one direction, inhaling on the first half of the circle and exhaling on the second half. Then repeat 5 times in the opposite direction. The circles will be only as large as you can make them while still keeping your hips still and your alignment controlled.

4. Bend your left knee to your chest, then extend your leg onto the floor beside your right leg. If you are doing the modified version with your right knee bent and the foot on the floor, rest for a moment by straightening that leg onto the floor, too.

5. Repeat Steps 1 through 3 placing your right leg overhead and keeping your left leg on the floor.

What to avoid:

- Rolling your hips side-to-side with the circling leg (make the circles small enough to avoid this)
- Tensing the upper body
- Drawing a jerky circle (remember that Pilates flows)

Rolling Like a Ball

Another classic move by Joseph Pilates has a very beautifully child-like feel. Kids can just toss themselves around at the whim of gravity. But you need to use your abdominal strength to master the control required. Figure 14-9 shows you how.

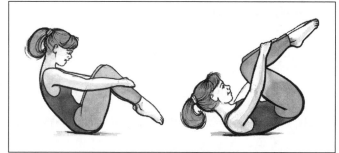

Figure 14-9: Rolling Like a Ball.

1. **Use Starting position No. 3 (refer to Figure 14-3).**

2. **Bend your knees in toward your chest, keeping your inner thighs glued together and your toes off the mat. Keep your entire spine slightly rounded. Rest your hands lightly on your shins. Find your balance before you begin.**

   To stay balanced and accomplish the rolling motion, really focus on tightening your abs. If you aren't comfortable holding your shins, then hold behind your knees to start.

3. **Inhale, and roll backward smoothly along your spine to the top of your mid-back. Keep your back rounded so your body rolls, rather than landing with a big ker-clunk. That would hurt.**

   Roll backward only to the top of your mid-back and not onto the base of your neck or your head. If you can't control the roll and stop there, decrease your momentum and use your abdominal muscles more (and your mental focus) to control the movement as much as you can.

4. **Now reverse the roll (like a backwards somersault) and let the change in direction bring you back up to the seated and balanced position. Stop in the upright sit. Now that's tough!**

If you have too much momentum on the swing back to sitting, you may likely go catapulting right past the seated upright position, stopping only with your toes.

5. **Repeat 5–10 times.**

What to avoid:

- ✔ Losing the curve of your spine
- ✔ Using too much speed and not enough control
- ✔ Swinging your legs open and closed

Single Leg Stretch

How many times can I call a movement "classic" Pilates. Okay, I'll stop. This one has kind of a funny name because you aren't really stretching the leg (as

---

Dead Bug Roll — the beginner's version of Rolling Like a Ball

Does it feel a bit weird, maybe even a little scary, to roll backwards from a seating position? Like Pin The Tail on the Donkey blindfolded? Here's a great little idea for a way to prepare both body and mind for the full Rolling Like a Ball movement. The Dead Bug Roll (you really have to love that name) was dreamed up by Cathleen Murakami, longtime Pilates trainer and owner of Synergy Systems Fitness Studio in Encinitas, California.

Pretend you're a bug on its back that can't get up.

Start on your back with your knees tucked into your chest and your chin pulled forward a little, still maintaining the space between the chin and the chest. Hold onto your shins with your hands.

Give a little kick with your lower legs upward to get your body to rock backward and forward

slightly, a bit like a teeter-totter. Feel the sensation as if the kick almost wants to pull you up.

Give another little kick with your lower legs, letting the rock pull your hips upward toward the ceiling a little (a little over your head). Let the weight of your hips pull you back down to the floor. The momentum should almost lift your upper body forward and off the ground.

Give a few more kicks, each time letting your hips lift a little more upward and allowing the momentum to carry your upper body forward and up slightly toward a seated position. Or the starting position for Roll Like a Ball!

Keep this little kick-and-rock routine going until you find yourself doing the whole roll. Then you can go ahead and try the Roll starting from the seated position.

if to gain flexibility), but you are *outstretching* the leg to further test your ab control and focus (see Figure 14-10).

1. **Use Starting position #2 (refer to Figure 14-2).**

2. **Pull your right knee into your chest (don't tuck the pelvis!), placing your right hand lightly on the outside of your right ankle and your left hand on your inner knee. Lift the left leg off the floor, keeping it extended and actively reaching away from you.**

3. **Lift your head and shoulders off the mat.**

4. **Now fluidly and with tempo, alternately pull in the left knee and extend the right knee, then pull in the right knee and extend the left knee, also exchanging the corresponding hand positions and keeping the extended leg off the floor.**

5. **Do 5–10 "stretches" per leg.**

6. **Finish by exhaling and bringing both knees to your chest, then return to Starting position #2.**

What to avoid:

✔ Tensing your neck (lower your head to the floor for the exercise if that helps)

✔ Losing your neutral spine

✔ Rocking your pelvis up and losing your ab control

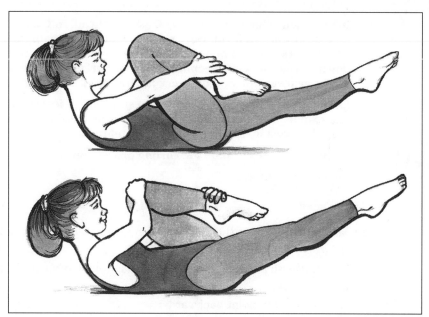

Figure 14-10:
Single Leg
Stretch.

Spine Stretch

You may be surprised how tight you are when you try to lean forward. But that's why you should do this. Tight backs and legs can lead to hurt backs and legs. Figure 14-11 shows you the Spine Stretch.

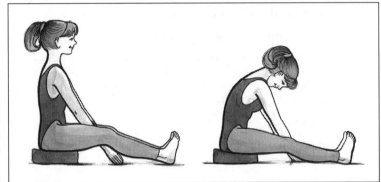

Figure 14-11:
Spine
Stretch.

1. **Use Starting position #2 (refer to Figure 14-2) but move your legs apart so the space is just wider than your shoulders.**

2. **Flex your feet so that your toes face the ceiling. Rest your hands palms-down on the mat between your legs.**

   If your hamstrings are too tight to sit comfortably, sitting on a small pillow or pad, as Figure 14-11 shows, can relieve some of the tension.

3. **Inhale, then exhale and, starting from your head, roll one vertebra at a time downward as if you were a flower wilting slowly in the heat. Walk your fingers outward between your legs away from you. Only go as far down as you can while keeping the pelvis upright and your abs tight. That may mean you don't go very far, but you'll still feel the stretch.**

4. **Inhale while down. Or if you want to stay there a few counts, inhale and exhale, then inhale again before coming back up. Exhale and roll the spine back up starting with the vertebrae in your lower back.**

5. **Activate your abs to start the curling process upward!**

6. **Repeat 6 to 8 times.**

What to avoid:

✔ Jamming the chin to the chest (remember to keep a tennis ball-size space between your chin and chest)

✔ Lowering with a straight back, rather than rolling through the spine

✔ Bending at the hips (sinking into your low back) so your pelvic bones at your back try to point backward

Saw

Now this is a funny name, but Joseph Pilates had a million of them. When you think about them, they all make sense though. Imagine that in the exercise I show you here that you're trying to "saw" off your toe with your hand as you reach it downward (see Figure 14-12).

1. **Use Starting position #2 (refer to Figure 14-2), but add some space between your legs so that your knees are as wide as your shoulders. Reach out your arms to your sides at shoulder height.**

   If your hamstrings are too tight to sit comfortably, sitting on a small pillow or pad can relieve some of the tension.

2. **Inhale and rotate the spine (not just the arms!) to the right, keeping the hips square to the front.**

3. **Reach your left arm forward and down in the direction of the *outside* of the right foot you are turned toward.**

   Keep your pelvis tall and not tucked or collapsed. The reach forward comes from back and hamstring flexibility.

4. **Roll upward, feeling as if you are stacking each of your vertebrae one on top of the other, and use your abs to initiate the roll up.**

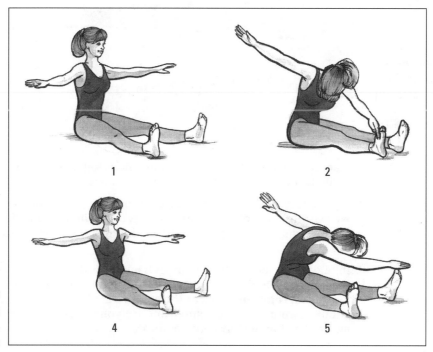

Figure 14-12: Saw.

5. **Rotate back toward center, and repeat on the left side.**

6. **Repeat 5–6 times on each side.**

What to avoid:

- ✔ Lifting one hip bone off the ground as you reach toward the opposite leg (Don't reach as far if you can't keep both hips on the ground.)
- ✔ Tensing your neck and shoulders
- ✔ Letting your toes relax forward

Breaststroke

If someone saw you doing the full version of this exercise, they'd think you were a fish out of water. But it's a bit complicated, too. So I offer an alternative that you can use to build up to the full version, which you may learn if you take more Pilates than I introduce in this book. I like the stepping stone this exercise gives you (see Figure 14-13).

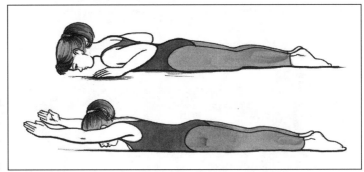

Figure 14-13:
Breast-
stroke.

1. **Start lying stomach-down with your thighs together. Place your hands, palm-down, on the floor underneath your shoulders.**

2. **Inhale, then exhale and reach (lengthen) your arms forward as if you were trying to stroke through the water, continuing to pull the top of your head away from your tailbone and turn the palms in to face each other.**

3. **Inhale while you circle your arms back toward your hips keeping them parallel to the floor (here it's like you're swimming along again). The palms rotate outward as the arms circle back, then return to the palms-down position. Lengthen and lift your upper back slightly, pulling the top of your head forward.**

4. **Finish by bringing your hands back down below your shoulders as you lengthen down onto the floor.**

5. **Repeat 8–10 times.**

If that's too complicated or difficult, then leave your hands on the floor and just practice lifting and lengthening your spine with the breathing pattern.

What to avoid:

✔ Tensing and lifting your shoulders, instead of smoothing the shoulder blades down along your back

✔ Letting your abdominals relax instead of maintaining the power

✔ Tightening your neck muscles

Cat Stretch

The starting position at least is very similar to Yoga's cat stretch, but everything after that is different, so don't get confused. In this version, you don't roll through the spine as much as in Yoga's version. Nevertheless, you may still look like a tomcat on Halloween, whichever exercise you do.

If at any time this hurts your back, stop doing it, or keep the range of motion smaller.

1. **Start on all fours, maintaining a neutral spine alignment (see Chapter 4 for an explanation of neutral spine), with your abdomen tight but not tucked.**

2. **Inhale, then exhale and lift your abdominals upward into your back, at the same time trying to spread your shoulder blades wide apart. Bring both the top of your head and the bottom of your tailbone toward the floor, as if they are trying to reach toward each other.**

3. **Inhale, and release the spine downward, opening the chest and ribcage while letting the shoulder blades slide back down your back. Reach both the top of your head and your tailbone toward the ceiling, as if they are now reaching away from each other. Continue to lengthen through the spine to achieve this reach.**

Avoid pulling your head back so far that you are crunching the back of your neck and spine. Instead, lengthen the neck, pulling the top of your head up and forward.

4. **Finish by returning to your neutral starting position.**

5. **Repeat 3–5 times.**

What to avoid:

✔ Collapsing through your center when you are in the swayback position

✔ Tucking your pelvis in the starting position

Spine Twist

This always reminds me of that drill we used to do in junior high school gym class: arms swinging open and closed, saying, "We must, we must, we must improve our bust." I know, Mr. Pilates, that's probably sacrilege, but I can't help it. In reality, this is a great movement if, you must, you must, you must improve your back's mobility. Hmm, not quite the same rhythm there, but you get the idea. See Figure 14-14 to get an idea of the Spine Twist.

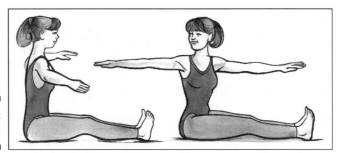

Figure 14-14:
Spine Twist.

1. **Use Starting position #3 (refer to Figure 14-3) with your arms reaching out to your sides at shoulder height.**

   If your hamstring flexibility makes it difficult to sit upright here, sit on a pillow or small pad.

2. **Inhale and rotate your torso to one side while keeping the hips square to the front and unmoving (that's the hard part, so focus, focus, focus). Be sure to carry your arms along with the shoulders.**

   Your eyes should follow your hands in the direction you are rotating.

3. **Exhale and return to the center and aligned position. Repeat to the other side.**

4. **Repeat 4–5 times each side.**

What to avoid:

✔ Moving your feet forward and back to compensate for not moving the hips

✔ Tensing your back and shoulders

✔ Losing the tightness in your abdominals

Side Kick

No, this isn't your partner in crime, but actually very much like the leg lifts to the side everybody used to do in the 1970s and 1980s. Anyway, they were pretty useless because people pretty much just sagged there on the ground and flailed their leg around without truly focusing on the muscle contraction or the work involved. This side kick exercise is a new animal (see Figure 14-15), making you focus and use your mind to become aware of your muscles, so that your butt feels the results. And it will.

1. **Lie on the mat on your left side with your left arm tucked under your head for support and your right hand flat on the mat in front of your chest for balance.**

   Your body will "hinge" forward slightly at the hips for additional balance. But avoid curving your body; it should be more like a very wide V, with the point of the V being your hips. Keep your right hip stacked right on top of your left; not leaning forward or backward.

   Don't let your middle just hang there. Keep your pelvis aligned, spine straight (no sagging), torso lengthened, and abdominals tight.

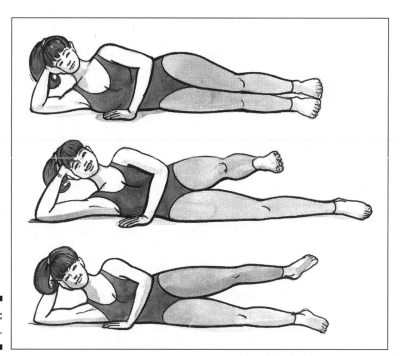

Figure 14-15:
Side Kick.

2. **Raise your right leg so that it's level with your hip. Then inhale and flex your foot (bend your foot at the ankle) while you bring the leg forward in front of your body slightly and *pulse* twice to the front. This pulse is like a little tiny, nearly stationary, kick to the front.**

3. **Exhale and bring your leg back behind your body a little with your toes pointed and pulse once.**

4. **Repeat 6–10 times, then switch sides and do the same with your left leg.**

What to avoid:

- Throwing your torso forward and backward when you move your leg (your torso should remain utterly still)
- Letting your leg sag lower, lift higher, or rotate in the hip joint
- Releasing your tight abdominals

Leg Pull Front

I'll never understand the name of this one, but it's Joseph Pilates at work again. You are actually facing **down** when you do this. But maybe the way he looks at it, your front is facing down, so you are pulling front? Whatever. . . . It's a pure strength move for your upper body and abdominals, as well as your hips and buttocks. (See Figure 14-16.) If you have trouble keeping your spine aligned and not moving during the movement, work on the other exercises, such as the Hundreds and Leg Circles before this to develop more core (or abdominal) strength.

Remember that Mr. Pilates always stressed quality over quantity. That tenet is evident here.

1. **Lie face down on the mat, with your palms directly below your shoulders, fingers pointing forward. Push yourself up into a pushup position. Keep your knees straight and lengthen your body. Tighten your abs, and keep the spinal alignment stuff going. Now you're ready to start.**

2. **Inhale and lift your right leg toward the ceiling (it won't go far!) and pulse it upward. (The pulse feels like a tiny, nearly stationary kick.) Lower it as you exhale. Repeat on the other leg.**

3. **Repeat 3–5 times on each leg, alternating sides.**

   You can also do fewer and rest between the repetitions by lowering yourself back to the floor.

4. **Finish by lowering yourself back to the ground.**

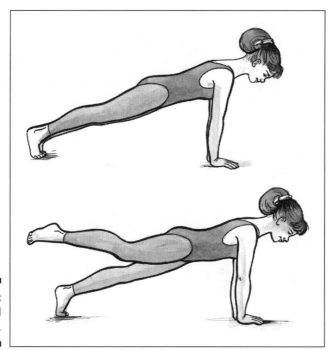

Figure 14-16:
Leg Pull
Front.

What to avoid:

- Lifting your buttocks upward with your leg lift
- Sagging in your abdominals or your head
- Twisting open the hips of the lifting leg

Side Bend

This exercise gives a wonderful tone to your arms and upper body, as well as a stretch through the torso (see Figure 14-17). Figuring out the position takes a little time though, so be patient. Other names for this movement may include Twist or Mermaid.

Tightening your abdominals in this exercise is extremely important because of the balance you need to maintain to keep from, well, teetering over and falling flat on your face.

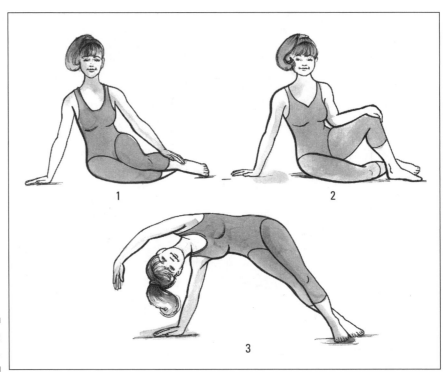

Figure 14- 17:
Side Bend.

1. **Find the starting position by kneeling on both knees, then allow your lower legs to pull out to the left so your right hip is on the ground as your right arm reaches to the floor to support your side-leaning position. Now extend your knees farther out to the side until they're bent at about a right angle.**

2. **Stay seated on your right hip, but now lift your top, left knee upward, opening the leg, and place that foot on the ground just in front of your right ankle. Rest your left arm lightly on your right knee.**

3. **Inhale and lift your left hip toward the ceiling, at the same time straightening your knees and lifting your left arm up and all the way over your head so that you end up in a big C-shaped position.**

Make sure that your weight is evenly distributed on both feet.

4. **Exhale and lower your right hip to the ground, returning to a seated position with your left arm resting on your left knee.**

5. **Repeat 3–5 times on each side, or fewer if you need to.**

As a modification, you can leave your right knee on the ground when you lift your hips up and just move your left foot out so the leg is straight. That gives you more points of balance.

What to avoid:

- ✔ Rolling your top hip forward or backward
- ✔ Tensing your neck and lifting your shoulders toward your ears
- ✔ Sinking into the lower shoulder

Pushup

This exercise challenges your upper body. Its name may sound familiar, and its directions may ring familiar, but with these pushups you put so much focus into each miniscule part that you can't just crank 'em out (see Figure 14-18). You can feel the few you do — if you do them with true mindful focus. Refer to Chapter 4 for basic information about focus.

1. **Start by standing in a good, balanced posture: Your abdominals tight, your pelvis aligned as it is when you are on your back, your arms relaxed by your sides, and your feet together with toes pointing straight ahead.**

2. **Inhale and roll forward, leading with the top of your head, unstacking one vertebrae at a time. Allow your hands to slide down your legs until your upper body is as low as you can go.**

   If this hurts your back or is in any way uncomfortable, bend your knees as your roll down. You can also stop the roll with your hands resting on your thighs. If you have a back injury, please consult your physician about doing this or any other exercises.

3. **If your hamstrings are flexible and your hands or fingers can reach the ground, walk your hands straight out into a pushup position. Of course, this is the Joseph Pilates pushup position with abdominals tight, pelvis aligned, neck straight out from your spine, and your body long.**

   If your hamstrings are tight, after you have rolled down as low as you can go, bend your knees and place your hands on the floor in front of your feet. Then walk yourself forward into the pushup position.

4. **Do one exacting and lengthening pushup, lowering your chest to the ground, then lifting your body back up to the pushup position, until your elbows are straight. You can do up to 4 if you are stronger. You can also lower your knees to the ground to do a modified pushup if you'd like.**

   If just maintaining this pushup position with good spinal alignment is hard for you, you may want to leave out the pushup itself and just hold the position for a second, then jump to Step 6.

5. Walk your hands back to the standing position (bending your knees when you need to, as above), then roll back up one vertebrae at a time, making sure to stack the head absolutely last.

6. Repeat 3–5 times.

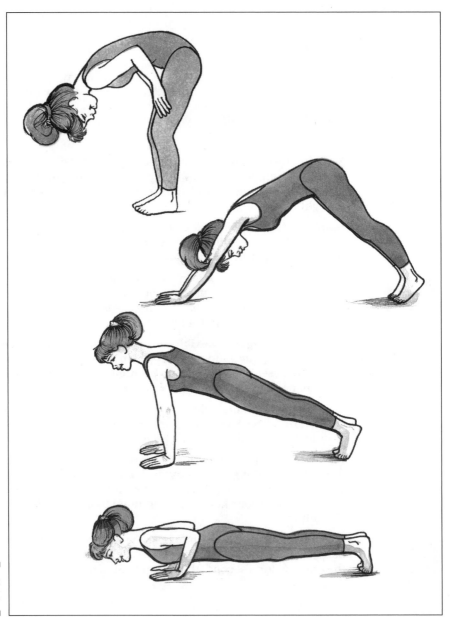

Figure 14-18:
Pushup.

What to avoid:

✔ Tensing your neck and not letting your head hang down in a relaxed position

✔ Losing your tight abdominals (Where did they go?)

✔ Sagging your head downward when you are in the pushup position

This completes the introduction to the mat exercises based on the work of Joseph Pilates. Next up, I introduce just a few movements using the Reformer so that you can see what these exercises look like. You may find the concept intriguing.

Trying Basic Exercises Using the Reformer

The Reformer is an interesting contraption. So low-tech compared to the gleaming iron plates, stacks of weights, soldered metal construction, and colorful weight-training machines of today. Yet it was far ahead of its time in the way it works the body and in its mechanical precision, using principles considered absolutely current even though it's decades old. The difference is, it doesn't do the stabilization work for you, as many machines of today do. You still have to hold firm to keep the sliding platform from, well, sliding where it shouldn't. Plus, this one piece of equipment lets you do multitudes of exercises for all body parts.

Getting acquainted with the Reformer

Many of the Reformer movements are similar to those you do on the floor, but are adapted to use with sliding platforms, springs, and foot rests. On a Reformer, you adjust resistance by adding and subtracting springs: The more springs or cords you attach, the tougher it is to pull or push against the increased resistance. (And of course, the fewer that you attach, the easier it is.)

Don't be shy about starting with fewer springs — or even none! You want to avoid struggling so hard against resistance that you can't focus your mind on your correct form so that you can get all the benefits you're striving for.

The Preliminary Exercises (see the section, "Mastering Preliminary Exercises on the Mat," earlier in this chapter) are still vital to doing any of the Reformer movements properly. So be sure to get familiar with those first because they can help you master the alignment and focus you need when you move onto a sliding platform.

I just introduce a couple of movements here. You can either read about them and look at the figures in this section to see whether you're interested in finding out more about them (refer to the Appendix to find out where you can do that.), or you can try the movements out if you *do* happen to have a Reformer close at hand, or can drop into a class at a local club or studio as a trial. Of course, you may already be planning to purchase one, so these can be your introduction. See Figure 14-19 to see how the Reformer works.

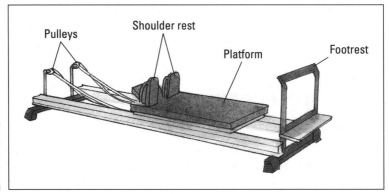

Figure 14-19:
The Pilates
Reformer.

Check out the "No Reformer Handy? Try a Stretchy Band" section later in this chapter, about a special adaptation of Reformer exercises that is a little more convenient. Why more convenient? Because instead of the mondo-Reformer machine with springs and platforms, you use only wide, stretchy, rubbery exercise bands of varying degrees of stretchiness (mo' stretchy equals mo' easy, of course). These are so compact, they can roll up and fit in a pocket. Can't do that with the Reformer! In the section, I describe the same two positions and variations I work you through on the Reformer so that you can see how the two compare.

Keep in mind these things to remember on all work on the Reformer. And normally a certified and trained instructor will show you what to do with the Reformer before you're on your own. If you choose to just buy one for yourself, do get some videos or take a lesson somewhere before just jumping aboard:

✔ Keep your spine in that ol' neutral position . . . as long as your abdominals are strong enough to support that position while you're moving. Refer to the basic concepts at the beginning of this chapter for details about alignment.

✔ Rest your arms on the carriage (that's the sliding platform you lie on that moves with you). Keep your palms facing down.

✔ Tuck in your ribs (no expanding up and out).

✔ Relax your shoulders and neck.

What to avoid during all this slipping and sliding:

✔ Rocking your pelvis forward or backward

✔ Relaxing your abdominals, even for a split moment

✔ Puffing out those ribs

✔ Allowing your knee caps to deviate from their position right over the center of your feet

✔ Banging the carriage back to its resting position without control

✔ Tensing your neck, arms, or shoulders

Okay, you're ready to slide.

Doing some fancy footwork

Ah, such a deceptive title for a series of movements that — trust me — work more than just your feet! For example, they also work your hips and legs from stem to stern. Lots of variations exist, including different foot, heel, and toe positions. I take you through two of them in this section.

First Position

This is called "first position" because it looks like the basic heels-together-toes-out position so often used by ballet dancers. Just holding the position demands your buttocks muscles to work hard.

1. **Lie on your back with the balls of your feet on the foot rest bar. Your heels need to be together and your toes need to be apart (like ballet's first position, if you ever took dance lessons). Make sure that your legs are rotated to the outside from the hip joint, not the knees.**

2. **Bend your knees outward (your kneecap needs to stay over the center of your foot) until they are just wider than shoulder width. The sliding carriage moves downward with the movement.**

3. **Inhale, hang onto that stabilized body with the spine neutral and abdominals strong, squeeze the heels together, and straighten your knees to push the carriage of the Reformer back upward.**

4. **Exhale, bend your knees, and return to the starting position with the carriage down again.**

5. **Repeat 10–12 times or until fatigue forces your form to falter.**

What to avoid:

- ✔ Lifting or dropping your heels
- ✔ Letting your heels slide apart

Wrap Toes on Bar

You can do many of the same movements with toes and feet in different positions. In this one, you work the feet and lower legs by wrapping the toes around the foot rest bar.

1. **Lie on your back with your legs parallel and your knees bent. Make sure your inner thighs are connected and touching, which requires you to use the inner thigh muscles.**

2. **Wrap your toes over the bar, and keep your heels pushed down.**

3. **Inhale, keep your heels where they are, and straighten your knees to push the carriage upward.**

4. **Exhale and bend your knees to return to the starting position. The sliding carriage now moves back down again.**

5. **Repeat 10–12 times, or until fatigue forces a form gaffe.**

What to avoid:

- ✔ Letting your toes come unwrapped
- ✔ Lifting your heels
- ✔ Allowing your inner thighs to drift apart

Back Rowing Preps

Who knows why they're called preps, since you're really working pretty hard — not just getting ready to! I introduce you to two of the numerous variations.

Pulling Arms Straight Back

This movement requires subtle stabilization through your abdominals to keep the arms controlled while staying in a seated position.

1. **Sit tall on the carriage facing the pulleys (which is a sort of backward position), keeping your legs straight with the feet on or between what are normally shoulder rests.**

2. **Hold onto the straps with your hands without gripping (try this while keeping your fingers extended instead of curling them around the strap handle). Your arms need to be long and straight in front of you with your palms down.**

3. Inhale, then exhale and use your back muscles and feel as if you are trying to slide your shoulder blades down your back. Feel as if you are trying to press your palms backward and your fingers toward the floor. Keep your arms straight. This moves the carriage upward.

4. Inhale, keeping those shoulder blades where they are, and reach your straight arms down again but forward, toward your toes, to allow the carriage to return to the starting position.

5. Repeat 5–10 times unless you tire earlier and your form collapses.

Curls

This sliding movement is about arm curls using your biceps in the front of the upper arm, not abdominal curls (see Figure 14-20). But of course, as usual, you still use your abdominals as you work to stabilize your spine during the movement.

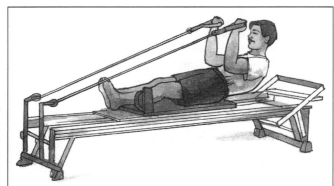

Figure 14-20: Doing curls on the Reformer.

1. Sit tall on the carriage facing the pulleys, keeping your legs straight between the shoulder rests.

2. Hold onto the straps with your relaxed-finger hands (as you did for Pulling Arms Straight back, above) but this time, turn your hands so your palms face the ceiling. Your arms reach straight out in front of your shoulders.

3. Inhale, then exhale, and curl your arms through the elbow to reach your hands toward your ears — here's the hard part — without dropping your elbows.

4. Inhale, and again without dropping your elbows, allow your arms to lengthen and straighten so your hands reach away from you again.

No Reformer Handy? Try a Stretchy Band

The exercise world has used compact and portable stretch bands for a long time to work muscles without a lot of gadgets. And the physical therapy and rehabilitation world used those rubbery bands for workouts long before the exercise folks stole them for theirs.

So, now how about a quasi-Reformer workout with a stretch band? This so-called Flex-Band workout was developed by Moira Stott, the president of Stott Conditioning, as an answer to the dilemma whose motto is, "I love the Reformer but it won't fit in my house." And a pretty cool answer to this workout is also, "Look, Ma, no Reformer." Or maybe, "Look Ma, my Reformer packs in my purse."

Try the same two exercises I describe on the Reformer (see the section, "Trying Basic Exercises Using the Reformer, earlier in this chapter) so you can compare the two and see how the band works instead.

One thing to be aware of: Be sure to hang onto the band tightly so that one end doesn't spring loose into your face or against your body. And check your band before each use to make sure you don't see any tears or holes that could make the band break. They are rubber, and they can break down with age, heat, or cold exposure, and just plain use. See Figure 14-21 for how to hold a stretch band.

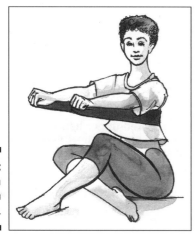

Figure 14-21:
Using a
stretch
band.

Footwork, First Position

As with the Reformer version of this exercise, you do this in what looks like the dancer's first position, with heels together and toes out. Hold the position strongly to recruit your buttocks muscles completely.

1. **Lie on your back, hold the band with one end in each hand and the middle part wrapped around the balls of your feet. Keep your toes turned out and your heels together.**

2. **Rotate your legs from the hips so that your knees are bent slightly but turned out with the knee cap over the toe.**

3. **Inhale, hang onto that stabilized body (meaning the abs are tight and spine aligned), squeeze your heels together, and straighten your knees against the resistance of the band, keeping the knees turned out from the hips even as they straighten.**

4. **Exhale, bend your knees, and return to your starting position so that the band loses some of its tautness.**

5. **Repeat 5–10 times.**

Footwork, Wrap Toes

Take a look at the Reformer version of this movement to get an idea of how it works. You're working your entire legs and hips.

1. **Lie on your back, with your knees bent and rotated inward so your knees and feet are side-by-side and inner thighs are glued together. Keep your feet flexed (so the feet are cocked into a right angle with the lower leg). Hold one end of the band in each hand and put the middle part around your heels.**

   Bend your elbows as much as you need to hold the band in this position.

2. **Exhale, and straighten your knees to push against the band. Let your feet move away from your body.**

3. **Inhale, bending your knees to return to the starting position.**

4. **Repeat 5–10 times.**

Back Rowing Preps, Pulling Arms Straight Back

In the next two exercises, if your hamstrings are tight, you can either bend your knees slightly or sit on a cushion to relieve the tension.

1. Sit tall on your pelvic bones with your legs straight.

2. Flex your feet (so the toes are pointing upward) and hold one end of the band in each hand with the middle part wrapped around your arches. (Make sure there's enough tension so that the band isn't just sagging there.)

3. Inhale, then exhale and use your back muscles to feel as if you are sliding your shoulder blades down while also feeling as if you are trying to press your palms backward and your fingers toward the floor. Your arms stay straight as the tension in the band increases. Reach backward only as far as your ribs and back remain neutral and you don't have to strain with any muscles.

   Inhale, keeping those shoulder blades where they are, and reach your straight arms down again but forward toward your toes to allow the band to relax a little bit of the tension you just added.

4. Repeat 5 times.

Back Rowing Preps, Curls

You use the arms and body in this exercise much as you do in the Reformer version of this exercise. Although it's called curls (for the biceps in your arms), you still work the legs and torso as you keep yourself stabilized.

1. Sit tall on your pelvic bones with your legs straight.

2. Flex your feet and hold one end of the band in each hand with the palms facing up and your arms reaching straight out in front of your shoulders. The middle part of the band is wrapped around your arches.

3. Inhale, then exhale, and curl your arms through the elbow to reach your hands toward your ears — here's the hard part — without dropping your elbows.

4. Inhale, and again without dropping your elbows, allow your arms to lengthen and your hands to reach outward.

5. Repeat 5–10 times.

Chapter 15

Picking a Pilates Lineup

• •

• •

*P*ilates movements can fit together in any number of ways, depending on your time, goals, and experience. You may just want a quick wake-up, a lunchtime stretch, or a pre-dinner power pick-me-up. You may want to focus on flexibility, or on fast-moving power positions that demand more strength.

In this chapter, I suggest some ways to put together your Pilates workout, as well as a few different combinations based on some of the most common goals. For now, I suggest only Pilates-inspired movements for your routine. But you may want to read more about other methods I present in Chapters 7 through 17. Then you can take a look at Part VII to see how you can pull together different ones in one lineup of moves that's designed by you and just for you and your own tastes and needs. After you have the knowledge of various mind-body movements, your workout may remain mostly Pilates, or you may make Pilates just a small part. Or that may change daily, too!

Picking Up Tips for Better Pilates Workouts

As with any type of workout, it's helpful to know a little bit about the hows and whys of movements and their progression so you can put them together safely and smartly. So that's where I start.

With Pilates, remember two things as you head off on your own to put together a workout from the exercises detailed in Chapter 14:

✔ Do movements where you both *flex* (bend forward) and *extend* (bend backward) your spine in each session so that you don't get all lopsided or tight on one side.

✔ Always do Ab Preps or Hundreds (which I explain in Chapter 14). These exercises are key to helping you focus on what's to come, to establishing your mental and physical alignment and to toning your abs. Even as you become more familiar with the physical alignment preferred in Pilates routines, the Ab Preps and Hundreds can bring your focus back and help you re-establish that alignment each time you start.

Each workout starts with a warm-up of sorts. In this case, that means a suggestion that you go through the Preliminary Exercises to get your spine, pelvis, abdominal muscles, mental focus, and everything else in the right place for the routine. (Check out Chapter 14 for more on warming up and on Preliminary Exercises.)

Although Pilates doesn't usually finish up with meditation or other relaxation exercises, each of these workouts finish with a mental cooldown of sorts. Consider that a mental transition to bring you back to your day at hand. Just top off your workout with a few of the Preliminary Exercises — particularly the ones you have the hardest time with. Doing so also helps you determine whether you now have an easier time with the Preliminary Exercises after doing the workout itself.

Take the Preliminary moves in your transitional cooldown a bit slower so you can bring your routine home peacefully and finish up in a calm state. Truly think about how your body is moving — here's where that mindful focus comes into play — and how your body has perhaps changed since you started the routine a few minutes earlier. Focus on your alignment in particular, including your spine, shoulders, head, and abs.

With these tips in mind, you are now ready to try your hand (and legs and arms and . . .) at some workouts. I suggest a couple of types of workouts — helped along in planning those first two by Moira Stott, program director of Stott Conditioning — then I suggest a couple of quickie exercise combos you can do when time is at a premium.

Of course, the workouts I describe in this chapter aren't law. The Pilates police won't come charging in if you do some movement twice or not at all. You can really do whatever you feel like.

And that's the beauty of all of this!

Facing the Basic Pilates Workout

A Pilates workout, as all workouts do, has three parts — the warm-up, the workout, and the cooldown.

Refer to Chapter 14 for the instructions, cautions, and tips for the following movements that you'll need as you do each one.

Warming up

Getting yourself ready for any workout starts with the warm-up. Just like a pot of water trying to boil, you have to simmer and bubble a little first. This is the simmering part.

Do all of these movements in the order presented since they start with the basics, then build.

1. **Breathing:** Use proper technique of rib inflation per Pilates' style as explained in Chapter 14.
2. **Body Positioning:** Move yourself slowly and carefully into the proper placement before you start any movements.
3. **Pelvic Placement:** Helps you make sure your spine is aligned well from your pelvis.
4. **Rib Cage Placement:** Double-check to see if your ribs are too puffed out.
5. **Shoulder Blade Placement:** Keeps your shoulders down and your chest open.
6. **Head and Neck Placement:** Be certain you maintain a long neck and comfortably aligned head on top of your spine.

Working the workout

After the warm-up, you move through the core of the workout. Here you work to find your pace — that is, the speed and rhythm you feel comfortable with — and do the main exercises for that day. Refer to Chapter 14 for instructional details.

The movements for this workout should be done in the order I present them. This doesn't mean that you can't skip one if you want. Or repeat one. But this order moves the spine and the body in the best and safest way.

I give you two basic Pilates routines, one for limbering your muscles and one designed to strengthen them.

The stretch workout

The stretch workout series focuses on stretching, although with Pilates you always get a good bit of toning, too. Take your time with each repetition and let your muscles relax into the position.

1. **Ab Preps:** Repeat up to 8–10 times. Keep your abdominals as flat as possible.

2. **Rolling Like a Ball:** Repeat up to 5–10 times. Avoid rolling back any farther than the top of your shoulders or back. Do the Dead Bug Roll to start if you like.

3. **Spine Stretch Forward:** Repeat up to 6–8 times. Stretch from your back, not from your neck or head.

4. **Saw:** Repeat up to 5–6 times on each side. Maintain good abdominal tightening to keep your back supported.

5. **Breast Stroke:** Repeat up to 8–10 times. Keep the extension (that's the upward lift of your back) as low as you need to keep good alignment.

6. **Cat:** Repeat 3–5 times. Allow the movement to roll through your spine.

7. **Spine Twist:** Repeat 3–5 times on each side. Sit on a bolster or pillow to help you sit up tall if your hamstrings are tight.

The power workout

You can do many of the same movements here as you can in the stretch workout. Here, though, your focus needs to be on tempo. Don't dawdle between repetitions. In other words, don't stop to rest too long, or decide to go put out the cat. Take a breath and just move on to the next movement. Push yourself a bit to do just one more. Think strong.

1. **Ab Preps:** Repeat 8–10 times. Keep your abdominals as flat as possible.

2. **Hundreds:** Repeat for 10 sets of 5 inhales and 5 exhales. Only tackle as many repetitions as you can handle without letting your alignment falter. If you want or need to take a break mid-set, go ahead.

3. **Leg Circles:** Repeat 5 times in each direction on each leg. Keep the circles as small as you need to so that your pelvis doesn't turn with your leg.

4. **Single Leg Stretch:** Repeat 5–10 times on each leg. Control the leg as it goes in and out. Avoid just tossing it around. The control comes from the abdominals, by the way.

5. **Spine Stretch Forward:** Repeat 6–8 times. Stretch from your back, not from your neck or head.

6. **Breast Stroke:** Repeat 8–10 times. Keep the extension as low as you need to keep good alignment.

7. **Spine Twist:** Repeat 3–5 times on each side. Sit on a bolster or pillow to help you sit up tall if your hamstrings are tight.

8. **Side Kicks:** Repeat 6–10 times with each leg. Hang onto your torso alignment, using your abdominals, even while you're swinging your leg back and forth.

9. **Pushup:** Repeat 1–4 times. Only do as many as you can. If even one is too many, lower yourself to the floor slowly, then come back up to standing by pushing your hips back and pushing yourself back onto your feet.

Cooling down

After you finish the hard part of the workout, it's time to allow your body to slow down and your mind to focus on what you've done and how you feel. Select your choice among the Preliminary Exercises below, which are the same as for the warm-up. Do the ones you choose in the order listed. Refer to Chapter 14 for detailed instructions for each.

1. **Breathing**
2. **Body Positioning**
3. **Pelvic Placement**
4. **Rib Cage Placement**
5. **Shoulder Blade Placement**
6. **Head and Neck Placement**

Trying a Couple of Mini-Workouts

So you don't have time for a full 30 to 60 minutes of rolling around on the floor? Then just try these quickie lineups in the morning, before bed, or anytime. If your mattress is firm enough, you could even do them on the bed, although on a mat or carpeted floor will do you just fine. No special clothes required. Refer to Chapter 3 for more information about equipment and apparel.

Each of these three sets is geared toward one particular goal and shouldn't take more than 2 to 5 minutes each, depending on how many sets and repetitions you decide to do. Mr. Pilates always emphasized quality over quantity. So only do as many as you can while keeping the technique flawless. Stop if you start to sag, sway, or falter.

As always, refer to Chapter 14 to read full and detailed instructions for each movement.

Give me abs

This set is all about toning your mid-section. Keep the alignment at all costs, calling it a day if you start to lose your spinal, abdominal, or rib placement.

1. **Ab Preps:** Repeat 8–10 times, or until you tire.

2. **Hundreds:** Repeat up to 100 times, which equals 10 sets of 5 inhales and 5 exhales, or until you tire.

Give your back a break

This set should help you build a little more flexibility into your back and help you loosen up any stiffness. Don't force these moves. But do breathe into each one and focus on the muscles trying to relax.

1. **Spine Stretch Forward:** Repeat 6–8 times.

2. **Spine Twist:** Repeat 4–5 times on each side.

Keep it strong, please

1. **Side Bends:** Repeat 3–5 times on each side.

   Make sure you are aligned and focused before you actually lift up into this one. Otherwise, you may just fall over.

2. **Pushup:** Repeat 1–4 times.

Part VI
Exploring More Mind-Body Methods

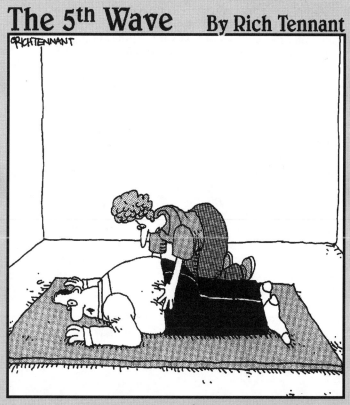

The 5th Wave   By Rich Tennant

ⒸRICHTENNANT

"I think I've found another energy point. It's at the end of an open ball point pen in my front shirt pocket."

In this part . . .

*A*ll the mind-body methods I cover up to this point are
fairly well-accepted and pretty widespread. Nobody
will look at you funny, raise an eyebrow, and say, "Huh?" if
you say you're doing Yoga — or even Pilates in most
cases. But the methods in this part are either esoteric or
unfamiliar enough — or just simply new enough — that
many folks may not know about them.

The fact that they're not at all mainstream can make them
all a heck of a lot of fun to try — even if you try a method,
say, "Huh?" yourself and move on. It's all about exploring
the mind-body horizon, and seeing what's on the other
side of the mountain, right? This dabbling is all a part of
the mindful journey you set out on when you picked up
this book.

This part is actually divided into two chapters: The first
presents methods that are about 50 to 100 years old, sort
of modern classics if you will. The second introduces you
to some of the "new kids" — contemporary methods that
are sometimes a composite of the well-accepted versions
in the first parts and the modern classics in Chapter 16.
Enjoy the trip!

Chapter 16

Trying Out the Modern Classics

- -

In This Chapter

▶ Training in precision with the Feldenkrais Method

▶ Observing your movement with the Alexander Technique

▶ Analyzing your body with Laban Movement Analysis

▶ Inverting your body for better circulation

▶ Considering some other forms you'd never think were mind-body

- -

So you think this mind-body workout stuff is just a trendy exercise thing? Well, think again. Not only do these modern classics I introduce you to here date back in some cases to long before our vault into the twentieth century, but they also are the foundation of many of the New Kids on the Mind-Body Block you read about in Chapter 17.

The New Kids had good reason to borrow from methods developed by the likes of Moshe Feldenkrais and Frederick Matthias Alexander: Many of these classical movement forms are not about doing a workout, but about *how* you do the movements of a workout or sport. This means no matter who you are, what you do, or which mind-body workout appeals to you, the concepts in these methods may just tickle your fancy to help balance you out before, during, or after other fitness routines, whether traditional or mind-body. Of course, some of these forms also stand alone, even as minute posture-correctors, stress-busters, or strengthening and calming experiences.

Ah, but compared to the New Kids, these classics took themselves pretty seriously. So if you get to play with a ball, or dance joyously around a room doing a New Kid method, you may in a classical form just walk upstairs thinking about the placement of your toes and fingers, or just hang upside down while meditating.

And these methods may not be as easy to grasp from a printed page because they can be so esoteric. That's why I work harder in this section to explain the philosophy and benefits, as well as who may consider doing one workout or the other. Of course, I still lay out some sample movements for you to try. That way you can figure out if you really want to dabble a bit further in mind-body exploration by perhaps heading off to find a certified practitioner or instructor. Feldenkrais certification and training takes at least 800–1,000 hours of work, so they are very detail-oriented sessions — much more than I can present in this sampler.

On, James, on to our mindful explorations!

Using the Feldenkrais Method

I start with correctly and precisely naming this method because the developer, Moshe Feldenkrais, would want it that way. The full name of this method is "The Feldenkrais Method of Somatic Education." Now you know. From here on out, I just call it Feldenkrais, a method developed by a Russian-born Israeli physicist who was "alternately warm and caring, critical and exacting, and even deeply disturbing to people," according to Michael Purcell, a Feldenkrais Guild-certified practitioner, worldwide trainer, and past president of the North American Feldenkrais Guild. Purcell studied with Feldenkrais, and everybody who trained with him or knew him alternated between being drawn to and recoiling from him, then being drawn to him again because of the way he forced them out of their comfort zones and into a learning zone.

Feldenkrais, who died at the age of 80 in 1984, developed these movement lessons after a doctor told him a knee injury he had needed surgery, but even with surgery, he might never walk again. That wasn't good enough for the physicist. After that doctor's pronouncement, he declined surgery and took it upon himself to study everything he could about the body and its movements — sucking up literature about and doing research in topics that ranged from anthropology and anatomy to neuro-physiology and psychology.

Out of years of study was then born his technique, The Feldenkrais Method, which has been called the anti-workout because of its lack of emphasis on muscular workout and instead on body awareness.

Doing Feldenkrais movements is all about observing your body and analyzing how it reacts or feels to you in different situations, and how various movement sequences dreamed up by Feldenkrais affect simple things, like the way you stand, walk, or even just turn your head! Feldenkrais is about becoming aware.

Exploring Moshe's philosophy

In 1975, Moshe Feldenkrais gave his first training in North America. And that lesson began with this statement:

"I am going to be your last teacher. Not because I'll be the greatest teacher you may ever encounter, but because from me you will learn how to learn. When you learn how to learn, you will realize that there are no teachers, that there are only people learning and people learning how to facilitate learning."

Read that quote again. Slowly. Let it roll around in your head a little, sloshing from side to side. Although a basic tenet of Feldenkrais — both the method and the man — it frankly could be a tenet of many of the mind-body exercises and practices presented throughout this book.

The Feldenkrais Method works with your nervous system with the goal of helping you to gain access to more of your body's potential. Long story really short: Feldenkrais helps you do other stuff better by straightening out what Moshe Feldenkrais was known to call "kinks in your brain." In fact, you discover as you move through this chapter that many of the Modern Classics are similar in their goals of helping you do other stuff better.

Throughout life, you develop habits — physical patterns of movement — that get in the way of optimum movement usually for one of two reasons:

- ✔ **Physical:** Some incident, such as a car accident or injury, shaped your movement pattern.

- ✔ **Psychological:** Something in your personality or social world taught you to move in a way that became part of who you are.

Both reasons are valid, but they may not lead to the best way to move. But these two reasons also represent ways in which doing Feldenkrais *lessons* (that's what Feldenkrais called the movements) can help you change:

- ✔ **Physical:** The lessons help you move better.

- ✔ **Psychological:** They help you gain a stronger sense of self because the way you use your body is stronger and healthier.

These two changes are pretty cool outcomes for simply putting some mind behind what you're doing. Basically, there is no right or wrong — just awareness of how it feels to you and what feels better.

I do hope that Moshe Feldenkrais won't turn over in his grave when I present a couple of basic concepts. You see, he had been known to say: "I have only one principle . . . There are no principles." Yipe!

The following principles then, with apologies to the man behind the method:

- ✔ You're in control of your own movements. No one can demonstrate a movement or tell you what it should look like. You do it the best way for you and your body.

✔ You pace yourself, doing what you can while still maintaining mental awareness.

✔ You breathe fully in and out throughout all the movements.

✔ You break down the movements into pieces as small as you need.

✔ You do one on one side only, until you're fully aware of what is happening. Then, and only then, do you go to the other side. Expect imbalances in awareness.

✔ You take everything very slowly. And I do mean slowly. Rest, even when you don't think you need to rest.

✔ You think about everything and how it feels. The purpose of some of the rest breaks between movements is to give you time to think.

Another Moshe Feldenkrais-ism: Most questions are silly questions because real knowledge comes from experiencing for yourself and thinking for yourself.

Feldenkrais, like all mind-body methods, is a process, not a goal; a time to be aware and not to try for a specific outcome.

Feeling the Feldenkrais effects

What you get from Feldenkrais is a mindful connection between your mind and your body. You discover how you do movements — from sitting in a chair to opening a jar — as well as what's going on in your body and how those goings-on affect your movements. You then learn to abandon negative habitual patterns and develop more flexibility, coordination, and awareness — or so Feldenkrais instructors hope.

Lessons, lessons everywhere

The Feldenkrais Method teaches what are called Awareness Through Movement (ATM) lessons. Note the use of the word "lessons." These are not exercises, oh no. Exercise conjures up images of mechanical repetition with a goal of trimming, toning, building, burning, stretching or pumping. Benefits here come not from the movement itself but what you notice — the lesson. "The movements themselves are not important," says Allison Rapp, a Guild-certified practitioner and worldwide trainer of teachers who trained with Moshe Feldenkrais himself. "What's important is that when we use our ability to become aware of what we are doing, we change *how* we do what we intend."

Here's the key to recognize: Feldenkrais is not an isolated routine, but something you do as a complement to whatever else you do. The "whatever else" can range from athletic pursuits to everyday tasks at home and at work to rehabilitation exercises.

Other benefits touted by practitioners, although mostly not scientifically proven, include breathing better, better digestion, more restful sleep, improved mood and self-confidence, increased alertness and energy, fewer headaches or backaches, and less stress.

I leave it to you to decide what you experience. Moshe Feldenkrais would want it that way.

Realizing personal gains

For anyone used to traditional exercise, Feldenkrais requires a real mental transition. You may find it difficult to not get fidgety during the slow process with all the rest breaks.

The slow, slower, slowest pace may present certain challenges at first, particularly to athletic types who are used to going fast, faster, fastest. But if you stick with it, breathe, allow yourself to think through what your body is doing, the rewards can be worth it. Heck, even successfully slowing down to go through some lessons is a reward!

Also, if you're used to traditional exercise methods where instructors always state the goal or demonstrate what something should look like, you initially feel a bit left in the dark doing Feldenkrais because you're never told how it should look or what you should feel. Purposefully so. Because being told or shown could bias your thoughts or feelings, the philosophy says.

To do Feldenkrais movement you need to be:

✔ Curious

✔ Willing to try new things

✔ Patient

✔ Ready to listen to your body

But wait . . . if you aren't any of those things, you may actually be an even more ideal candidate because you may have more to learn about your body if you stop and truly listen.

Patience is a virtue here though because you're often told to think about how something feels. Period. That's it. Then you go on. You have to be able to think about it, to tune in, to check in, and to try to feel.

Doing without stuff

As long as you have a small carpeted space or a comfortable chair, you can do any these sample movements. That and some comfy clothing to accommodate any bending or twisting. More advanced movements, which I don't cover, may require more space, more rolling around on the floor, and even more twisting or turning. Feldenkrais lessons often use the floor or a wall so you have a reference point for your movements.

Sampling Some Feldenkrais Lessons

In this section, I take you through three basic lessons. But I start with an illustration so you can see by example how difficult small changes can be for you.

Interlaced Fingers

First challenge: Interlace your fingers, palms together, as if you were going to pray, or beg for forgiveness. Super. Look down and see which of your thumbs is on top and which is folded underneath. There's an illustration of habit since you didn't have to think about which one went where, but just did it.

Second challenge: Shift all the fingers so they are directly opposite of what you had positioned before, in other words, so the thumb that was on top is now shifted underneath and all the fingers of that hand are shifted backward.

Most people have to think pretty hard about doing this in the opposite way of their habitual placement.

Michael Purcell, the past president of the Feldenkrais Guild, noted that Moshe Feldenkrais in the 1980 training he took from him at that time said, when the students couldn't handle the switched interlacing of the fingers: "You see, you're so cuckoo in your head that a silly thing like this throws you all off kilter."

No, I wouldn't call you cuckoo. Purcell said he felt as if he had two left hands all of a sudden. I did when I tried it. Perhaps you did, too. But if you think about how it feels, then do it the opposite way, pretty soon both ways feel comfortable. That's the theory of doing Feldenkrais movements: Think about what you do, and if you think about it enough, you can change them for the better so you can choose which way of doing something is better for you.

Stand and Be Aware

Stand upright with your weight on both feet. Don't try to stand any way in particular, such as taller, straighter, more balanced, or in a way you think is right. Just stand there as if you'd just gotten up from a chair.

Now start at the top of your head and think about every part, all the way down to your feet. Close your eyes if you'd like. Take time to really consider whether:

- ✓ Your head is straight
- ✓ Your chin pokes forward
- ✓ Your shoulders are hunched
- ✓ Your fingers are relaxed
- ✓ Your hips are push out to one side
- ✓ Your knees are straight
- ✓ Your weight is more on your heels or toes, or evenly distributed

Work your way through your entire body. Avoid passing judgment. Just become aware of what is and how it feels and what may feel better. Always take a moment to "pause and observe," as Moshe Feldenkrais wrote in his book *Awareness Through Movement*.

You can also do the same lesson, for example, sitting, lying down, walking, or running. But always: Pause and be aware.

Sit, Turn, and Look

This is a classic Feldenkrais lesson (shown in Figure 16-1) that you can do simply sitting in a chair if you prefer. I explain it, however, in the more classic position on the floor, where Moshe Feldenkrais taught it.

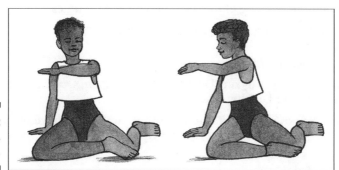

Figure 16-1: Sit, Turn, and Look.

Sitting

1. Sit on the floor.

2. Bend your left leg backward to the left so that your foot is behind you and your knee rotates inward.

   If you have knee problems, you may choose to do this in a chair.

3. Bend your right leg so the knee is turned outward and the sole of your foot is close to the top of your left knee. Position the lower part of your leg so that it's parallel to a wall in front of you so you can easily return to this same position.

4. Put your right palm on the floor to the right and a little behind you and allow your body weight to lean on it as needed.

5. Raise your left arm so that your forearm is almost parallel to the ground and your shoulders, but at about shoulder-height and about a foot from your face. Let your hand relax comfortably without effort.

6. Close your eyes.

Turning

1. Turn yourself to the right with your left hand leading. Allow your head to follow the thumb of your left hand in its movement to the right.

2. Move to the right only as far as your body and back are comfortable and can move with ease and without strain or effort, then stop.

Looking

1. Open your eyes. Notice what you are looking at that is directly beyond your thumb, perhaps on the wall across from you.

2. Now leave your body and arm where they are, and turn your head a little bit farther, as far as is comfortable, while scanning to the right with your eyes.

3. Return your head and eyes to the place you found in Step 1 of Looking, above.

4. Repeat the turning of the head and eyes 8–10 times.

5. Return the entire body to the front. Rest.

Doing it again and being aware

1. Close your eyes again. Turn to the right again. Open your eyes as in Step 1 in the Looking lesson, above.

2. Are you now looking at the same spot on the wall beyond your thumb? Is the spot farther back than before? How does your back feel?

3. **Return to facing the front. Then return to a standing position as in the first "Stand and Be Aware" lesson. Check your body from head to toe, slowly. Are there any differences in how you're standing? How does that feel.**

4. **When you're done on one side (feel free to repeat this), try it on the opposite side if you'd like.**

In contrast to other methods that ask you always to do both sides for balance, Feldenkrais only asks that you do what feels right at that moment. And that may not be doing both sides!

Bringing Head and Knee Together

I know, you aren't supposed to be exercising when you're doing Feldenkrais lessons. But be aware of how a simple move uses your muscles and how that feels. Remember to do this lesson slowly, exhaling on the upward movement, and without any strain or tension. Relax, and rest between every 4–8 movements. Figure 16-2 shows you the particulars.

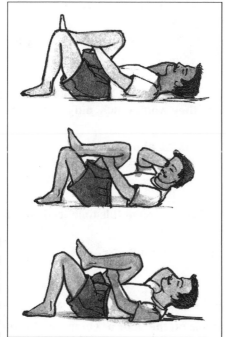

Figure 16-2:
Bringing
Head and
Knee
Together.

Preface

1. **Lie on your back with your arms at your side and your legs extended. Check your body from head to toe, becoming aware of how each muscle and limb feels and how it is lying against the ground.**

2. **Get ready to move.**

Positioning

1. **Bend your knees so that your feet are flat on the floor, shoulder-width apart.**

2. **Lift your right knee toward your chest and hold it behind the thigh with your left hand with thumb turned parallel and held together with your fingers.**

   If this isn't comfortable, use a towel or strap to hold your leg.

3. **Put your right hand behind your head and rest your elbow on the floor with the arm opened and out.**

Flex I

1. **While holding your knee, lift your head and slowly guide your elbow toward your right knee, and your knee toward your right elbow. They won't touch, just move toward each other.**

2. **Repeat 4–8 times, then rest. Be aware of how your body feels.**

Flex II

1. **Do the same move as in Flex I, except this time guide your chin toward your knee. Again, they won't touch, only move in the direction of each other.**

2. **Repeat 4–8 times, rest, and think about the movement's effect on your body.**

Flex III

1. **Do the same move a third time, except this time lead your forehead in the direction of your knee.**

2. **Repeat 4–8 times, rest, pause, and observe.**

Finish

1. **Stretch out both legs and relax your arms.**

2. **Notice how your body feels on the floor as compared to when you began.**

You can now do the whole series again, do it on the other side, do one part of it again, or even do it on the same side again. You can also go back to earlier lessons and see whether any of those movements have now changed their pattern or if your awareness during them has changed in any way.

When you're done doing movements sitting or on your back, stand up and walk around to see if you notice anything different in your walk, your hips, your back, or any other part of your body.

Observing the Alexander Technique

The Alexander Technique is in some ways very similar to the Feldenkrais method and in many ways very dissimilar. It involves subtle thinking about the way you do things. But it is concerned less with what you do than with *how* you do it.

Where the Feldenkrais system prescribes certain movements, then asks you to think about them so you can influence how you move in daily life after that, the *Alexander Technique* has you do your normal movements mindfully and asks you to focus so you can influence your body immediately, perhaps making changes as you go along.

The bottom line for both methods is to use your mind to improve how you use your body, whether in day-to-day activities like carrying a toddler, or in sports and fitness activities where the goal may be fitness, health, or performance. That's how these rather esoteric concepts fit into a book on fitness. Apply them properly, and your fitness activities of mind and body may become more successful, too.

I suppose the other similarity is that both were developed by a man after whom each method is named. Each man questioned something about his own body and became frustrated with traditional ways to heal or fix it. Both used that curiosity to come up with a solution — a solution about which each began to spread the word because each believed his method could help others also.

In Feldenkrais's case, it was a physical injury. In Alexander's case, it was chronic laryngitis that threatened his profession as an actor and Shakespearean orator. Frederick Matthias Alexander — all his teachers and students called him simply "F.M." — lived from 1869 to 1955. When he developed laryngitis, F.M. Alexander questioned what he may be doing to prompt it. He focused inside, observed himself consciously, and found that he commonly tensed his neck and pushed his head back.

The big ah-ha moment!

It wasn't long before he began to teach to others his technique of observation to influence physical change.

Call him Coach Alexander. That's all he did really, was coach people as they moved. Thanks, Coach.

Getting down to Alexander basics

Alexander is known to be fond of saying, "Anyone can do what I did, if they will do what I did."

Dang, these developers can lead your mind in circles. But think about it. If you take time to observe your physical habits, you too can recognize the habits that may be harmful or painful, and then fix whatever may be causing you that discomfort, pain, injury, fatigue, or stress. Somehow, such a simple concept is so difficult to grasp, yet it is the heart of the Alexander Technique.

You have ingrained physical habits, as we all do, imprinted starting when you were a toddler and promoted by both physical or cultural influences. These habits affect how you hold your body and how you move it, as well as how you react to life's demands.

One man I know says he invariably stands up from the computer after a few hours with his head protruding forward on his neck. Everybody looks at him and says, "So you've been at your computer again, huh?"

That's where the Alexander Technique education starts to happen — during your everyday physical habits, says Nicholas Brockbank, an Alexander teacher and author in England. Lessons can be maddeningly simplistic because they may be only about sitting or standing while you (or a teacher, if you're in a private lesson) observe what you're doing and try to correct it. You try to stop abusing your body by releasing unnecessary tension and odd postures. That takes being present. No making out the grocery list in your head during an Alexander session!

Then, the technique moves into real life, which is where the real learning occurs. And is also the most difficult to do because all those old habits sneak back again. You can apply the Alexander Technique of mindful observation to anything you do. Brushing your teeth? Look at how you're standing. Dancing a waltz? Think about the carriage of your back. Running an interval? Observe the way you hold your neck.

The essence of the Alexander Technique? Going about your daily life and thinking about what you're doing while you're doing it. You may be asked to think about the smallest curl of a little toe, or how you hold a knife. But those little movements may be influenced by something else going on in your body.

Gleaning gains from Alexander's ways

The Alexander Technique is not a *workout* for your heart, lungs, muscles, mind, and body, but work that can help you get a *better* workout for your heart, lungs, muscles, mind, and body. And isn't that what we all want in the end?

When you spend time observing and moving in the Alexander tradition, you should be able to:

✔ Rid yourself of physical tension that causes you problems.

✔ Allow your head to float freely on top of your spine. (This was a real key issue for F.M. Alexander, who found head and neck movement and tension caused his problems.)

✔ Move any body part freely without unnecessary involvement from unrelated body parts.

✔ Breathe fully and comfortably, which also helps release tension and frees movement.

But you only get these things if you use the technique as the filter through which you put your everyday habits.

You don't use the following Alexander exercises to treat a specific condition, but indirectly you do indeed treat specific conditions by becoming aware of them. You may in fact become aware enough to find relief from back pain, neck pain, tension headaches, and any repetitive strain injuries, not to mention physical idiosyncrasies that affect sports performance.

Sort of like Heathrow Airport's air traffic control, Alexander's *Primary Control* is the relationship between the head and the neck and its influence on the entire body. Alexander believes that nearly everybody has an unhealthy relationship between head and neck and the carriage there. Get your head resting freely on the top of your spine and neck, loosening it from its unhealthy relationship with your back and the rest of the body, and you can notice the benefits from ankles to eyelashes.

Nicholas Brockbank, the England-based Alexander instructor and writer, relates a story of a mini running lesson he and other Alexander teachers experienced a number of years ago:

> "We all legged it back and forth across the park and the teacher yodeled out to us to do — or rather, to think — typical Alexander things such as "free your neck," "lengthen up," et cetera. What astonished me at the time was how simply thinking differently while running alone changed the nature of the way I ran completely. I became lighter and easier on my feet, and just felt better in myself."

Discovering whether Alexander is really for you

I suppose if you want to be in good company, practicing Alexander Techniques certainly puts you there! The Alexander Technique has been taught at the Juilliard School of Performing Arts in New York, at the Royal College of Music and the Royal Academy of Dramatic Arts in London, at Boston University, the Stratford Shakespearean Festival, and to Olympic athletes around the world. It has also earned praise from actors, performers, and authors including Kevin Kline, George Bernard Shaw, and Aldous Huxley — an impressive roster!

Now that you're duly impressed, let me also say that if you are willing to use your mind, to focus on what your body is doing, then work to mindfully alter it for the better, the Alexander Technique is indeed for you. You must also be able to focus on very small movements, repeat them constantly, and have a heck of a lot of patience as you await change.

Considering that much of this can be done either while you do other activities, and in brief moments here and there, you don't even have a reason to slap your forehead and moan about adding another task to your day.

Typical students fall into several categories. You may have:

- ✔ A specific pain, injury, or chronic dysfunction (like F.M. Alexander's laryngitis).
- ✔ General tension or stress that leaves you tight and nervous. Well, that includes almost everybody!
- ✔ A problem that affects your work, daily activities, fitness, or sports performance.
- ✔ A chronic condition such as asthma or arthritis. Be sure to talk to your physician first!

Wearing what you will

This simple method requires only that you wear comfortable clothing. That can even mean normal street or work clothes, as long as you aren't confined in any way. No tight belts, collars, or ties, please!

Moving the Alexander way

The difficulty in coming up with a few sample Alexander movements is that, well, there really aren't any! As I explain in the previous section, you mostly just observe what you do in daily life.

But, yes, I can still guide you through some lessons, which is what I do in this section. The reason for a lesson is to help you develop an awareness of your body so that you can more fully observe it all the time. If you take a lesson from a certified Alexander teacher, you start at the beginning, breaking down old habits and learning new ones. The teacher may have you stand, sit, or walk around in a room while he or she observes you and comments about what he or she sees. Sometimes having that neutral person on the outside looking in can help you sort of look inside yourself later.

Making a video tape of yourself in motion can help you become your own Alexander teacher — making you your own observer.

The lessons I present were developed by Alexander instructor Nicholas Brockbank and are displayed on the best one-stop Internet shop for information and resources about Alexander, www.alexandertechnique.com. This site is run by Robert Rickover, also an Alexander teacher in Nebraska and author of *Fitness Without Stress: A Guide to the Alexander Technique.*

Sit to Stand I

This exercise is so simple, but so telling. Do this exercise, then do Sit to Stand II for a really revelatory moment.

1. **Sit on the edge of a chair or other firm surface. If your seat is too squishy or low, it affects your muscle action, so choose something like a kitchen chair.**

2. **Think relaxed, then rise as if you were standing to greet somebody.**

3. **Think about your body, your head, and your neck. Did you activate any muscles besides your legs and lower body to propel you from sitting to standing?**

4. **Try the same routine quickly and more slowly, all at once and in small stages. Whatever you do, pay close attention to the muscular activity in your Primary Control. (That's what Alexander loved to call the area where your head sits on top of your neck, as I explain earlier in this section.)**

You're likely to notice nothing or nearly nothing, and think, "Man, this is weird. Why am I doing this?" But wait before you pass judgment. Go to the next version first.

Sit to Stand II

1. **Sit as in Sit to Stand I on a relatively firm surface.**

2. **This time, place the palm of one hand on the back of your neck and let it rest there heavily so that your arm is relaxed.**

3. **Do the standing routine one more time, leaving your palm on the back of your neck.**

4. **Let your hand tell you what's going on in your neck.**

Notice anything different? Do you feel extra muscular tensing or neck movement? Is your neck tensing? Where? Is your neck sort of goose-necking forward as you stand? At what point is the activity most noticeable? What is happening to your head and neck at that point?

Your Primary Control, my friend, may be out of control, or at least that's what F.M. Alexander may have said.

Does this extraneous activity such as tensing or goose-necking in your head and neck area coincide with a tendency to:

✔ Lose your balance?

✔ Hold your breath?

✔ Hike up your shoulders?

✔ Swaying your low back more than you should?

✔ Tighten your stomach?

✔ Let your knees fall together sort of knock-kneed?

✔ Let your ankles cave inward?

After you become aware of your extraneous movements, you can work on eliminating them whenever you move from a sitting to standing position.

Variations on the Sit-to-Stand Theme

The concept of noticing what you're doing applies to every movement you make. You can observe other movement sequences also, for example, standing to sitting; lying down to sitting up; walking up or down stairs; running, whether to catch a bus or for fitness.

The list is actually endless. Just notice.

Head Turn — Relax

Ever see a star basketball player spin a basketball on the tip of a finger? Well, imagine your head is the basketball and the tip-top of your spine is the tip of the finger. That ball (your head, in other words) is sitting loosely and freely on the top of the finger (your spine). If the ball were glued down, it wouldn't spin and it wouldn't be so easy to bend the finger to get the ball to move.

Alrighty then, with that introduction, you're ready to turn your head on the top of your spine. Keep thinking about that basketball spinning. You want to avoid in these moves letting your head rock or tip in the neck itself.

1. **Sit down on a firm chair.**

2. **Place the palm of your right hand on the back of your head just above where the base of your skull meets the top of your neck.**

   You can feel where your skull ends.

3. **Place the palm of your left hand on your forehead, as if you were feeling for a temperature.**

4. **Using your hands to move your head, rotate your head to the left to look off your left shoulder.**

   Your neck muscles of course do some work, but try to let them relax as much as possible and use your hands to move your head. This takes some focus and effort, some thought, and perhaps some readjustment of your hands.

5. **Switch the placement of your hands so that you can look over your right shoulder.**

6. **Use your hands to tip your head forward.**

   You're moving from the base of your head. Tip your head forward as if looking at something you dribbled on your shirt right below your chin.

7. **Use your hands to tip your head backward.**

   You may feel as if you're standing with the back of your head and your back against a wall (you can actually try this!) because your head doesn't fall backward but tips from its base.

8. **Repeat all the above actions several times — a couple of times each to the right, to the left, then forward and backward.**

You need to consciously think about not using your neck. Your neck muscles follow, not lead, the action, and your head is still that basketball balanced kind of precariously on the tip of a finger.

Head Turn — Resist

Do the same movements as in the preceding lesson, but this time let your neck muscles resist the turning movement of your hands. Don't clamp down and turn the movement into a huge tug o' war. Just resist.

If you have a neck or spinal injury, consult with your doctor before adding tension.

Imagined Head Turn — No Hands

Do this less after you try the preceding two (the Head Turn, Relax and Head Turn, Resist) which have you use your hands, trying to relax your neck muscles and then trying to resist with your neck muscles. Now, without using your hands, repeat that process. This time totally relax your neck muscles, just as you did when you used your hands the first time. But just imagine your head turning — don't actually move your head at all!

Actual Head Turns — No Hands

Here we go for the big finale of head turning. After you do the preceding three lessons — turning your head with your hands, without your hands, relaxed, resisted, and just imagined — turn your head as in the first progression but utterly relaxed in the head and neck (Primary Control). You may still have to fight the tension that tries to creep in.

Moving and Motivating with Laban Movement Analysis

If you read the preceding two sections about two other Modern Classic mind-body methods, you can see a bit of a trend when you dive a little more into Laban Movement Analysis (or LMA, as the inside lingo goes).

Just as Moshe Feldenkrais and F.M. Alexander did, Rudolf Laban developed a theory of movement that looks at your whole body and how the parts interact in their relationship to each other and their surroundings. Sounds like a TV sitcom plot! That's because the goal here is to get the mind and body to get along better. Just as with Feldenkrais and Alexander movements, Laban movement analysis can help you do other things better, from athletic performance to fitness activities to life's everyday doings, such as carrying groceries or getting out of a car. LMA is the means, not the end.

Laban is a little different from Feldenkrais (with its movements where you are told to just think about what you feel) and Alexander (where you try to increase awareness in everyday movements). *Laban movements* are very specific exercises and drills designed to let you feel and become more aware of how the body should move in different situations. Note the word "should." In this method, you are actually told what you want to feel and how it should affect what you are doing.

Laban, who lived from 1879 to 1958, shared nearly the same era with Alexander. Plus, heck, they were both real thinkers. Who else would slap you down on the ground and have you rolling around so you could feel your body? Laban, a Hungarian choreographer who taught in Berlin, developed theories about the nature of movement and created a system to record and analyze movement of all kinds, including dance and martial arts.

Certainly, Laban is key to the analysis of what the body is doing and making it better. But it was his protégé, Irmgard Bartenieff who died in 1981 at the age of 81, who designed the fundamental exercises that help with the movement analysis. In fact, as a physical therapist in New York, Bartenieff founded the Laban Institute of Movement Studies to promote the method and her teacher's theories. Laban Movement Analysts are actually the only certified Bartenieff Fundamental practitioners. Oh, and the Institute is now called the Laban/Bartenieff Institute to honor all her contributions.

After you figure out the LMA philosophy, the method's movements can help you understand why you sometimes just can't get your body to cooperate with what your mind is telling it, sometimes even begging it, to do. That enlightenment can at least begin with a sampling of exercises, which I present in the section, "Sampling the Movements," but can of course be furthered by visiting a certified practitioner. These practitioners also study many long hours to fully understand and teach the method.

Understanding Laban's hows and whys

Irmgard Bartenieff considered her fundamental exercises the building blocks of all human movement. They may have kinda funny names, such as Pelvic Lateral Shift and Vertical Body Half, but each has a goal of affecting four components of the movement, as described by Janet Hamburg, a professor of dance and an author at the University of Kansas and a certified Laban Movement Analyst. These fundamental exercises try to encapsulate the following areas of human movement, answering the questions that are posed about each:

- ✔ **Space:** Where does the body move?
- ✔ **Shape:** What shapes does the body make in space?
- ✔ **Effort:** Which dynamic qualities are clear in the effort?
- ✔ **Body:** How does the body start and move through each action?

Oh, and let me get the terminology correct now. These are not exercises, but were called *sequences* by Bartenieff because she wanted to emphasis the connection of each movement to the next and the necessity to truly think about what you ask your body to do. Count repetitions? Nope, never. Instead, do what you need to do in order to understand . . . as long as you can still think clearly enough to make the movement productive.

This is where the mind-body aspect now enters.

Take a look at traditional Western exercise again. There, you normally get a piecemeal approach. Do biceps curls; ignore your legs. Do leg lifts; let your upper body just be there. Ride a bike; don't think about what your shoulders are up to. You don't do this with Laban analysis or Bartenieff movement. Your mind doesn't just come along for the ride and put up a closed sign. It's an active participant.

Gaining the goods from Laban

If you assemble the sequences properly (sort of like doing your piano scales), you should be able to restore *efficient neuromuscular pathways.* Translation? Your muscles, nerves, bones, and breath are able to talk to and understand each other. That's when you're playing a piano concerto.

To get to where you can play the concerto, you have to practice the sequences (or scales) so that you can:

- ✔ **Use the deep muscles in your core.** Those are the ones that because of their deepness often get ignored in traditional exercise. For one thing, strengthening them doesn't give any aesthetic feedback. (Oooo, what strong erector spinae you have! . . . I don't think so.)

- ✔ **Use your breathing to support the power and flow of the moves.** If you hold your breath, which is not uncommon, your muscles and any intended movement is weaker and less effective.

- ✔ **Understand where the movement initiates in your body and how it ripples through your body.** Think your toes are responsible for propelling you through space in a walk or a run? Wrong. Try your torso and hips.

- ✔ **Release tension from your muscles.** Both Laban and Bartenieff found most people floundered in successful and pain-free movement partly because they clamped down too hard on their muscles.

As with many other techniques, scientific proof of the benefits is lacking. But practitioners say that they see the benefits in their practices. So I leave it up to you to decide. Janet Hamburg, the Laban Movement Analyst in Kansas who has trained athletes using Laban sequences, has seen her students go from also-rans to U.S. Olympic Track & Field Trials competitors.

Successfully understanding the whys and wherefores can help you move forward to:

- ✔ Moving more easily and expressively

- ✔ Improving your athletic performance

- ✔ Reducing your risk or number of injuries

- ✔ Adding greater clarity and expression to performances, practices, or competitions

✔ Rehabilitating injuries and other conditions that limit mobility

✔ Experiencing joy and ease in your daily movement

✔ Becoming an Olympic athlete (Oops, just kidding. Well, unless you're already on the way.)

Discovering whether Laban is really for you

Yes, I won't deny it — Laban, like the other Modern Classics, is a slow and repetitive process involving deep analysis. But take a look at the preceding section where I discuss the benefits that can be gained as a way to decide if Laban is for you. Then try a little.

If you're eager to make any of these changes due to frustration with your performance, pain or injury, or if you have a bent toward joy of the analytical, then Laban may be just your ticket. I always figure it can't hurt to give it a whirl!

This method was originally developed for actors, dancers, and other performance artists. But it has also been used successfully by:

✔ Athletes at all levels

✔ People who suffer from chronic physical limitations

✔ People recovering from injuries

✔ People wanting to improve coordination or daily function

Well, hmm, that covers just about everybody, doesn't it?

Note that athletes in particular can find great performance gains by tampering with the smallest bit of muscle awareness. Five-time Olympic Gold Medallist in the discus, Al Oerter, used Laban as a part of his training. For example, if a runner comes out of the starting blocks with greater ease, that hundredth of a second can make the difference between winning and losing. Tennis players who need to shift their pelvis to make quick and fluid moves can find themselves nailing that game point. Volleyball or basketball blocks may happen more adeptly because of smoother weight shifts.

Getting your gear bag packed

Ah, the beauty and simplicity of the Modern Classics. A carpeted floor or other open space with some kind of mat or blanket is all you need. Because these movements do involve some rolling around on the ground, and doing moves on your back and knees, you also want to make sure your clothing is loose and doesn't bind. And if you have long hair, it may be best to pull it out of the way so you don't ruin a moment of enlightened muscle awareness because you need to flip hair out of your face.

Sampling the movements

Bartenieff Fundamentals are straightforward and exacting. Oh, certainly there are variations, but the basic six include what are called: Thigh Lift, Pelvic Forward Shift, Pelvic Lateral Shift, Vertical Body Half, Knee Drop, and Arm Circle. All certified practitioners use these six to at least begin to analyze movement. Then comes the creativity seen in variations that are and have been developed to address particular needs, goals, or problems. That's not to mention the different demands on the body and mind when you vary the tempo, direction, dynamics, or phrasing.

Be forewarned, dear reader, that these movements look and sound simple enough, just like that aggravatingly simple head turn in the Alexander method. But when you apply your mind to concentrating intensely, you can do these for years and learn something new every time.

I don't present all the Bartenieff Fundamentals. I cover one Fundamental of the basic six, then take you directly to two more advanced moves that are directly applicable to walking, running, and other forward movement. These can be found in the book by Bartenieff called *Body Movement,* including instruction and illustrations for all the fundamental sequences. (Check out the Appendix for more info on the book.)

Pelvic Forward Shift (Fundamental #2)

The purpose of knowing how to shift your pelvis forward is to prepare you to move your entire body forward and backward. Because you don't spend your life just standing in one place, to be able to move from sitting to standing, or just walking in a straight line can be a boon to all aspects of your life. Figure 16-3 shows you how to do it.

1. **Lie on your back with your knees bent and feet flat on the floor. Place your arms on the floor comfortably at your sides, hands relaxed.**

2. **Exhale fully and deeply, including the air in your belly as much as possible.**

3. **As a part of the exhale, slowly raise your hips off the floor by shifting the center of your weight toward your feet and up into the air. Your tailbone should feel as if it's moving toward your heels, and your head, shoulders and feet are still on the floor. Keep your buttocks relaxed.**

CAUTION!

If you have back problems, consult with your doctor before trying this kind of spinal roll.

4. **Inhale and on the next exhalation, slowly lower your hips back to the floor. Instead of rolling through the spine, try to lower in one piece. Just let your hips soften and place them back onto the floor. While lowering, extend your low back.**

5. **Repeat a few times.**

What to avoid:

✔ Using your arms and hands for support by pushing them into the ground.

✔ Overusing your buttocks muscles.

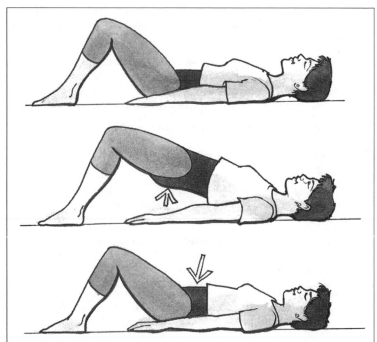

Figure 16-3: Pelvic Forward Shift.

Think about:

✔ Opening the front of your hips — basically the belly area and the area where your leg creases when you lift your thigh.

✔ Pressing your heels into the floor to engage your hamstrings (the muscles in the back of your upper legs) for support.

Preparatory Exercise for Creeping to Standing (Sequence #8)

Creeping? Translate that as "moving consciously." This preparatory movement helps you focus on going to a standing position using the deep muscles of your hips and power center (abdominals and the like in your core). It's not about grabbing with the muscles in your abdominals and buttocks. You definitely want to get this one down before you go onto the next one. Don't just go through the motions as much as this is seemingly childlike rolling around. Use your mind to focus on awareness in your muscles.

Position

Start in the same position as in the Pelvic Forward Shift — on your back, with knees bent and feet on the floor. In this case, however, extend your arms out at shoulder-height on the ground so you look a bit like the letter "T."

First step

1. **Roll over onto one side, curling your entire body softly into a ball with knees folded high and arms pulled in to your chest. Call it the fetal position, if you will.**

2. **Roll back to starting position on your back, allowing your arms to spread back to the "T" position when you are there. You get your arms there by one circling above your head, sort of tracing a half-circle, and just extending the other outward at shoulder level.**

   Initiate the rolling maneuver from your hips and your power center.

3. **Repeat this first half several times.**

Second step

1. **Do the first step where you fold softly onto your side. But don't just come to a rest there.**

2. **Continue the roll to the side into a total shift of your body weight so you keep right on going up onto your knees and elbows, while looking down at the floor.**

3. **Straighten your arms directly beneath your shoulders into a hands-and-knees position. Keep your chin dropped so that the back of your head and your spine are on one plane and you're looking at the floor.**

What to avoid:

   ✔ Jerking up or stopping the movement part way. Make sure the movement flows.

   ✔ Tensing your neck or shoulders when you straighten your arms.

Creeping to Standing Level for Locomotion (Sequence #11a)

Ah, here's that creeping again, but this time you do the creeping stuff and actually get ready to move forward. Use this sequence to discover and use the deep muscles in your power center in your hips and pelvis as you transfer your body weight forward and up. Bottom line: This sequence, shown in Figure 16-4, can help you move from sitting to standing with ease. Or it can help an athlete perform if that performance involves rising to a standing position or rising to a movement.

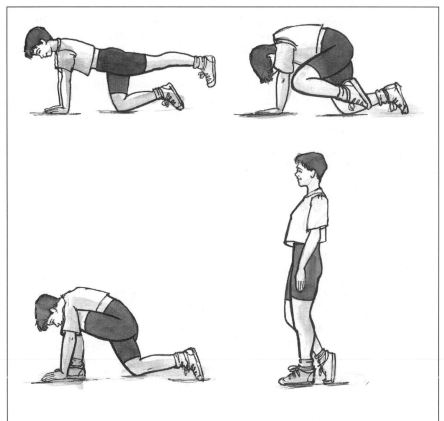

Figure 16-4:
Creeping to
Standing
Level for
Locomotion.

Position
Start where you finished in the previous prep sequence (on all fours).

First step

1. **Exhale, and initiate this movement from your groin (the area of the crease when you lift your thigh). Swing your left knee forward to your chest, allowing your back to round as much as you need and your head to drop as your knee approaches your nose.**

2. **Then swing your left leg backward as you inhale, extending it straight out behind you, with the heel pushing outward and away.**

3. **Repeat this swing from nose to leg-extension several times to find your muscle sense of both ease and power.**

Think "knee forward, heel back." Flex your ankle so your toes point toward the floor and not back or out.

Second step

1. **After repeating a few swings on your left side, on a forward swing, plant your foot with the toes pointing forward between your hands, allowing your pelvis to shift forward. Your right hand may want to come up from the ground, but try to keep it down.**

2. **Without stopping your forward weight-shift, continue forward and up onto that foot, releasing both hands and rising up to an upright stance. Use the momentum of the shift to simply walk forward a few steps.**

3. **Repeat on the right side, and continue several times, alternating sides.**

One side may be more difficult than the other because everybody is a little unbalanced.

What to avoid:

✔ Tensing your neck, back, or shoulders as you begin to use your hands to come to a standing position.

✔ Jerking your leg forward during the swing. Find the easy rhythm of the forward motion as you exhale.

✔ Straining your back as your place your foot between your hands. Your back should round a little bit as you place your foot.

✔ Fighting the leg action as you place your foot between your arms. Slip it smoothly into place.

Changing Your Perspective through Inversion Therapy

Inversion Therapy sounds way too clinical to me. So I like to call it Going Upside Down, because that's what you do. But you need to know the technical name.

Going Upside Down is a mind-body workout? Definitely, and it dates back not only decades but hundreds and thousands of years. I don't address the head-down stuff in the Yoga section, but it is a key part of Yoga. Think about head-stands. Think about bridges. Think about just sticking your butt up in the air when your hands and feet are on firm ground. Even that's a kind of inversion that's a part of a Yoga practice. Supposedly, Hippocrates, the father of medicine, used to go head-down regularly. And that was in 400 B.C.

Heck, think about all the inversion you did as a kid. Cartwheels, bridges, hanging from your knees on tree branches (as long as mom didn't catch you), or swinging upside down from ropes or from someone's jungle gym. Of course, you didn't go upside down to reverse the forces of gravity, turn back the aging clock, reduce mental negativity, or any of the other acclaimed benefits I explain in a bit. You did it because it felt weird and kind of cool all at the same time. Hmm, guess that's what adults like about it, too — it's sort of weird and cool all at once.

Kids are the grandest of master teachers. Watching their actions can teach us adults a lot about life, and that includes the joy of going upside down.

Turning to upside-down philosophy

Inversion is just about going topsy-turvy. Period. You go upside down. You get the benefits — some proven, some not — that I discuss in the next section.

Looking at the world upside down is all about reversing gravity's forces on your body, which allows your lymphatic system, vertebra, muscles, heart, and circulation to function from a different angle. Edging into the esoteric, yogis have been known to go upside-down for hours on end as a way to control the mind, facilitate meditation, and eliminate restlessness while bringing on a focused calm necessary for better fitness and health of both mind and body.

No, I won't ask you to stand on your head for hours. Really, no one should do that unless they are truly advanced practitioners of a mind-body method and fully in control of their bodies, and definitely do not have any medical complications.

But I do suggest that you try a few semi-inverted, or recumbent inverted poses to experience some of the effects.

Remember, because of additional and varied forces on your heart and head, anyone with high blood pressure, cardiovascular disease, or eye diseases such as glaucoma, or anyone who is prone to these conditions, should avoid inversion. If you're uncertain, consult with a physician to make sure that you aren't prone to any of these conditions. Pregnant women may find comfort with a recumbent-like inversion (not a full inversion), but only for the first trimester. After that, doctors advise against lying on your back for more than a minute or so because of pressure the developing fetus can place on veins and arteries. If you are unsure, always consult your physician.

Enjoying the benefits of inversion

What can you get out of inversion? Depends on your outlook (oh, I'm so funny). No, really, it depends on what you put into it and what you want out of it. The following list highlights a few of the benefits you may experience. Remember, some of these have been scientifically researched, some have not. Most of the benefits that have been researched involve back pain relief from less pressure on the discs:

- **Reduce back and muscle pain, or decompress your spine:** If you've ever had any back pain, due either to a bad disc or muscle spasms, you know how traction or just hanging your weight from a bar can provide relief. The release of gravity's pull and the force on your feet can decompress your vertebra and allow your muscles to relax. Even the beginner inversion poses can work wonders in pain relief. I can personally vouch for that. And if you pound, pound, pound, then you need to release, release, release. Inversion can stretch muscles that are tightened in other workouts, too.

- **Cleanse your lymph system and stimulate your circulation:** Yoga practitioners and others may tell you that the lymph fluid (a mix of a type of white blood cells and fats) needs to periodically drain in the opposite direction.

- **Reduce gravity's aging effect:** Effects can include less loss of height because the discs in your back are able to regenerate themselves. None of this is truly scientifically proven.

- **Decrease stress and improve mental focus:** Heck, if your back and neck muscles aren't tense and overworked, you're less stressed. Being able to relax and meditate calmly while upside down may help you focus better in other situations, too.

Discovering whether inversion is really for you

When it comes to going upside down, you and your doctor need to give the final word on whether you should try inversion.

Without things like music or choreography to influence a decision, your answer about trying inversion comes strictly from your medical history or genetics, as well as your comfort factor in being topsy-turvy.

Even if you don't go all the way over, however, the simple semi-recumbent poses are usually okay for most anyone to dabble at.

Using the extra baggage

Ah, another simple mind-body workout that doesn't — at least for novices — require a lot of gear and gadgets to get you started. For the simplest of poses, you want a mat or carpet to cushion your back, a chair or bench to raise your legs (or even a stack of pillows), or maybe a wall to prop up your feet.

If inversion is something that your doctor approves for you and you're not freaked out at seeing the world upside down, then you may decide to go for fancy chairs, racks and boots, or tilting tables. These can run from $100 to upwards of $400, depending on the degree of complexity, materials, company, and whether it's motorized or not.

If you're going all the way upside down, you definitely want snug clothing or at least something that's tucked in, rather than something that can billow back down over your face. Suffocation is not part of this workout. Same goes for your hair if it's long. Tie it out of the way.

Sampling Inversion

Avoid just flipping onto your head or jumping onto a tilting table. Try the simplest poses first, which can be an especially good way to meditate or relax after you finish another workout.

In all the positions — be they semi-recumbent or totally inverted — practice deep breathing, especially trying to exhale into your back muscles and feel them give up the tension they may be holding. Visualize your vertebra separating and releasing.

You also want to limit how much time you spend in a certain position at first. Even minutes can be plenty. As you get more experienced, you can shoot for 10 to 30 minutes.

If you ever begin to feel dizzy, come up out of the position slowly and consult with your physician. In the next sections, I set out some techniques for novice inverters to try.

Going Horizontal with Pillows

This may seem simple, but it works. When I had back pain, I used to tell my husband I needed to "go horizontal," which was a simple way of saying I needed to lie down on my back. The difference in this type of stretching out is the pillows and the deep breathing.

1. **Lie on your back on the floor or on a firm couch or bed.**

   Place several firm pillows or rolled up blankets and pads underneath your knees so they are bent, completely relaxed, and your feet aren't resting on the floor or couch.

2. **Place your arms at your sides, and let your shoulders roll back to open your chest.**

3. **Relax, and practice deep breathing.**

Going Horizontal with a Chair

Heck, I've done this one at trade shows in side hallways to release my back and relax and regenerate for a few more hours. Try it before bed or after work.

1. **Sit on the floor with the side of your right hip up against the center of the chair (or whatever firm object you're going to use).**

2. **Place your hands behind you to support your torso as you begin to lean backward, lift your knees and legs, and pivot on your buttocks so your legs rest on the chair seat with your knees bent. Slide your buttocks close to the chair so you don't have to extend your legs at all.**

3. **Place your arms at your sides.**

4. **Relax, and practice deep breathing.**

Going Horizontal with Legs on a Wall

This takes you one step farther toward true inversion. You need to relax in the position and let the calming effect happen. This is super when you're traveling by plane because the reverse position can help travel-induced swelling become less bothersome.

Getting into the position is much like the one above.

1. **Sit on the floor with the side of your right hip against the wall.**

2. **Place your hands behind you to support your torso as you begin to lean backward and, at the same time, swing your legs and heels up onto the wall.**

3. **After you're on your back with your legs up, arrange yourself a bit by pushing your buttocks up as close as possible to the wall.**

4. **Place your arms at your sides.**

5. **Relax and breathe deeply.**

   Place a folded towel or small pillow under your head if the floor is too hard.

Try the following intermediate upside-down techniques only after you're comfortable with semi-recumbent poses. With these, a doctor's clearance is particularly important.

Half Shoulder Stand with the Wall

This pose, shown in Figure 16-5, gets you higher up on your shoulders, but with the security of a wall so you don't fear tipping all the way over.

1. **Lie on your back with your feet away from the wall and the top of your head toward the wall. You should be about an arm's distance from the wall, more or less — if you extend your arms overhead, your fingertips would touch the wall. Put your arms at your sides, palms down, for support.**

2. **Bend your knees with your feet flat on the floor close to your hips.**

3. **Lift your knees toward your chest and place your hands on the back of your hips or in the small of your back.**

4. **Continue to lift your knees toward your nose, using your hands on your hips and back to support and assist in the lift.**

5. **Extend your legs so your toes are reaching toward the wall slightly behind you.**

   Keep your upper back and shoulders on the floor so you don't strain your neck.

6. **Remain there as long as you're comfortable, even just 30 seconds or so.**

7. **Use your hands to help lower your hips toward the ground to come out of the position. Bend your knees as you lower your hips.**

Figure 16-5:
Half
Shoulder
Stand with
the Wall.

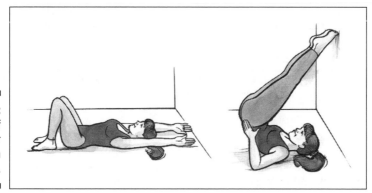

Lying Backward over Something

I know, I know, that sounds odd. But this backward bend position — if you don't have any back injuries and your doctor is okay with it — can be done over a stack of firm pillows, an exercise ball (those large inflatable things), or specially made half-circles. Figure 16-6 shows this using one of these half-circles. This position can be a nice relief from all the bending forward you do all day.

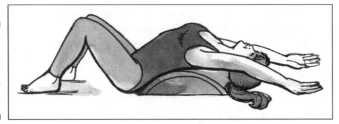

Figure 16-6:
Lying
Backward
over
Something.

When you first try something like this, make sure that the back bend is very minimal.

1. **Sit at the base of whatever object you're using.**

2. **Release yourself backward slowly, using your hands on the floor for support of your back and torso as you lie backward.**

3. **Let your head relax backward and your arms lie at your side or dangle down slightly as gravity pulls them.**

4. **Relax and breathe.**

I have two bright red inflatable exercise balls. Sometimes in the evening, I lie over one with my face down, breathe into my back and let it relax, then I lie face up to get an additional release, stretch, and calming moment.

Advanced Upside-Down Technique

In the advanced techniques you can find the full gamut of headstands and other bridges, none of which I go into. I do explain how to use an inversion table.

This tilting table looks something like a sleeping cot tipped up so it stands vertically. You back yourself up to it and slip your head between a couple of rests and your feet between two holds that keep you from sliding over on your head when you go upside down. Figure 16-7 shows a person on one of these tables.

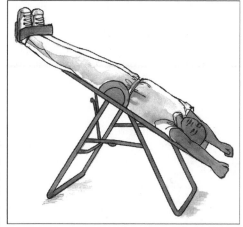

Figure 16-7:
Someone on
a tilting
table.

Then, lift your arms up toward the ceiling and let their weight tip the finely balanced table. If you let them go all the way over your head, you can hang nearly all the way upside down. Or you can stop yourself part way and just hang out there. Pretty simple stuff.

Check out the Appendix for resources, look in the yellow pages for back-care stores, or search the Web for other information on these tables.

Introducing a Few More Modern Classics

The methods in the previous sections aren't the only ones out there. In this section, I present a few others that can fit into your exploration of the mind-body methods. These methods date back to 10 decades or more, although a couple of these can perhaps be considered Early Classics instead of Modern Classics.

Getting into Ethnic Dance

Dance born in Africa or the South Pacific often involves low-intensity movement, distinct breathing, focus, and even a meditative aspect. Try these ethnic dances to round out your mind-body exploration.

Capoiera

Perhaps the most well-known of ethnic dance among fitness aficionados, Capoiera was developed by Brazilian slaves in the 1500s out of a need. What was that need? Their owners forbade practice of any martial arts, so the Afro-Brazilian slaves came up with this form that disguised the martial techniques. It is a pulsating dance-like movement with acrobatic moves even for more advanced dancers. Capoiera combines the movement with music, drums, and song. Dancers usually switch off with each other between dancing in the middle of a circle and playing drums on the side.

Afro-Haitian dance

Whatever the form, there is often a similar thread of movement, breath, and beat — all of which can lead to wonderful mind-body awareness. Sometimes finding these forms is a trick. Try private dance studios, community colleges, and adult education centers.

Walking Meditation

I discuss Qigong walking in Chapter 11. But Walking Meditation — practiced by many cultures for centuries — doesn't have to be anything in particular except:

- ✔ Walking without a goal of arriving anywhere
- ✔ Walking without any special effort to increase heart rate
- ✔ Walking with a focus on how your body feels
- ✔ Walking with a mindful effort to breathe deeply and fully

During walking meditation, focus as you do during a sitting or standing meditation — avoid planning your next vacation, or thinking about yesterday's discussion with a friend. You just want to be in the present.

The Rosen Method movement

Marion Rosen (yes, it's named after her) developed her own method after studying breathwork and relaxation in the 1930s in Germany. Like Feldenkrais, Laban, and Alexander work, Rosen movements are designed to improve alignment and flexibility, increase ease of breathing, and deepen body awareness. It, too, can complement other physical exercise so you can do it better, or a healing program to help you relieve stress and increase mindfulness. It is taught worldwide by teachers trained by The Rosen Institute.

Chapter 17

Meeting the New Kids on the Mind-Body Block

*B*eing members of an innovative society, who among us is going to just stop and be happy with the tried-and-true classics? People always want to find another widget to invent or, in this case, another method to mold. Everybody has a better idea, it seems, not just big car companies. In the following methods, it just took one person taking the time to feel how his or her body liked to move and what his or her body needed to feel good and to be healthier for the proverbial light bulb to go on: Ah-ha! So, from such inauspicious beginnings come all of these new kids on the mind-body block whose founders are taking their methods to the masses.

Interestingly, many of these forms incorporate some of the essence of the classics — both Early and Modern — such as Pilates, Yoga, Tai Chi Chuan, and Feldenkrais. Then they apply a new idea, or a different way of moving the body to make their method individual. Or the founders just link together and mix up bits and pieces of several classic methods all together. Voilà! A new exercise is born.

The following types of fitness and exercises are all great ideas, although be forewarned that not every one is for everybody. I may think Body Rolling is the cat's meow; you may think it's silly playing with a ball. I may think NIA is a fun way to reconnect with my spiritual side while getting a great workout; you may feel downright goofy dancing around like that. I may love the way the aromatherapy of a Chi Ball lights up my senses; you may consider the smell an assault on your nostrils. And what about all the others that exist in water, on land, with new machines that I introduce only in concept? I may find getting wet, or twisting in that new way odd, but you may love the concept and want to find out more. Such is the delight of these contemporary methods — there is something for everybody.

These aren't the only ones out there, either. More are coming along everyday as exercise and health professionals begin to think outside the box and explore other ways to work out. These just happen to be spreading more widely now.

What's really cool about many of these New Kids on the block is their playful nature. Many of the classic methods took themselves awfully seriously, which is just fine since they served their mind-body workout purpose well, and still do. But there is something to be said for being allowed, for example, to roll around on the floor on a ball, don't you think? Especially if it's a bright red ball.

Rolling Around with Body Rolling

Yamuna Zake (pronounced *yah-mah-nah* <u>*zah*</u>*-kay*) is a woman whose name alone is enough to make you want to try her method. She'll throw you on the floor in a second, hand you what looks like a kid's rubber ball, and next thing you know, you're sitting on it, then rolling your body around on it. And you're really glad no one is watching.

But leading you through the essence of her routine isn't enough for Yamuna. She doesn't believe in just *fixing* you, which simply makes you reliant on her. She wants to *educate* you about her technique so that you can do it on your own, any time, any place, and feel better any time you need it.

Body Rolling takes a softer approach to exercise, so anybody can do at least some part of it. But this isn't just for wimps. A good, smart session really uses your muscles, too!

Playing ball: Body Rolling basics

You may think that you're moving through the world just fine. But you may actually be moving in a way that isn't best for your body. Many of us are moving unhealthily, Yamuna Zake believes, and because the body is an intelligent thing, it may be fighting with you. It has an inner memory. It knows what's right — if you only give it the freedom and space to do it. (Can you hear it yelling at you now to sit up straight?) With the right information, it can actually heal itself. With healing, you move and feel better in any exercise or in day-to-day life.

Whoa! My body is fighting with me? Heavy stuff. Body Rolling, if you do it correctly and safely, helps your neuromuscular system (you can call it the nerves and muscles) and your skeletal system (your bones, of course) move together in the way they are supposed to. At least that's what Yamuna Zake found in the last decade or so that she's been working with the ball and seen the relief her clients have found.

Body Rolling uses a 6- to 10-inch specially designed thick rubber ball. When she first started, Zake tried using regular kid's balls from the corner department store, but a few blow-outs showed her they weren't necessarily strong enough to hold up under 200 to 300 pounds of either a really muscle-bound guy or someone who was overweight. Now that's a blow to the self-esteem, to try an exercise and have the ball explode under you!

The ball works as sort of a self-massage as you sit on it, lean on it, press against it, or hold it. To take that concept of massage a step farther, the pressing even acts like a bit of self-acupressure, since the method targets the ball onto some very distinct points on the body that can release pain or tension if pressed. (*Acupressure* is sort of a kinder, less intimidating version of the ancient Chinese medical treatment called *acupuncture* that uses needles in different points of your body to release pain or disease. Acupressure uses pressure by the fingers or an object on the same points.) Some of these points are mid-muscle, but some are aimed specifically at the muscle attachments, either at one end or the other, where the muscle becomes tendon and attaches to the bone.

Massage therapists have found that working the ends of a muscle often releases the entire muscle. Have you ever used that theory when you suddenly got a cramp in the middle of the night and leaped out of bed hopping and dancing and grabbing at your calf? Don't massage the cramp mid-muscle, but instead rub the ends of the muscle; then that bulging, lumpy cramp smack in the center of your calf should relax. Ball Rolling uses that theory again, this time in a modern-day, mind-body method.

Yamuna Zake also tries to get you to tune in to your body, and to stop and sense what is tight, what is off-kilter, or what is relaxed. Feel what's wrong, she says, and you'll eventually be able to feel what's right. Learn to breathe into that area — or even just to breathe more deeply and fully — and you'll feel better.

Rolling out the benefits

Rolling's benefits come directly from the philosophy of muscle release that says if you relax and unclench your muscles, everything simply works better. Body Rolling's philosophy then, according to Yamuna Zake, may be in part scientifically unproved, but states after practicing the method you can:

✔ Create space between your bones and vertebra by allowing the muscles to release, which can eliminate compression. Less compression can equal less pain.

✔ Give muscles length, which can eliminate tension. And we all carry way too much tension in all of our muscles.

✔ Stimulate the bone, which can create more blood flow and bone growth. Bone stimulation may help counter the thinning of bones, called osteoporosis.

✔ Learn to move every joint in its full range of possible movement, rather than cramping its style after sitting or standing a certain way all day.

The first time I got on the ball I felt a little weird. The next day — and I am not kidding — I couldn't wait to do it again. I felt longer, more relaxed, massaged, looser and freed in my spine, and ready to tackle the day, or maybe even a long run or other hard workout.

And what about the mind-body connection? No, you won't get all spiritual with this workout, but it teaches you to tune your mind into your body and, as we said earlier in this section, not to disconnect the two parts. If you connect, you may be present and feel what that smart body is asking you to do or not to do.

Doing Body Rolling

You can do most mind-body methods either as a full routine all on their own, as a warm-up or cooldown in another program, or as one of many parts of another routine, which is also where Body Rolling fits into your program.

Try Body Rolling for many purposes — both to remedy certain ills or and to add something different to your exercise. You can use Body Rolling:

✔ **If you are less fit:** With Body Rolling, you can teach your body better alignment, more relaxation, and a mental connection, which may be the first step to exercising safely and staying uninjured in more aerobic workouts.

✔ **If you cross-train:** Body Rolling can be a cross-training tool on off days from different workouts that are more aerobic.

If you're recovering from an injury: Body Rolling can help with your rehabilitation or help you learn how to move in such a way as to avoid further injury, assuming your physician says this kind of activity is okay.

✔ **If you don't want or like impact:** Body Rolling is an impact-free way to use your body.

✔ **If you don't like trends:** Does the hip fashion scene or keep-up-with-the-Joneses aura at health clubs turn you off? Rolling needs no big iron dumbbells, sweaty weight rooms, or trendy clubs.

✔ **If you are more fit:** The uses of Body Rolling get broader when you're fit. You may use it as a warm-up, a cooldown, a way to stay stretched out, a way to stay uninjured, or as a complete secondary workout on a hard workout day. You may also pick out one or two movements and do them only on certain days — for example if your hamstrings are particularly tight.

Rolling out your equipment

Body Rolling does need a specific ball. For starters, you could try the exercises using a kid's rubber ball rather than the specific Body Rolling ball I mentioned earlier in this section. But the kid's dime-store ball may not support you (beware of the blow-out factor), and may not be able to hold enough air pressure to get the results you want. Still, there's certainly no harm in trying so you can figure out if you like this!

If you want to try some foot massages in the Body Rolling way, you could use a racquet ball instead of the little pink Body Rolling balls, but racquet balls may be just a little too hard to be comfortable for everybody.

Oh, you may likely want to wear tight clothing since the ball can catch and pull on loose clothing as you move it along your body. You don't want to have to stop and re-adjust. The ball rolls well on skin, too, so shorts (and a sports bra for women) may work well, also.

Other than the ball, though, you don't need any special mats or other gadgets. Just a small space on the floor, and you're ready to roll. Literally.

I tell you more about equipment in Chapter 3 — small stuff, big stuff, and other stuff that may come in handy in general for mind-body routines. And, you can take a look in the Appendix under Body Rolling to find out more information about books and other specialized information.

Trying some rolling routines

I introduce two exercises for the body — one for the upper body and one for the lower — plus another exercise for your feet. These are three basic Body Rolling moves that come illustrated and with instructions on a sheet of paper when you buy the ball itself for a simple introduction.

Remember, if you have any injuries, diseases, or any back, neck, or other orthopedic problems, or are pregnant, you should always consult a physician before trying these movements.

Ready to rock . . . and roll?

Up Each Side of the Spine

Your spine is of course a major conduit — this exercise, as shown in Figure 17-1, is a low-impact way to help keep things loose and flowing.

1. **Start by sitting on the ball on the floor and placing it at the tip of your coccyx between the two sitzbones.**

The *coccyx* is what most of us call our tailbone. It's the slightly bony piece at the base of your spine. It's bonier or more prominent in some people and if you're one of them, take special care. The *sitzbones* are actually the *ischial tuberosities,* those slightly bony prominences on the base of your pelvis that bear your weight when you sit down. A lot of muscles attach there — like the hamstrings — which is why massage therapists may work on that area. Remember that working the attachments of a muscle helps to release it.

Just sitting on the ball may be an interesting trick. You can just stay on the ball for awhile and get used to it, sitting tall, but kinda rolling your buttocks back and forth, or 'round and 'round.

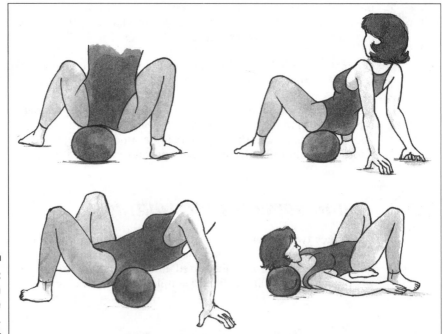

Figure 17-1:
Up Each
Side of the
Spine.

2. **After you're used to sitting on the ball itself, roll your left hip slightly off the ball so that the ball is below your right sitzbone only.**

3. **Place both hands on the floor behind you for balance, and gently curl your pelvis and tailbone upward.**

4. **Slowly begin rolling the ball up the right side of your spine, starting at the coccyx, moving to the *sacrum* (just above the coccyx where you feel sort of a flat spot at the base of your spine), then along the out-side of the *vertebral spine* (the bony prominences on the spine).**

   You kind of walk with your feet as you begin to lie backward.

   Do not actually roll the ball on these bony prominences, but along the muscles and other soft tissue just alongside them.

5. **Move very slowly, only about an inch at a time. Then stop at each place and take a deep breath. Inhale so you feel the inhalation expand out against the ball. Then exhale very deeply and fully. Try to feel the breath going to the place where the ball rests. Try to sense it sinking into that muscle on the exhalation.**

   If you were with Yamuna Zake, she'd say, "Now sink, . . . and sink, . . . and sink, . . . and sink, . . ." So do just that at each stop!

6. **Trace the ball all the way up the spine, breathing and sinking along the way for 1–3 long, deep breaths at each stop.**

   If your neck begins to feel uncomfortable from the weight of your head, use one hand to support it rather than holding it up tensely or letting it hang down.

7. **After you are comfortable with rolling up the *lumbar* (the low back) and *thoracic spine* (mid-back), you can take it up to the *cervical spine* (the neck area), as long as you don't have any neck problems.**

8. **After the ball moves into the lower part of the neck, work more on relaxing and elongating your entire neck.**

   Allow your neck to be supported by the ball as you relax your upper body, shoulders, and arms downward as if they were wrapping down around the ball. Keep your back and buttocks off the ground, however, for better ball control by using your feet on the floor as if you were cre-ating a mini-bridge.

   If you have long hair, you may want to tie it up on top of your head so it doesn't get caught under the ball and yank at your roots. It hurts. Take my word for it.

9. **Try to lower your shoulders to the floor, releasing the tension. Move the ball slightly up the neck and into the lower part of the skull.**

   The lower part of the skull is another key place where people hold stress. Have you ever had a massage therapist or friend put his or her fingers at the base of your skull and massage or even just press? You want to melt into their hands it feels so good. And so does the ball pressure here!

   Be sure to also relax the jaw and eyes.

   You may want to support or hold the ball with one hand as it moves toward your head to keep it from popping out abruptly.

10. **Support the back of the head and neck with one hand, while the other hand slowly removes the ball. Lower your head to the floor.**

11. **Take a couple of deep breaths and connect with how your body feels.**

12. **Oh, and now repeat the whole thing on your other side!**

Basic Hamstring Rolling

If you have a desk job, you may experience a lot of tightness in your *hamstrings,* which is the group of three muscles that go up the back of your upper leg, because of all the sitting you do all day long. If you are active, you may have pulled this muscle in the past. Because the hamstrings are so tight in many people, it's a common place for a muscle strain to occur.

Follow these steps to try Basic Hamstring Rolling.

1. **Start by sitting on the ball on one sitzbone (see the "Up Each Side of the Spine" exercise earlier in this chapter to clarify the location). Use your fingertips on the floor beside you for a bit of balance and support.**

2. **Roll the ball around on the sitzbone to begin to massage some of the hamstring attachments that are in that area.**

3. **Sit tall, feeling as if you are lengthening the spine. Then slowly start rolling the ball down the back of the leg. And I do mean slowly.**

   Use the breath — both the full inhalations and exhalations — to feel the ball and connect with your body to release the tension and separate the tissues (see the exercise, "Up Each Side of the Spine," earlier in this section).

4. **Stop about three or four times between your sitzbone and your knee. At each point, breathe and "sink, . . . sink, . . . sink, . . . sink, . . ."**

   Do not stop with the ball directly behind your knee because that puts pressure on the knee joint.

5. **At each point where you stop, roll side-to-side slowly with the ball to release the trio of hamstring muscles.**

6. **After you reach your last spot just above the knee joint, roll back up to the sitzbone.**

7. **Finish by leaning your weight over to the opposite hip and releasing the ball into the same hand as the hip resting on the ball. Lower yourself to the floor.**

   Take a minute to stand up, shake out your legs, and walk around the room, before doing the same thing all over again on the opposite side.

Pinky Ball Foot Rolling

Massaging a little ball around under your foot may sound simple, but you'll find that it isn't so simple! It's amazing how much tension our feet put up with, especially when most of us wear shoes that are too small, or we pound them during exercise and never pamper them.

Whenever I get a massage, I'm surprised how many times I say "ouch" even to the lightest touch at the start. Using the Pinky Ball can release some of that tension so that your feet are ready to succumb to the benefits of rolling or any other mind-body exercise.

1. **Start standing, preferably next to a wall, desk, or something else that you can rest one hand on for balance and support.**

2. **Place the ball on the ground, then place one heel directly on top of the ball. Now — get ready — let all of your weight, or as much as you can stand, relax down into the ball. And wait. (or, should I say, sink, and . . .)**

   Be sure to keep you arch and ankle lifted upward and not collapsing.

3. **Roll the ball around to contact all the points on the bottom of the heel, making sure your body weight is still sinking into the ball.**

4. **Roll the ball from your heel bone into your arch. Wait. And sink. Place as much body weight on it as you can. Relax your jaw! And breathe.**

5. **Shift your weight so that the ball moves to the outside of your arch. And wait.**

6. **Now shift your weight so the ball moves to the inside area and hold that position. Still sinking.**

7. **Move the ball forward on the foot a bit toward your toes, and repeat the same pattern shifting one way, then the other. Work your way down the foot that way.**

   You may find three or four spots to stop and move the ball back and forth as you progress along the foot — more if you want to take more time.

   You can also use the ball to roll around under your toes and into the toes for an additional massage.

Feel all rolled out?

You could be happy just doing the three exercises in this section for a while, but you may get hooked and want more, either for an entire workout, or as part of another workout.

Integrating NIA

The first thing to discover about **N**euromuscular **I**ntegrative **A**ction (see where the NIA comes from?) is how to pronounce it. Try _knee-ah_. That's it. You got it. This is the only time I use this rather lengthy and esoteric name. Now, I want you to just forget it — nobody uses it anyway.

The developers of this method, Debbie and Carlos Rosas, came up with this nifty tongue-twister to explain the principles of NIA, which they began nurturing in the early 1980s. NIA attempts to help participants combine (that's the "integrated" part) their minds and the mind's tie with the nerves. (that's both the "neuro" and "muscular" parts) in a moving dance (the "action" part). Dancing and moving.

NIA didn't always mean Neuromuscular Integrative Action, though. When the twosome began working together, the acronym meant, simply enough, _non-impact aerobics_, which was useful because the early 1980s were, of course, the beginning of the group-exercise era. That was enough at that time to mean a softer, gentler approach to fitness — a movement without impact that would bring results without pain and stress.

But as the Rosas duo developed the form, it took on more depth and more flow.

Getting to know NIA

The Rosases move beyond physical directives such as "move your right foot to the right." Instead, they try to nurture purpose, feeling, passion, uniqueness, and even an electricity and connection with the fluid movement method.

Nia in Swahili means "with purpose." That alone sums it up a bit. And that's why NIA is a mind-body method.

Interestingly, as with many new kids on the mind-body block, NIA has tastes of many other mind-body methods from both Eastern and Western cultures that you read about in this book. If you look closely, you can recognize touches of Yoga, Tai Chi, Qigong, Alexander, Feldenkrais, and many other forms, too, all steeped in a base of jazz and modern dance.

Finding a purpose with NIA

Aside from all of the basic benefits shared by most mind-body methods (see Chapter 2) that include aerobic fitness, strength flexibility, spinal alignment, balance, inner calm, and the like, NIA has its own list of what it calls *awareness ingredients* that are a part of how you benefit from it.

The awareness ingredients of NIA include:

- **Rooting yourself:** Connecting your physical body and your energy to the ground through your feet.

  The foundation of NIA movement teaches you to be "fully in your feet." That means stepping rhythmically and working with gravity, not against it, and allowing yourself to feel the ground with every inch of the soles of your feet, rather than just floating above them.

- **Balancing:** Recognizing the polarity of opposing movements such as open-closed, in-out, tight-loose, and using it to your advantage.

- **Centering:** Using the body weight evenly over your feet to encourage balance of body and mind.

- **Developing awareness:** Perceiving movements with all of the senses and connecting with the flow of energy that comes from the awareness.

- **Finding intention:** Knowing what you want from a movement and getting it.

- **Focusing:** Being conscious of every body part through a concentrated focus on what a limb is doing.

- **Softening:** Replacing effort and tension with ease and relaxation.

- **Using energy:** Using and feeling the energy channels so they fill with energy, called *chi*. Refer to Chapter 4 for more information about chi and the energy channels.

Oh, and NIA offers one more thing — individuality of movement. In most workouts and methods — most all Western ones and even some mind-body and Eastern ones — you are told exactly what to do and all students mimic an instructor or illustration. NIA encourages you to experiment with different arm and leg movements, different speeds of gliding around a room, and different music so you can discover what feels right to your body. In a NIA class, the teacher almost always incorporates a section where she or he encourages the students to just move however they want to for a few minutes so the room becomes a free-for-all of flowing bodies.

My first NIA experience

In the mid-1980s, I took a NIA class from Debbie and Carlos personally. The class was in a small, very stuffy room in a convention center at a conference for fitness professionals. The room was small — that was the era when most teachers only cared about how hard a class was or how many high kicks they could do. Not many of us were drawn to that strange-sounding name, NIA. Although that class was one in many, many classes I have taken over the years, it touched me profoundly. Both Debbie and Carlos ooze a passion, warmth, and spirit that infects you as the rhythms of their movement engulf you. Debbie gracefully slides from one pattern to the next; Carlos, in his delightful Latin American accent, coaches and cajoles you to breathe and feel as you let your body go while staying grounded. Their passion and belief for this method of exercise has driven them over the years to stick with it, even when many students originally turned away, because it wasn't the intensely impactful aerobics that other instructors taught. Today, their belief in NIA has taken hold. Hundreds of teachers in the United States, Mexico, Canada, and Europe now teach NIA in clubs and spas, as well as in hospitals and prisons.

The caution here, of course, is that if you aren't really comfortable "doing your own thing," or "letting it all hang out," this can feel a little odd.

You can also take the offering of spirituality in NIA to whatever level you choose. You can, for example, just treat a NIA class as a nice, flowing, connected dance-like workout. You can also go deeper into using the moves as almost a prayer-like offering of spirit and a way to seek clarity in your life.

Truly experiencing the advanced and more spiritual levels of NIA from a printed page is difficult, so I encourage you to try the introductory movements I present and to try to apply the "awareness ingredients" I talk about earlier in this chapter. If you want to learn more, area classes and videos are the way to go. Refer to the NIA Web site listed in the Appendix for resources, classes, videos, and a directory of teachers around the world.

Deciding on NIA

You can pick and choose from all of the methods I present throughout this book and put them together in a way that best suits your needs, be it for strength, weight loss, or even athletic performance. NIA is a very distinct method, however, that demands some interest in free-flowing, dance-like, circular movements, rather than the linear moves of running or traditional dance aerobics. NIA at least requires a willingness, or a desire, to try to just let your body go. If nothing else, try not to be self-conscious, or find a room where you can close the door if you are!

The NIA method also relies heavily on imagery. So if you really are a left-brained person who likes spreadsheets and detailed 1-2-3 instruction in black-and-white, you may feel a little uncomfortable with being told to "feel like a kite" or "to let the skin on your leg melt like candle wax over your bones into the earth." But that's the beauty of these mind-body methods, which even have huge differences in characteristics, methods, and goals among them.

More practically speaking, NIA movements can serve:

- As an active warm-up before more stretching and stationary postures.

- As the aerobic section of a session to get your heart rate pumping a little bit.

- As the freely moving or releasing part of a session after you have perhaps been more controlled in what you do with other types of analytical exercises.

- As a short interlude in a day to just dance around a little bit to some favorite music.

Were you one of those kids who played imaginary games, or who put on music and just jiggled around the room? Were you a teenager who liked free-style dance rather than choreographed partner dance? If you were, you may really enjoy NIA.

No equipment required

You don't really need any stuff to do NIA.

The only thing you really need for NIA is music. That's it. Just music. And really, whatever moves you best, not anything in particular (although there are special NIA music CDs). But remember not to make music a crutch. With NIA, music is just a way to learn to listen to and play with your personal rhythms, the ones that are inside of you day in and day out.

You can also wear whatever you want, as long as you're comfortable and your movement isn't inhibited. Some people's tastes here lean toward snug clothing, like dance leotards. Others want baggy and loose, like martial arts pants.

Doesn't really matter with NIA. Whatever floats your boat — that's the beauty.

Finding your NIA moves

Because NIA is so free-flowing, basically, anything goes. In this section I roll out some guidelines for experimenting a bit, then introduce two ways to move your feet, and a handful of movements you can dabble at in your living room. Remember, the individual beauty of this: Even though I'm introducing you to only a handful of moves, when you vary their direction or flavor, or combine them with each other in different ways, you'll actually have dozens of moves!

Steps to NIA-ism

You don't try to build an entire house for your first carpentry project, but construct small pieces — a deck, one room, a roof, a door, and such — until you have enough to put together the house. Same with NIA!

✔ **Bit by bit:** Tear apart the movement and do one piece at a time, in isolation. Repeat it until it feels comfortable. Forget about what the rest of your body is doing while you practice that one itty-bitty chunk. Once you get each piece separately, trying linking them together for a short sequence.

✔ **Go short:** Use a workout session to practice one sequence, repeating it over and over, adding new flavors or directions as you are moved to do. Keep it short, maybe just five minutes at first.

✔ **Link 'em:** After you have the pieces, and put them together, and you've gone short, it's time to try to go longer by linking together different movements. Shoot for 15 minutes at first, then add a few minutes at a time.

You can actually do short NIA interludes of three to four minutes during the day. Are you walking to the post office? Try the footwork. Are you vacuuming? Make it flow and dance. Are you driving in your car? Just feel your body moving to the rhythm (just don't take off your seat belt or get up on the seat — you don't want to have to explain: "But, officer . . .").

Fancy footwork

Bet you don't really think about how your feet are moving when you just stroll around. Experiment with these two ways to plant your feet, then add them to the moves to come (or moves in other methods even), playing with each way, or both ways, to see how planting your feet affects the movement.

With these exercises, lower your center by bending your knees slightly and let them feel springy as you move. This method strengthens your feet, ankles, and lower legs, which gives you better balance and helps your strength in other activities.

Heel Lead

You focus on your heel and allow it to lead your entire foot and body into a step when you do this.

1. **Step out with your toes lifted so that you land heel first with each step.**

   Try moving sideways or forward.

   Try keeping your weight over your supporting leg as you move.

   Try moving your body and its weight with your moving leg.

2. **Roll down with your forefoot and as that foot is fully in contact with the ground, let the other foot release from the ground behind you and plant in front of you with the heel leading.**

Whatever way you do it, stay grounded and feel your feet fully roll along the ground. Use the ground to move yourself, pushing with your feet with each step.

Whole Foot Lead

In this exercise, you focus on your entire foot leading you forward into the step.

1. **Step out with your entire foot, but not with either your heel or your ball.**

   Feel your entire foot, both the inside and outside edges, plant into the ground.

   Try shifting your weight from one foot's edge to the other to sense the ground under your feet.

2. **As one foot is fully in contact with the ground, let the other foot release from the ground behind you and plant it in front of you, stepping with your entire foot.**

Try applying this sensation of the entire foot to other activities, too, such as running or step aerobics.

The ups and downs

Here I present another two ingredients to try alone or use in combination with some *traveling sequences* — a series of steps that move you across the floor in some way or some direction. Your goal, again, is to feel the earth and to use your feet against it, as well as to feel the earth's energy moving upward through you and strongly in your legs. You can strengthen and tone your legs and hips, as well as teach your body better balance with this kind of focus and work.

Sink Step

The Sink Step is a basic NIA move. Figure 17-2 shows both the Sink Step and the Rise Step, which follows this one. Both need to be part of a sequence, or you can simply do the one step, return to a center position and repeat it.

1. **Start with your feet in a narrow stance. Inhale, then exhale, and step into a wide stance leading with your right foot.**

2. **Bend your knees so that you sink into a squat that is as deep as comfortable.**

   To protect you knees, don't bend them more than 90 degrees or farther than a right angle.

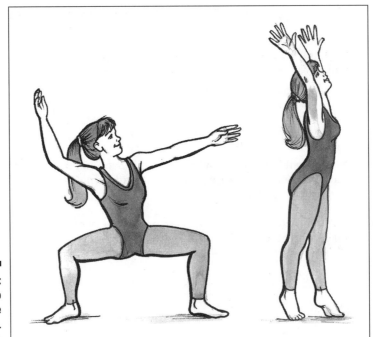

Figure 17-2:
Sink Step
and Rise
Step.

3. **Step back into a narrow stance.**

4. **Step out on your left side into a wide stance to repeat this on the other side.**

Although I haven't mentioned arms, feel free to add a few movements after you have the stepping-sinking motion down. For example, as you step out, you can spread your arms wide, reach them upward, push them down, or move one arm one way and the other arm the other way.

Rise Step

Just as you may suspect, the Rise Step is the opposite of the Sink Step (see the preceding section, "Sink Step," and Figure 17-2).

1. **Start with your feet in a wide stance.**

2. **Inhale, then exhale, and step into a narrow stance bringing your right foot in. This time, push into the ground and lift your body's energy straight up to work against gravity, straightening both knees to reach your body tall toward the ceiling.**

3. **Return to a wide stance, sinking low again.**

4. **Step back in with the left foot to a narrow stance to try the move on the opposite side.**

You can raise both arms and look up as you rise up, or you can drop them both and look down. Try different variations.

Pivot and Sink Stance

This takes the basic moves of stepping out and back, and adds a little turn with the body. See Figure 17-3.

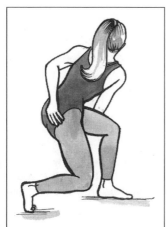

Figure 17-3:
Pivot and
Sink Stance.

1. **Stand with your feet in a wide stance, slightly larger than hip-width apart.**

2. **Shift your weight slightly forward onto the balls of your feet.**

3. **Pivot on the balls of your feet to the right.**

4. **Sink toward the ground bending both knees.**

5. **Unwind yourself back to a standing wide position, facing forward.**

6. **Pivot and sink to the left side.**

Wanna try some arms? Push out to the side with both, or try wrapping them around your waist with the arm to the side that you're turning going behind you and the opposite arm wrapping to the front.

Be sure to keep your abdominals tight and your torso upright to protect your back. You can also place your hands on your thighs to support your torso as you sink. You can take a few steps in between alternating sides to see how some movement feels, too.

I'm a traveling (wo)man

With both the footwork and the sinking and rising motions, you're mostly stationary. Now I show you a couple of NIA movements that move you across the floor. Depending on your space, you can keep the steps small, or you can really reach out with your feet and legs and move farther. You can also link together the sinking and crossing steps, as well as the pivot steps, to the end of this simple traveling move.

The larger the space you cover, the higher your heart rate goes up, and the more aerobically intense the movement becomes.

Travel 1-2-3

The Travel 1-2-3 actually has a "4" with this move, but the four is whichever movement you want to tack on to it. So it's 1-2-3-foot touch, 1-2-3-knee lift, 1-2-3 sink, or 1-2-3-kick, for example. You can cover lots of territory to really heat yourself up, or you can keep it tiny for a less intense movement.

Try the move first without a tacked-on ending by just walking forward and touching your toe to the ground.

1. **Start by standing with both feet together. Step forward with your right foot, then your left foot, then your right foot, then just touch the floor with the left foot. Don't put your weight on that left toe, just touch the**

ground lightly, so that you're ready to reverse the step going backward.

2. **Because your left foot doesn't have any weight on it, you are ready to start moving backwards on it: Step backward with your left foot, then your right foot, then your left foot, then just touch the floor with the right foot. Just like in Step 1, above, don't put any weight on your right foot.**

Continue this step forward and backward with the simple touch, smoothing out the rhythm.

3. **Continue the forward and backward walking, but instead of a touch step, lift your knee. So you step forward with your right, then left, then right, then lift your left knee. That leaves that foot free to start the same progression moving backward.**

4. **Lower your left knee and step backward with that foot, then step backward with your right, your left, then your right.**

5. **Repeat as desired. You can also move the pattern side-to-side instead of just front-to-back.**

Other variations you can try: *Sink* on the 4th step, either straight forward, to the side, or crossed-over. *Rise* on the 4th step, also in any direction. Try a *kick* with that 4th foot, either to the side or forward. If you get really daring, you can also try a *pivot-and-sink* on the 4th step, turning out toward the leg that took the 3rd step.

Just with these few feet, body shift, and traveling moves, you could keep yourself busy for a long time, especially once you add arms in different ways, experiment with different musical rhythms, different speeds, or varying degrees of space covered.

Choosing the Chi Ball Method

Take a Texas grapefruit-sized rubber ball that smells nice. Mix it with the essence of Yoga, Tai Chi, Qigong, Pilates, the Feldenkrais Method, aerobic dance, and the best of both Eastern and Western exercise philosophies. That's the Chi Ball Method. *Chi* means "energy" or "basic life force." Refer to Chapter 4 for more information about chi. Yes, this chi is the same chi you tap into with Tai Chi Chuan and the same qi (or chi) you try to move in Qigong. But this time you have a colored ball in your hand wafting various aromatherapy scents.

How did such a thing come about? From a bad experience in life that was turned around into a good thing. Chi Ball developer Monica Linford was the epitome of an aerobic-dance enthusiast — a long-time master instructor who bopped between Australia (her original home) and England (her second home). She crammed life full, never stopping to take a vacation, and laughing at people who said she needed to slow down and rest a little now and then.

Frequent bouts of colds and flu didn't stop her. She often pushed herself through high-energy classes, then didn't have an ounce left for herself. I tell her story briefly in Chapter 6. Long story short, it all began to catch up with her in 1991 when a shooting pain up her right side left the doctors thinking she'd had a stroke. All the tests came out negative. In 1992, she was diagnosed with chronic fatigue syndrome. She closed her business and went home to Australia to try to get well and figure out life and her future.

And figure it out she did. Chinese medicine helped her recognize a drain from her system's energy that she began, little by little, to replenish by doing non-strenuous Qigong and Yoga. It was the prescription for meditation that at first did her in. Sit still for 10 minutes? You've got to be kidding?! "It was torture," she wrote in her book *Awaken Your Body, Balance Your Mind*. (Refer to the Appendix for information about the book.) "All the emotions I had denied feeling or expressing came bubbling up."

But it started healing her health. It took three years, but she says she learned to be aware of her emotions and control them, facing the day with calm, not stress. "The key to my recovery," she wrote, "was to allow these feelings space for expression."

As a longtime fitness professional, she didn't just keep her discoveries to herself. Out of the ashes a Phoenix was born — a gentle mind-body method she called Chi Ball because it combines the best of what she learned, uses a ball, and tries to help participants tap into their chi. She now teaches it — and trains teachers to teach it — in several countries.

And she makes sure she takes a rest whenever she needs to.

Divining the purpose of Chi Ball

Feel good. That's founder Monica Linford's philosophy in two words: Feel good.

Isn't that what we all want? Fitness should feel good. Fitness should bring peace, contentment and happiness. But, does it? Not always, because so many of us start fitness because of fear, not fun — fear of not losing weight, fear of a high blood pressure, fear of not looking as good in jeans. Just fear. Plus, fitness has become too much like work, instead of a pleasurable game that we want to "go and play" more often. Linford's theory is that many people still think a workout should hurt and leave you feeling drained.

Wrong, she says. You should finish your workout feeling uplifted both physically and emotionally. That's why it's so vital that the routine you choose incorporate both mind and body. The unfortunate thing is, most people have no idea how stressed they really are, or how much it is affecting their overall health, happiness, and inner being.

The purpose then of the Chi Ball Method is to let each person develop his or her own sense of well-being, balance, and self-awareness. That can lead to a more satisfying, well-rounded way of life. Oh, and you'll enjoy the movement too as it helps you along a path to complete fitness.

Benefiting from Chi Ball

Fitness, meditation, relaxation, energy release, stretching, release of your back muscles and tension — all can be benefits because the Chi Ball program mixes up, well, all kinds of things. That leaves you to choose the flavor you want to get what you're looking for.

The method aims to be a holistic approach to exercise, with five major components, each fulfilling a different need. As usual, none of this in this combination has been proven by those researchers out there. What else is new?

- ✔ **Energy flow, internal health and balance:** This comes from its mix of moves and concepts from traditional Chinese medicine and healing arts, such as Tai Chi and Qigong. It is called *energize and tone* in Chi Ball.

- ✔ **Strength, flexibility, and physical balance:** As compared to internal balance of spirit and energy, this comes primarily from its dash of Yoga postures.

- ✔ **Core stability and control:** This part comes from the Pilates-inspired movements mixed in to the routine.

- ✔ **Relaxation and tension-free movement:** Feldenkrais techniques, which I cover in chapter 16, are a part of Chi Ball to bring you these benefits.

- ✔ **Deep relaxation and well-being:** This comes from visualizations and meditations, as well as its emphasis on full and deep breathing.

These benefits come from Chinese mind-body and healing arts:

✔ **Balance:** Monica Linford intends a class to flow rhythmically so you move from yin, or soft movements and use of inner energy, to yang, or more active and expressive movements. Using both types of inner energy, or chi, balances you in both body and mind, she says.

✔ **Inner energy:** Using both breathing techniques and muscular movements, the class tries to regulate your energy flow so it's neither too high nor too low.

✔ **Revitalization:** In Chapter 4 as well as in Part IV, I talk about the meridian system where your chi flows and how your chi can be blocked like the water in a kinked hose. The Chi Ball method attempts to get your system flowing and revitalized.

Now whether you get all of these things from trying the Chi Ball method is a different matter, of course. That depends on how you approach it, how ready you are, and if you can get the feel from these introductory movements I show you.

Getting the most from the Chi Ball Method

The interesting thing about the Chi Ball Method, as with the other New Kids I present in this chapter, is that these methods are often a mix of old and new, so almost anybody can find something they like. Plus, the new methods are couched in a format that may appeal to our modern minds more than a very early form like Qigong.

The Chi Ball Method may be for you if you want:

✔ **Simple:** The movements are not highly choreographed and may be repeated quite effectively. Beginning exercisers won't have a problem learning it.

✔ **Gentle:** It is entirely non- or very-low-impact.

✔ **Varied:** That's from that mix of methods put together.

That's not to say Chi Ball has to be low-intensity. It's your choice whether you want to keep the intensity very, very low, take it to a moderate range, or allow the movements in "yang" portions to bump the intensity up a notch.

You still do it barefoot, like many of these methods, but, heck, Monica says if you want to keep your shoes on, that's okay, too. It's a flexible and adaptable method.

I found the aromatherapy essence in the ball as I carried it back and forth, overhead, down, around my body, or side-to-side, a wonderful addition. Without the scents, the ball may seem gimmicky. With the scent, you want to keep it moving.

Finding a chi ball

Hmm, well since this is called Chi *Ball,* that does kind of imply you need the specific aromatherapy ball. I'll tell you about it in a minute. But — here's that flexibility again — if you don't have one or don't care to run out and get one right away, you can do two things:

✔ Do the movements without one. It won't feel quite the same because of the coordination of moving the ball around, having it in your hand, or smelling its scent. But you can do it.

✔ Do the movements using a bunched-up towel — perhaps a hand towel. At least then you have something in your hand. You can even apply a scent to the towel if you want.

I've selected three sampler movements that you can do either way. If you decide to try more, some movements have you lie on the ball (with it in different positions along your spine) or to sit back on it. If you don't have the right type of ball, you should probably avoid those moves. You'll see why when I describe the ball. Also, don't use a small ball like a tennis ball because you won't be able to pass it around yourself very well, and you definitely shouldn't sit or lie on such a hard object! If you have a towel bunched up, unbunch it so it's a softer shape when you lie back, or just put it aside.

Taking the ball by the horns

This simple little ball about 6 inches in diameter took three years to research and develop. That's because it had to be the right sticky texture to stay in your hand comfortably, the colors had to be altered since the fragrances changed the dyes, it had to be able to be inflated and deflated easily by participants (you may change its pressure during a class), and it had to be just the right size to safely sit or lie on it so you wouldn't put undue pressure on your spine.

Then there's these fragrances, which are based in the aromatherapy world's concept of how a smell affects your feelings and mood:

✔ The orange ball is a sweet orange scent. It is associated with happiness, joy, playfulness, and spontaneity.

✔ The yellow ball is a lemon grass scent. It is associated with self-esteem, ability, self-discipline and personal courage, and helps to clear the mind and enhances the ability to concentrate.

✔ The green ball is a geranium scent. It is associated with our capacity for compassion. It enhances emotional sensitivity to build more stability and tranquility.

✔ The purple ball is a lavender scent. It is associated with the desire for knowledge and intuition, helps release suppressed emotions, and calms the body and mind.

Other than the ball — or not — you need only a medium-sized area and perhaps a mat for any work on the floor.

Checking out Chi Ball Method movements

With flavors and tastes from so many different mind-body methods, you could actually hold a ball while doing some of the Qigong and Yoga moves that I present in other sections. Chi Ball doesn't try to be any of those, mind you, but takes a hint from each. So feel free to experiment once you try these!

Butterfly

This reflects the Tai Chi element of the method and is shown in Figure 17-4. You can use it to increase your yang (active, expressive) energy.

1. **Stand with your feet hip-width apart with an open chest and aligned spine.**

   Make sure you knees aren't locked.

2. **Hold the ball in your right hand with your arms hanging relaxed at your side.**

3. **As you inhale, raise your arms out to your sides to about shoulder level. Keep your elbows soft and rotate your palms (and the ball) upward.**

4. **Exhale, let your arms float back down to your sides.**

5. **Gently put the ball in your left hand and repeat the motion several times, alternating sides.**

Think about your breathing, which is the key aspect of this movement.

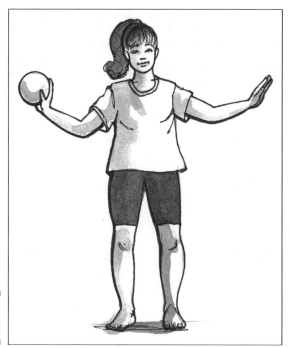

Figure 17-4:
Butterfly.

Chi Ball Triangle

This posture, shown in Figure 17-5, reflects the Yoga element of the method and stretches your hips, back and legs, as well as massaging your spine and the nerves that run through it.

For additional tips on this position, refer to the Yoga posture instructions in Chapter 9.

1. **Hold the ball in your left hand.**

2. **Stand in Tadasana or Mountain Posture (check out the Cheat Sheet at the front of this book for a reminder). Spread your feet about 3–4 feet apart, or about the length of one leg.**

3. **Turn your right foot out about 90 degrees, or so it's pointing straight out to your right side.**

4. **Turn your left foot out between 30 and 45 degrees (whatever's comfortable for you).**

5. **Lift your arms out softly to shoulder height at your sides.**

6. **Inhale, and shift your pelvis to the left as if you were trying to bump someone out of your way with your hips. Then exhale and reach your**

right arm down to the right shin. If you're comfortable you can also grab the ankle or even put your hand on the floor. You can even leave your right elbow resting on your bent right knee.

7. Reach your left arm and the ball up toward the ceiling. If it's comfortable, look up toward the ball; otherwise, look down.

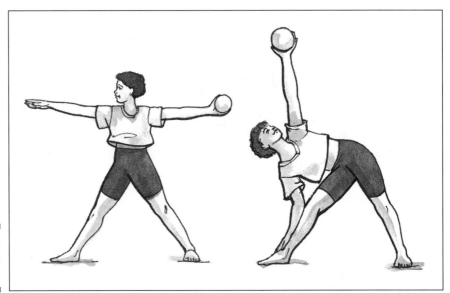

Figure 17-5:
Chi Ball
Triangle.

8. When you find the position, try to flatten your body as if you were doing the position with your heels, buttocks, and shoulders flat up against a wall behind you.

9. Hold for 3–5 breaths, then return to Tadasana by bending your front leg and lifting your torso as you also lower you arms and the ball to your sides. Be sure to lengthen your spine rather than sink into it.

10. After repeating this posture several times, do it on the other side, switching the ball into your right hand.

Spinal Twist

This reflects the Pilates-inspired element and strengthens the obliques (these muscles are part of your abs but run diagonally from your sides to your front). This may also provide some relief from an aching or stiff back if you do it gently. Figure 17-6 shows the positions.

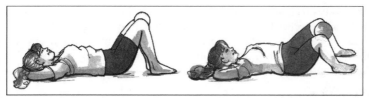

Figure 17-6:
Spinal Twist.

If you have a back problem, consult with your doctor before attempting any twisting movements.

1. **Lie down on your back with your knees bent and your feet flat on the floor about hip-width apart.**

2. **Place the ball between your knees and press gently in with your legs to keep it from escaping.**

Apply the tips on spinal alignment I discuss in the Pilates section in Chapter 14, as well as in the section on mind-body basics in Chapter 4.

3. **Place your hands behind your head, letting the weight of your head relax back into your palms and open your elbows wide.**

4. **Inhale, then as you exhale, press your left shoulder into the ground as you roll your knees (and the ball) to your right side. Your left foot lifts off the floor slightly so that your knees stay side-by-side.**

If you can't keep your shoulder on the floor, your knees are twisted too far over for your level of flexibility. Lift them a little until you can keep your shoulders down and relaxed.

5. **Inhale again, then exhale as you press your navel to your spine and use your abdominal power and the muscles in your sides (those oblique things) to return your knees to their upright position. Continue to press your left shoulder to the floor as you do this.**

6. **Repeat 6–8 times on each side, maintaining your full breath in and out.**

Avoid just yanking your buttocks back to the ground and leading with your hips since that can strain your back. Be sure to use your waist muscles to unfurl yourself to the floor.

Introducing a Few More New Kids

The neighborhood has a lot of New Kids. And there are more and more moving in everyday. That's probably because of the burgeoning interest in mind-body movement, which means a growing number of people discovering other ways to use and combine classics and ancient styles. I can't begin to name or describe them all. So I've picked a few to describe and others I just name or define — just so that if you read the name somewhere you'll recognize it. You can find information or contacts for many of these New Kids in the Appendix.

This is in no way an attempt to be a complete list since methods are being bred and born daily in clubs and facilities all over the world. Oh, and do note that most of these methods are trademarked by their developers, who teach and train others to teach.

Gyrokinesis

Juliu Horvath suffered through chronic low back pain for 25 years as a professional ballet dancer in Romania. But enough was enough after about four decades. The pain was too much, so he quit and began to look into Yoga and other mind-body movement. Through observation of how the body moves and how the mind interacts with it, he came up with a method that is sort of combines the essence of Tai Chi, Qigong, Yoga, and dance, with the fluidity required of moving through water while swimming.

The style is based on what Horvath discovered as six possible movements of the spine: forward, backward, side-to-side, spiraling (twisting like a corkscrew), circling (as if you were drawing a circle above your head), and rippling (like a snake). "Everything else in the universe is just a combination of these six moves," said Horvath, who started teaching the movement in his New York studio in about 1980. It wasn't until nearly 18 years later that he broke it down enough to help beginners to movement, and not just more advanced movers.

Horvath, who now is pain-free, says the goal is to obtain full function in all of life's requirements and to tap into the full capacity of every part of the body. Rhythmical breathing helps create an energy that spreads throughout the body. The movement itself is slow, gentle, and undulating.

Gyrotonic Expansion System (GXS) is similar to Gyrokineses in style and method, GXS uses a machine that Horvath himself developed that guides the body through spiraling and undulating movement. Dancers in particular are drawn to this, but Horvath is also using it with senior citizens and others with needs for gentler movement.

Tai Chi Chih

Although the name is similar to the ancient Chinese mind-body art of Tai Chi Chuan, Tai Chi Chih really is only a distant relative. It was developed in 1974 by Justin Stone as a way to make the long and complex forms and associated benefits of classic Tai Chi Chuan easier to pick up and more accessible to the public.

Instead of dozens and dozens of forms to learn, Stone's method has only 19 followed by one held pose. It is a much more gentle method (Tai Chi Chuan can be quite intensive), so it's great for seniors, people with disabilities, or anyone who just needs or wants very soft and easy movement. Stone tried to keep the essence of meditation, energy flow, and relaxation found in Tai Chi Chuan.

In Tai Chi Chih, you'll find forms with names like Daughter on the Mountaintop and Working the Pulley — sort of modern-day adaptations of Tai Chi Chuan's forms names the likes of Wave Hands Like Clouds and Repulse the Monkey.

E-Motion

Standing for "Energy in Motion," the E-motion program is another composite developed by Laura Sachs in an attempt to bring the benefits of Eastern mind-body movement to Westerners with a style they could more quickly appreciate. The class has three parts:

- ✔ A sensory-directed warm-up that uses visualization and Tai Chi-like movement
- ✔ A low-impact cardiovascular section using the beats of various drums and an ethnic flair.
- ✔ A yoga-like relaxation and cooldown with some traditional postures.

Sachs, who lives in San Francisco, says any part of the program can also be used separately. "In our hectic lives, any activity that gets us to breathe and that puts our attention inward," says Sachs, "is worthwhile."

Brain Gym

This program is used to enhance learning ability with improvements in things like concentration, coordination, and listening, which uses concepts of focusing and centering. Brain Gym grew out of research started in 1969 by Paul Dennison, Ph.D. It's all about how coordinating physical movement is necessary for brain development.

Yogarobics

One of the first mind-body programs that ventured into the fitness world, Yogarobics is pretty much what it sounds like — an upbeat Yoga workout intended to become more of an aerobic workout. Developer Larry Lane still teaches and trains others in this technique.

Aquatic mind-body

Just about any form of movement can get all wet — you can choose from water aerobics, water running, water walking (yes, even meditative if you want), and others. So what surprise is it to see Aqua NIA or Aqua Tai Chi?

Both are similar to their land-based versions, but use the resistance of the water to create even more internal focus. Of course, the water's reaction to movement means the methods also have some of their own movements, too. So don't expect just NIA or Tai Chi or Yoga or whatever to be thrown overboard.

Water, for those of you who haven't tried it, is a wonderful womb-like experience for movement that leaves you feeling as if you've had a whole-body massage.

What else?

As I said earlier, it's impossible to name them all. Here are a few other names and concepts you may bump into. Again, some of these are trademarked and proprietary names, so they aren't just up for grabs.

- ✔ **The Five Rhythms:** Think dance. Think moving meditation. Think free. Think . . . stop thinking. Just move.
- ✔ **Mindful Weight Training:** Some purists argue about simply taking a mindful element and overlaying it onto traditional Western exercise. But sometimes adding a focus, a few visualizations, or a touch can make the whole difference. You be the judge and jury.
- ✔ **Soul Sensation:** A combination NIA, Tai Chi, and general body awareness.
- ✔ **Watsu:** A more therapeutic movement in the water done mostly at spas. Other offspring include WasserTanzen (also called WaTa or Water Dance) and Aqua Soma, done with underwater music.

The methods listed below are fairly obvious combinations. You can see the possibilities are endless. Oh, and these New Kid methods aren't just being birthed in the United States. Look for new and different ideas coming out of all corners of the world, from Monrovia to Czechoslovakia to Slovenia.

BODYFLOW	Yin-Yang Walk
Chi Motion	Yin-Yang Water
Flow Motion	Yo-NIA
Mindful Riding	Yo Chi
One With Nature	Yoga Spin
Power & Flow	Yoga Water Stretch
Somatics	

Maybe the next new mind-body method will have your name on it!

Part VII
Pulling It All Together

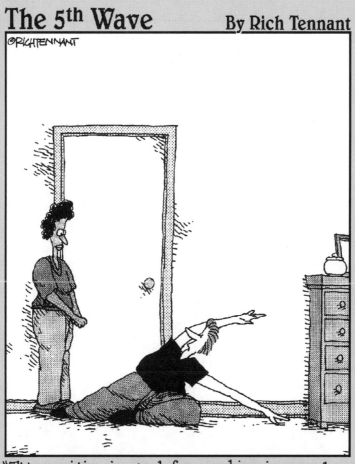

"This position is good for reaching inner calm, mental clarity, and things that roll behind the refrigerator."

In this part . . .

*I*n this part, I give you pointers on how to make mind-body methods a part not only of your fitness lifestyle, but also of your everyday life. I guide you with tips, examples, and suggested times for a little bit of mindfulness. In Chapter 19, I show you how the different methods fit together — either with your traditional exercise or with each other.

This is playtime, folks! A time to use your creativity, your imagination, and a time to tap into what feels good to you. Then to do it!

Chapter 18

Making Mind-Body Your Fitness Lifestyle

In This Chapter

▶ Embracing mind-body every day

▶ Living healthfully

▶ Taking time for a mind-body minute

*N*otice the word "Fitness" in the chapter title. I'm not talking religion here. You don't have to go live in some secluded community to truly experience the mind-body lifestyle. Oh, sure, you may find yourself so drawn in that you want to experience living in an ashram (that's a live-in community) or going on some extended retreat to deepen your practice. Those experiences can prove truly enlightening. But you don't have to go that far. You can continue doing what you're doing, and living where you're living and still start a mind-body lifestyle.

What you *do* want to concentrate on is *how* you do what you do and *how* you live day-to-day. You may discover improvements to your life that can make you a happier person, your heart a calmer place, your mind more at ease, and your body a more holistic center.

With all the following advice solidly in place, you may have an easier time really integrating mind-body fitness into your life.

Fitting Mind-Body into Each Day

You may spend only a half-hour or an hour a few times a week doing traditional fitness. With mind-body fitness, however, the patterns become a part of you every minute of the day, whether you're actually doing your routine or not. Or at least they should become more a part of you in order to derive the greatest benefits. Again, you don't have to munch on bean sprouts for lunch or meditate in the Lotus position on your office chair. Mind-body exercise just means looking at and reacting to things a little differently.

Take a close look at your day to see where you can best apply some mind-body techniques. You may want to pencil a few ideas into each time slot about specific things you can do or think about.

At sunrise

There is something magical about watching the sun rise — the colors, the majesty, the power, the reverence — as warm oranges and reds wash over you and the surroundings, painting everything in preparation for the day, prompting a wake-up to people still at rest. Sunrise has a stillness — even in the heart of most cities — that can create an oasis in a normally frenzied day.

If you aren't used to being awake at sunrise — or you're awake only in the grumpiest of moods and not usually at your choice — try it. *Choosing* to get up early makes all the difference in how you feel about it. (But make sure to get enough sleep the night before.)

In the morning, go out onto a deck, a patio, or into a quiet room near a window. Go someplace where you can see the sun rise. Face the east if you can. Let the light wash over you. Just sit and experience the sunrise. Even if you don't have time to do your full routine, just take five minutes to meditate a little, to go inside yourself and feel a little, and to just experience the quiet. This time may be your only chance before the alarm clocks go off, the kids race through the hall, your roommates pound on the bathroom door, or your spouse starts asking you about the evening plans.

If you are used to being up at sunrise, take time to look at what you see. Use the time to fuel yourself for the day with some mind-body activity, such as 10 minutes of Yoga.

Sometimes writing down your ideas helps you to organize your time more easily. Try jotting down your answers to the following questions.

  ✔ Where can I go to watch the sunrise?

  ✔ How much time can I spend there?

  ✔ What exercises can I do?

  ✔ How many times a week can I do this?

  ✔ On what days?

During midmorning

Sometimes as midmorning hits, your speed picks up as you race toward lunch meetings, or home from school projects, or off to another class. This time is often bad for people to practice mind-body exercises because they are in the middle of a period of higher activity. But that activity may be even more reason to take a few short moments for yourself. (See the "Taking a Mind-Body Minute" section later in this chapter.)

No matter where you are, you can find a secluded bench, an empty corner office, a spot behind a building that no one frequents, or even an empty stairwell. Instead of running for a cup of coffee, do some meditation walking or some Qigong movements to re-energize you for an upcoming meeting or the rest of the morning's flurry.

Consider these factors:

 ✔ At what time of the morning can I take a break?

 ✔ How long can the break last?

 ✔ Where can I find a quiet space?

 ✔ What activity or method best fits my location and time frame?

At noontime

Sometimes when noon rolls around, you hurry off to lunch and eat on the run, or grab a bite in the car, or at your desk. Slow down. Take time for yourself away from your daily routine. Taking even a short break can re-energize and refresh you. And it may be the perfect time to actually do your routine. You can go to a mind-body class, or pop in a video, depending on where you are and if you aren't home to do your own routine.

You need to do some homework by either planning your schedule (for example, calling around for a studio or class near your office), or having a video ready to pop in at home.

Think about your answers to these questions:

 ✔ How much time can I take at noon?

 ✔ What movements can I do to fit that time?

 ✔ Do I want to practice alone or with a class?

 ✔ If with a class, is there a studio that I can get to easily?

In the midafternoon

Most people enter a slump period around midafternoon. Researchers even found that about seven to eight hours after you get up, the body slows down. So for many of us that time falls between about 1 and 4 p.m. — just when a large coffee mocha sounds really appealing as a pick-me-up. Stop. Forget the large mocha. Go for 5 to 10 minutes of mindful moving about instead. This time of day may be great for a simple brisk walk, but be sure to use it to open your mind and clear your head. You may just need five minutes of a standing meditation. Or you may want to practice some quick Yoga standing postures.

Even if you're stuck at a desk and can't get away, you can probably sit back in your chair for a couple of minutes and breathe consciously and fully. You can also take the long way to the bathroom or lunch room, making an excuse for some meditation walking.

Evaluate these points to help decide the best plan for you.

- ✔ When do I usually experience an energy slump?
- ✔ How do I usually get through it?
- ✔ What mind-body techniques can I try instead?

At sunset or in the early evening

Ah, another beautiful and peaceful time of day, especially in the late spring, summer and early fall, when the days last a bit longer. (In the dead of winter, however, sunset may come too early to truly enjoy it because it may fall practically at midafternoon!)

In contrast to sunrise, when you energize yourself for the day, at sunset or in the early evening, you want to find peace with your day and slow down your pace. Sunset or early evening can be a grand time to take 30 minutes before dinner or after work to go through your mind-body routine. If you have a family, ask them to have a snack because dinner won't be happening for another half-hour. If you're hungry, have a light snack (such as some fruit or granola) an hour before your practice so that you won't just be listening to your grumbling tummy while meditating. Boy, can that be a distraction!

Just as at noon, you want to do some homework either planning your routine, calling around to find a convenient studio, or having a video ready to pop in.

Other factors to consider:

- ✔ How much time can I take for mind-body exercise?
- ✔ What techniques can I do to fit in that time period?
- ✔ Do I want to practice alone or with a class?
- ✔ If with a class, is there a studio nearby that I can get to easily?
- ✔ What kind of snack do I need to have handy for myself (or my family)?

Before bedtime

Perhaps bedtime is the first time you can find for yourself during the day. So be it; bedtime is a great time. Just avoid what many of us commonly do: Rush, rush, rush all day until bedtime comes before we know it, then collapse into the sack, only to start the rush-rush schedule as soon as the sun rises the next day.

You may find you can sleep better (and more peacefully) if you've had some time to practice your mind-body movements during the day. If you can't get in a little exercise earlier, then take 10 to 30 minutes at bedtime. The only caveat is this: Right before bedtime, you don't want to do anything that is high-intensity and gets you so hyped up that you can't fall asleep.

Living the Yoga lifestyle

Taking on a mindful lifestyle may not be the main reason you begin one of the methods in this book, but sometimes it just happens. Richard Miller, Ph.D. and co-founder of the International Association of Yoga Therapists, took his first Yoga class in 1970 after moving to San Francisco. He used the class as a way to meet people, although he also harbored a little bit of fascination about Yoga teachings. Still, it was — at first — primarily just a Yoga class.

"Over the next several years, my life changed slowly, but quite dramatically. I stopped smoking and began eating less red meat and consuming less alcohol. I became increasingly

more flexible, both physically and emotionally. Old internal and external conflicts and angers dropped away, and I felt more peaceful within myself, and in the way I faced challenges that arose in my daily life. I began daily meditation, exploring and actualizing the rich spiritual dimensions of life," recalled Miller, who after three decades of practice is now considered an expert and master in the fields of Yoga, breathwork, and Yoga therapy.

"I slowly moved from taking Yoga classes," said Miller, also a clinical psychologist, "to living a Yoga lifestyle that became integrated into all facets of my daily life."

A few other aspects to think about are:

- ✔ How much time can I devote to mind-body exercise at bedtime?
- ✔ What type of routine works best at bedtime?
- ✔ Where can I find a sanctuary to do my exercises?

I give you some tips about creating your sanctuary in the very next section. Then in Chapter 19, I give you some sample routines and ideas for creating your own combinations. So, start thinking about what time of day you prefer and what exercises fit best into your schedule.

Creating a Sanctuary

This section talks about how to find your sanctuary where you can feel safe to go away into your mind-body routine for 10, 20, or 30 minutes.

- ✔ **Find a place where you can focus.** Focusing on yourself is hard enough, without having a place to call your own. You don't want to look at a cluttered desk, the kids' toys, the piles of dishes or laundry, or the great balls o' dust in the corners when you try to do mind-body exercises.

- ✔ **Add items that help you forget distractions.** Room dividers or screens can help you block out the family, the mess, or the chores you need to do. (And they can be really attractive, too.) Candles and lamps can also help set the stage, or give you a light to focus on for any relaxation or meditation. Pillows can help you get into the safest and best positions for your body. A mat can make your bones more comfortable. And, a soothing picture on the wall can help you feel as if you're really on a true retreat. See the Appendix for some resources for accessories like these.

- ✔ **Preserve your sanctuary.** Even if this space can't be permanent, look around for a corner and mentally claim it. You can then keep your "sanctuary supplies" in a drawer, on a closet shelf, or folded up under the bed. When you're ready for your mind-body retreat, just pull out the dividers, candles, music, and incense, and set yourself up in a flash.

Extending Mind-Body 'Round the Clock

As I mention at the beginning of this chapter, mind-body fitness doesn't stop when you roll up your mat and put it away. This section gives you some ways to take your lessons — and the wisdom you have gathered through them — along for the ride as you cruise through your day. You're likely to find other ways that work for you, too.

Concentrating on breathing

In all situations, breathe. Train yourself to be aware of your breathing. You may be surprised at how often you catch yourself holding your breath. Really. Especially if you're writing at a computer on a project deadline!

If you're in a conversation, debate, discussion, or even an argument with someone, take a moment to breathe before you respond. Breathing alone can help slow your pulse and blood pressure. (See Chapter 6 for more on the physical benefits of mind-body exercise.)

Looking inside yourself

Think about how and why you feel and react the way you do in certain situations. Is it really something about yourself or your own frustration that you take out on the other person? Let yourself feel all during the day, in everything that you do, by looking inward in short meditative moments.

Observing the world around you

Observe both yourself and others in daily interactions. But remember that mind-body fitness is nonjudgmental. So observation doesn't mean thinking, "Oh, what I just said was so stupid," or "How could she ever have worn those odd shoes?" Observation just means noting things around you and how they affect you, then acknowledging that reaction or affect. After some time practicing mind-body fitness methods, you find more calm and peace day-to-day.

Sending healing energy

Really. Don't laugh. Use the awakened mental powers you develop from mind-body exercise to "beam" positive energy to someone else. Perhaps a colleague is angry, or a cashier you encounter is having a bad day, or the airline ticket agent is acting like you are a nightmare-incarnate when all you want to do is change your seat. Think healing energy that can envelop that other person, doing so can make their day (and yours) better.

Being nice

Okay, being nice is a simple one, I suppose. But how many times do you find yourself being a snip or a grump to someone who has no responsibility for your snippiness or grumpiness? What did he or she do to deserve such treatment? Probably nothing. So take a deep full breath, center yourself, and be nice.

Taking 5 (Or 10, or 20 . . .)

No time for breaks, you say? Look, that excuse doesn't work. Everybody —
and I do mean everybody — can find at least five minutes in the day for him-
or herself. Writing down your daily schedule to figure out where those extra
minutes get lost may be helpful. (For more suggestions about finding time,
see Chapter 2.) You can even pencil in a time you intend to take a break, or
set an alarm on your watch so you don't get so wrapped up that you forget.

Find five — make that your motto. At least five.

You can find a minute or two to do a quick balance pose, stretch, alignment
drill, or standing meditation many times during the day. But also look for
practical times when you're just waiting for something. How about when you
fill your car's gas tank? That's the "Gas-Station Moment." You can do a standing or breathing exercise. See how easy it is to find a couple of dangling minutes in your day?

Playing music

This idea varies depending on the individual and the music choice. Certain
music may calm some people while it pumps up others. For many people,
however, a calming mind-body-appropriate choice of music can encourage
you to breathe deeply and center your thoughts. Appropriate music changes
based on your taste and the type of movements you're doing. You can listen
to tapes of chirping birds and fluttering leaves, or you can try the peaceful
flutes and wind instruments often used in recordings like these. You may find
you like vocals, although many people avoid lyrics because they can be distracting. Usually a more mellow tune helps you get in the mind-body mood.
Take a look at the Appendix for some places to look for music you may want
to try during your workouts or routines.

Setting up your surroundings

When I talk about surroundings, I don't mean the area where you actually do
your mind-body exercises. What I mean is your day-to-day environment.
Make your bathroom, bedroom, or work cubicle smell nice with candles,
flowers, or leaves. Have incense handy in the living room. Burn candles for
that touch of flickering light dancing on a wall. Your environment can really
affect your reaction not only to mind-body practices but also to your everyday life. So set yourself up for success from the start.

Trusting your intuition

Trust is the first word I learned in an intuition class I once took. In fact, we wrote the word in block letters (in any style we wanted) on a piece of blank paper, then colored in and around it — also in any way that suited our fancies. Then to continually remind ourselves to go with our gut feelings, we posted the drawing in plain view where it seemed best for each of us. Mine was on a file cabinet beside me where I could see it many times during the day.

For about four years, I looked at that word in bright little-kid Crayon colors on my office wall. Trust. And every time I looked at it, the word reminded me to go inside, to listen, and to believe.

Taking Care of Your Body

Much of this book talks about your mind, your mind's effect on your body, and how you can adjust your movements to suit your body's needs. But what about what you put *in* your body as fuel? Or how you sit? How you stand? If you get enough rest?

This section provides a brief look at some of the other ways you can take care of your body, because if you take care of your body, it will take care of you. Of course, for more in-depth or individualized nutrition and lifestyle advice, you want to find other books or consult with a specialist. Check out *Nutrition For Dummies,* 2nd Edition, by Carol Ann Rinzler.

Eating smart

I'm not going to tell you that you have to become a vegetarian, shun all refined foods, eat organic, and avoid alcoholic beverages (or drink only moderately). Some people may tell you that. I won't. These lifestyle changes are your own choice. You may, however, find yourself drifting that way if you decide to deepen your mind-body practice. Eating healthfully makes you feel better and focus better when practicing mind-body techniques. That means you need to eat a diet with low fat, high fiber, moderate protein, whole sources of carbohydrates, and plenty of fruits and vegetables.

Research shows that most people know what they *should* eat, but most don't heed the advice. Doing so takes a bit of effort sometimes. Eating healthfully may mean stocking up on healthy snacks to put in your briefcase, desk drawer, or even your car so that you don't so easily succumb to vending machine munchies or fast food out of desperation. That also means drinking plenty of water, even keeping a water bottle with you so that it's easily accessible.

My dad used to joke that he liked driving my car when he came to visit because it had a snack bar. I suppose he was right. I hate being caught with a growling stomach and an impending headache, knowing I had no food except what was in the 24-hour market at the corner. I know from experience that such junk doesn't satisfy me long-term, so I kept a supply of healthy munchies in the car.

No demand being made here to flip-flop your eating habits from today to tomorrow. I just want to nudge you to start thinking twice when you fill your grocery cart or peruse the menu in a restaurant.

Sleeping well

Okay, a show of hands, please? How many of you get enough sleep most of the time? Just as I suspected. Just that one man in the back of the room. So, the rest of you feel a little sleep-deprived; doesn't everybody at least some of the time? Sleep studies show that most of us walk around pretty sleep-needy.

Two things to note if you're sleepy a lot:

- ✔ **You may end up just going to sleep during your deep relaxations.** Doing so can prove pretty embarrassing, especially if you're in a class or if you have a tendency to snore. You also won't reap the benefits of a normal meditation if all you do is nap.

- ✔ **You may have a hard time finding the time and energy for your fitness routine, either traditional, mind-body, or both.** Your sleepiness makes you want to just flop in a chair like a big sack of potatoes.

You probably know how much sleep you need to feel good. Try to get that amount of sleep every night so that you can actually enjoy the day, function at a productive level, and feel good about finding time for fitness.

Standing up straight (Your mama was right)

Whether you're meditating or standing in line at the bank, if you stand up tall, you not only feel more confident, but you can also "unkink" your energy hoses. (I introduce these energy channels, called meridians, in Chapter 4 and discuss them more thoroughly in the Tai Chi and Qigong chapters — 10 and 11.) Your mama probably wasn't thinking about your energy flow, though, when she nagged you about standing up straight.

Standing tall doesn't mean a strained military posture, but a relaxed and spine-straight position. Your chest should be open, shoulders back and down but easily in place, your teeth unclenched (your dentist thanks you), and your head tall on your spine.

Standing straight makes you think more clearly, focus more easily, and meditate better.

Sticking to a sane work schedule

This crazy world sometimes seems to encourage and bless those people who work insane hours, forgoing all time for family, fun, and freedom. Just say no. Doing so doesn't mean becoming a slouch. It just means knowing when enough is enough, and when to go home or to take a day off. Work isn't a substitute for other entertainment. Go find other entertainment. Work is only one part of your life. Balance is what keeps people sane.

Taking a Mind-Body Minute

Have a minute? Take a mind-body adventure. Keep it simple. Allow it to take you where it does each time. For example, you can use your mind-body adventure to:

✔ Explore what burbles up on its own

✔ Get in touch with a feeling you didn't realize was so strong

✔ Re-energize yourself by filling yourself with chi

✔ Meditate to clear your head

✔ Calm yourself. You can take many roads to get to your destination. That's the beauty. The route you choose is the best part, especially because you can change it each time.

The following steps give you one way to enjoy a short mind-body ride.

1. **Sit comfortably on a firm chair with a straight back. Sit up tall, but relaxed so that your spine is straight and comfortable. Put the soles of your feet flat on the floor.**

2. **Place your hands on your knees, palms turned upward if you are in need of gathering more energy in, or palms turned down if you need to calm down and ground yourself more.**

If you take a moment in an office or someplace with people around you, just leave your arms relaxed on your legs (if you don't want to stand out).

3. **Close your eyes, if you're comfortable with doing so. Otherwise, leave them open, especially if you're around other people. If your eyes are open, turn your mental focus inside away from the bustle around you.**

4. **Now, inhale fully and exhale fully, then let your breath return to a regular pattern, but still deep and regular.**

5. **Feel any heat or energy you can coming up through the soles of your feet; follow the energy with your mind as it travels up your legs, and your spine, stopping to circle around your heart.**

6. **Send the energy circling up into your head, then back down the front of your body, letting it pour out toward your hands, before returning back to your torso.**

7. **You can pull more energy in through your feet and let it cavort around your body again, or even several times.**

8. **To finish, acknowledge that presence of energy and calm, inhale fully again and exhale fully, and come back to the present.**

That's Therese's Mind-Body Minute! I often use this before regular athletic workouts, before meetings, or when I'm a little tired.

Chapter 19

Fitting Mind-Body Methods into a Complete Picture

In This Chapter

▶ Measuring the levels of intensity of mind-body exercises

▶ Incorporating traditional exercise into mind-body methods

▶ Trying out some mind-body exercise combinations

A s with traditional exercise, mind-body methods provide you with a variety of choices. And that variety is a good thing! The different methods that I introduce to you in this book can fit together very nicely — either all at once or gradually over time. You can use one method or the other for a complete routine, for just a warm-up, for just a cooldown, for relaxation, for small meditative moments in the day, or as a way to revamp your entire lifestyle. Or you can do all of the above on different days, depending on your mood, mixing and matching them as you feel best suits you so you end up sequencing several forms or applying just one. You can even try doing some of these methods as a part of traditional workouts.

You see, all you have to do is know which piece or method fits where, and off you go! The beauty too is that many of these methods can vary from the lightest of intensities to quite vigorous ones. It all depends on whether you choose to do them:

▶ Quickly or slowly

▶ With very bent knees (so you stay low and use more muscle) or nearly straight knees (less demand on your muscles)

▶ Expansively covering space with large movements or staying very stationary

▶ Using many repetitions with little rest in between (so you work harder) or fewer repetitions with more rest in between (so you work less intensely)

The decision on how to do these exercises is all up to you.

Matching Up the Levels

First, you have to know which methods can give you a low-intensity workout, which can apply to moderate routines, and which can be more vigorous. Understanding these levels can help you figure out which method is best for you.

I rate these levels in two different ways:

- ✔ **MET:** A MET, or metabolic equivalent, is a multiple of resting metabolism based on the amount of oxygen a body needs per minute to support an activity. One MET is equal to just sitting or lying down (being at rest) and doing utterly nothing. Sports medicine experts rate activity based on how much (metabolic) energy an activity takes compared to being at rest. Four to seven METs is considered moderate activity.

- ✔ **Sense of Effort:** This number relates to how you rate an activity on a scale of 0 to 10, with 0 being equal to the 1 MET rating above and 4 to 6 considered moderate. This is all about how activity feels to you and not how some exercise physiologist says it should feel.

Following, I introduce a very preliminary and general classification system for the intensity and physical effort of the mind-body methods in this book. Because this type of classification has never been thoroughly investigated, the categories that these methods fall under may change over the next few years. For now, this system, adapted from work by Ralph La Forge at Duke University, gives you some idea about how to choose and combine methods.

Easing in: Level 1

This level of mind-body method is very, very low-intensity aerobic activity to almost none, depending on which exercise you choose and how you do it.

You can do many mind-body methods at Level 1. Table 19-1 covers only those methods I address in this book.

Here is a key to the column headings in Table 19-1:

- ✔ **All movements:** means *all* of this method's movements are the corresponding intensity.

- ✔ **Most/modified movements:** means *most* of this method's movements are the corresponding intensity, or are this intensity if they are done in a *modified* format that de-emphasizes speed and repetitions and emphasizes rest.

- ✔ **Some movements:** means *some* of this method's movements can become the corresponding intensity.

Hey, what about heart rate?

If you exercise at all, you've probably heard about taking your heart rate. Maybe you're wondering why I haven't talked about that. Because many mind-body methods are based on the benefits you reap from being mindful and focused. Also, because they concentrate on a sense of effort, taking your heart rate may not be as telling as listening to how you feel. Or as necessary.

That said, you can choose some more highly aerobic forms (or forms that can become more aerobic) of mind-body exercise where taking your heart rate can prove beneficial, especially if you wear a wireless heart rate monitor and don't have to stop and put two fingers on your wrist and count. That process may be a bit of an interruption to your flow, eh? Taking your heart rate may also be advised by your physician for maintaining appropriate intensity.

So, how do you know what heart rate is right for you? The simplest way (although the number is truly a rough estimate) is to take your age and subtract it from 226 for women, 220 for men. That number is your maximum heart rate. Now, multiply it by the desired target percentage (which the next paragraph can help you determine) to get your target heart rate. If you are under a physician's care, he or she can advise you about the best percentage.

A low-intensity workout should raise your heart rate to less than about 55 to 60 percent of your maximum heart rate. A moderate workout raises it to about 60 to 75 percent, depending on your fitness level. A vigorous workout is anything above that, again depending on your fitness level (and vigorous workouts are in fact not truly advised to achieve mindful benefits). Most beneficial mind-body routines fall between about 55 and 70 percent of maximum heart rate.

For example, a 40-year-old woman has a maximum heart rate of 186. She wants to work out moderately, or at about 70 percent of her maximum. She multiplies .70 times 186 for a result of 130. Her target heart rate therefore is approximately 130, if she chooses to use heart rate as a way to measure her effort.

Know that you can have a margin of error of up to 10 to 15 beats in either direction using this estimate. So using a number that corresponds to your sense of effort can be very helpful and perhaps better for most mind-body methods. To find stories about heart rate as well as a heart rate calculator (to make your life easier), go to www.totalfitnessnetwork.com, where you can find a whole section on this subject, written by yours truly.

Table 19-1	Mind-Body Methods That Contain Level 1 (Low) Intensity Movements	
All Movements	*Most/Modified Movements*	*Some Movements*
Alexander	Meditation Walking	Chi Ball Method
Body Rolling	Qigong, standing forms	E-Motion
Brain Gym	Tai Chi Chih	Hatha Yoga
Feldenkrais	Tai Chi Chuan	Laban
Watsu	Rosen Method	

Measure the intensity using the following criteria:

- ✔ **METS:** Less than 4, which is about the effort you expend just walking casually, like through a shopping mall when you're just browsing.

- ✔ **Sense of Effort:** Less than 4 on a scale of 0 to 10. Should feel very easy or quite light.

Raising the bar: Level 2

This level of mind-body method is moderate activity. If you already do traditional exercise, this is likely the level you are familiar with during that activity. You may also want to try to reach a moderate intensity in some of your mind-body exercises. Table 19-2 lists exercises that qualify, broadly, as Level 2, using the preliminary classifications as I explained earlier in this section. The table also includes only the methods that I have addressed in this book.

Here again is a key to the column headings in Table 19-2:

- ✔ **All movements:** means *all* of this method's movements are the corresponding intensity.

- ✔ **Most/modified movements:** means *most* of this method's movements will be the corresponding intensity, or will be this intensity if they are done in a *modified* format that de-emphasizes speed and repetitions and emphasizes rest.

- ✔ **Some movements:** means *some* of this method's movements can become the corresponding intensity.

Table 19-2	Mind-Body Methods That Contain Level 2 (Moderate) Intensity Movements
Most Movements	*Some Movements*
Aqua exercise with mindful element	Capoiera & other ethnic dance
Five Rhythms	Chi Ball Method
Gyrokinesis/Gyrotonic XS	E-Motion
Meditation Walking	Hatha Yoga, NIA, Pilates-inspired exercise
Qigong, Moving Forms	Tai Chi Chih
Yogarobics	
Tai Chi Chuan	
Traditional exercise with mindful element	

Measure the intensity using the following criteria:

✔ **METS:** about 4 to 7, or the effort it takes to walk briskly on level ground, as if you're late for an appointment. About a medium level.

✔ **Effort:** about 4 to 6 on a scale of 0 to 10. Should feel moderate or about halfway between what would be very low intensity and what would be very, very hard.

Pumping it up: Level 3

This level of mind-body method is moderate- to high-intensity activity.

Table 19-3 covers only methods discussed in the book. You may see quite an overlap in some methods on Levels 2 and 3. The reason for that is that you can do most of what could be Level 2 faster or without as much rest to make it harder, and thereby push it up to level 3.

Here again is a key to the column headings in Table 19-3:

✔ **All movements:** means *all* of this method's movements are the corresponding intensity.

✔ **Most/modified movements:** means *most* of this method's movements will be the corresponding intensity, or will be this intensity if they are done in a *modified* format that de-emphasizes speed and repetitions and emphasizes rest.

✔ **Some movements:** means *some* of this method's movements can become the corresponding intensity.

Table 19-3	Mind-Body Methods That Contain Level 3 (High) Intensity Movements
Most Movements	*Some Movements*
Aqua exercise with mindful element	Capoiera & other ethnic dance
Five Rhythms	Chi Ball Method
Gyrokinesis	E-Motion
NIA	Hatha Yoga
Tai Chi Chuan	Pilates-inspired exercise
Traditional exercise with mindful element	Yogarobics

Measure the intensity using the following criteria:

- ✔ **METS:** higher than about 7, which is equivalent to hiking uphill. More than a moderate level. Usually hard to very hard.

- ✔ **Effort:** higher than about 6 on a scale on a scale of 0 to 10. Should feel comfortably hard to very hard, if you really want to push it over the top a bit.

Applying the Levels

Applying the different levels of mind-body exercise to your routines is easy. In this section, I give you an overview of how to choose which level is most suitable for each part of your daily workouts.

Selecting any one of these levels for a fitness routine is a means to a mindful end. Never feel as if you must combine Levels 1, 2, and 3, or put them together in any particular order. Doing all Level 1 movement is just beautiful, as is a combined routine, too. The ratings by level are only to help you decide which is best for you.

- ✔ **Choose Level 1 activities** to start your routine as a warm-up, to finish it as your cooldown, or if you want very low-intensity activity overall. For example, use Level 1 if you want only to become more body aware, are rehabilitating from an injury or a heart attack, have a particular disability or disease, are a senior who needs low-intensity movement, seek only functional training, or just want relaxation or meditation. Your complete routine can be Level 1.

- ✔ **Choose Level 2 activities** for a transition between your warm-up and an even more vigorous tempo (if you choose to do that), or if you want moderate activity and are an average and healthy exerciser. Your complete routine could be Level 2.

- ✔ **Choose Level 3 activities** for the middle section of your workout after being thoroughly warmed up, or if you want a very vigorous workout and are already exercising and fit or athletic. *Note:* You should normally precede Level 3 activity with some lower-intensity movement as a warm-up because of its higher intensity.

If you have a special physical or health situation such as a disease, injury, or disability, or if you are recovering from a heart attack, you should see a physician to get his or her approval before beginning any physical activity.

The other thing to note is that I have described only low-intensity, stand-alone movements for some methods in their respective sections, or I may have described only moderate movements because of the limited space in this one book to describe all of these great methods. To discover the full range of each, or how to link many movements together, or how a sequence can flow, explore further on your own, using the Appendix of resources in the back of the book. You can also try moving faster, taking fewer rests, or doing more repetitions to make your workout more intense. Just use common sense when you modify your fitness program.

Integrating Mind-Body with Traditional Exercise

Many a mind-body purist may pooh-pooh the idea that you can experience true mindful benefits by overlapping some meditation or mind-body move-ments with your traditional exercise. But that is one way to begin to dabble at mind-body movement, so you can start to feel your energy flow or find the contemplative moments in a familiar practice. Everybody has to discover for themselves what combination of exercise and workouts is right for them. Try these ideas on how to combine mind-body with traditional exercise, if that sounds like your idea of a great workout.

You may find success, as others have:

- ✔ Doing easy runs or walks while focusing on your muscles and your breathing
- ✔ Riding a stationary bike while meditating on the repetitive motion of your feet
- ✔ Ending (or starting — or both) a traditional routine with some mind-body movements, meditation, or centering

You may want to dabble in all three of those examples to see which — if any of them — work for you.

Adding mindful centering

Who hasn't heard about zoning out on a run and not even remembering those last few miles? Have you been there?

Studies show that physical mind-body benefits (see Chapter 6 for a detailed breakdown and summary of the benefits) come when your workout intensity is not too vigorous, but rather a low to moderate intensity. So, no, that relaxed feeling you get after puffing and groaning vigorously on a fast hike up a steep hill is probably only from endorphins and other neuro-active substances and not from any particularly mindful component.

Neuroactive substances, or neurotransmitters, the naturally occurring chemicals in the brain (a couple of well-known ones are adrenaline and endorphins) are responsible for altering brain function, perception, and behavior by transmitting messages between brain cells.

But if you keep your intensity lower, you may be able to incorporate a contemplative element with your traditional workout and finish feeling your calm and peaceful center.

To see what I mean, try this combination: Do your regular workout, be it a run, walk, hike, walking on a treadmill, riding a stationary bike, or whatever. Keep your effort level below 6 on that scale of 0 to 10, meaning that you are exercising only moderately. Rather than tuning out or distracting yourself with reading or the TV, tune into your body. Think about keeping your breathing regular and deep, and concentrate on how your muscles are working. Just like with meditating, staying focused may be difficult at first. But experiment with doing this combination for even 5 minutes, then try 10, or even 20. See if trying this helps you to experience any additional feelings of calm, centering, focus, or relaxation.

Integrating meditation

You can compare this combination to meditation or Qigong walking in some ways, but you can also do it with aerobics, riding a stationary bike, or even jogging. (Refer to Chapter 11 for more information about Qigong walking, and to Chapter 16 for a description of meditation walking.)

For example: Do your regular workout. Again, keep your effort level below 6 or at a light to moderate level. Try to meditate while you move, by tuning into each step (or pedal, or push, or whatever) and letting the energy flow through the limbs of your body. Try to empty your mind, and consciously let your breaths move fully. If a stray thought wanders through, acknowledge it and let it pass. Try this combination for only a short period of time at first because it takes some practice.

Make sure this combination is safe for the type of workout you plan. For example, try it indoors on stationary equipment, or in a safe place to walk or run without rough terrain. I don't want you to fall off a real bike while meditating!

Incorporating mindful starts and finishes

This idea is a more traditional way of being . . . well, less than traditional. You find more and more people, including fitness instructors, simply starting a session by doing some simple Tai Chi Chuan, Qigong, or Yoga movements that center you and bring you to the present place. Adding mind-body methods to your traditional workout lets you look forward to your familiar aerobics segment and also allows you to dabble in something new without feeling as if you have to give up a routine you love.

Try this combination: Start your regular routine, from a run out the back door to a step-aerobics class, by first taking 5 to 10 minutes to do some Yoga, Qigong walking, or even just repeating a couple of Tai Chi forms on each side. Use your breathing techniques while you go through these movements. Then go ahead and do your regular workout thing. When you finish, take another 5 minutes to do the same mind-body method that you started with, or maybe even try a deep relaxation in the yogic Corpse pose or a semi-inversion with your legs up on a wall.

Sampling Some Pure Mind-Body Combos

Here comes the fun! This section gives you about a half-dozen sampler mind-body combos — some developed by experts especially for you! After you see how endless the possibilities are, you can devise a couple of routines on your own.

Look for combination names like Yo-Chi or Yo-lates or Yo-NIA. By the way, Yo-Chi is a combo of Yoga and Tai Chi, Yo-lates is a combo of Yoga and Pilates, and Yo-NIA is — you guessed it — a combo of Yoga and NIA.

I won't rewrite all the instructions in this section, but I do list the movements. (Check the Table of Contents or the index to point you to the actual exercises.) In some cases, I also give you tips on transitions or intensity.

Sampler combo #1 — mind-body circuit

This combination is for those days when you have at least 30 minutes, want it all, but just can't decide which method to choose. Do the preliminary movements, then continue through the circuit (a series of movements done either one after the other), repeating each movement as often as you like before moving on. After you finish with the entire circuit of movements to the extent you have time, go to the closing.

Preliminary movements

1. **Stand and Be Aware** (Feldenkrais).

2. **Open the Door** (Tai Chi Chuan): **Repeat 1–4 times, or more if you like.**

Circuit

1. **Grasp the Bird's Tail** (Tai Chi Chuan): **Once on each side, using a Centering Step to change sides.**

2. **Warrior** (Yoga): **Return to Mountain Posture after one Warrior to be able to turn and do the posture on the other side, too.**

3. **Travel 1-2-3** (NIA): **Moving both forward and back, and right and left, using a toe touch at the end, or a knee lift, or a high kick. Repeat as desired, alternating endings to the 1-2-3 as you like. Cover more space if you want it to be more intense aerobically. Slow it down and cover less space for a couple of minutes before concluding this movement.**

4. **Triangle Posture** (Chi Ball Method): **Once (or more if you want) on each side.**

5. **Pushup** (Pilates).

Closing

1. **Hundreds** (Pilates): **For abdominal work.**

2. **Corpse posture** (Yoga): **For relaxation.**

Sampler combo #2 — Tai Chi and Yoga

Tai-Ga or Yo-Chi — whatever you want to call it — these methods fit naturally together in many ways. For example:

✔ Starting with gentler Tai Chi, move into Yoga, then close with Tai Chi.

✔ Starting with standing and warm-up Yoga postures, move into Tai Chi, but push yourself more, then close with a relaxing Yoga meditation.

✔ Starting with either method in a gentler form, alternate with five minutes of each, then close with a slower version to cool down.

David-Dorian Ross, a Tai Chi instructor and long-time Yoga practitioner (who also advised on the Tai Chi Chuan chapter in this book), put together this short set for you to try. Do each movement on both sides, more than once if you like. This set is, of course, only one example of the vast array of possibilities.

In this set, you test your balance, both moving, standing, and leaning forward.

1. **Open the Door** (Tai Chi Chuan): **Stand calmly to find your alignment, breathe, then begin.**

2. **Play the Pi'pa** (Tai Chi Chuan): **Hold the position for a moment to test your balance. Breathe please! Do this several times, gently at first so you can warm up a bit.**

3. **Step Up and Kick** (Tai Chi Chuan): **Try to keep your alignment and get your leg a little higher each time you do it.**

4. **Triangle Posture** (Yoga): **For stretching, balance, and strength.**

5. **Tree Posture** (Yoga): **Hold the pose and breathe.**

6. **Warrior** (Yoga): **To challenge both strength and balance.**

7. **Mountain Posture** (Yoga): **To return to a centered state. Use this position to breathe and calm yourself after the set.**

If you want, do movements in Steps 2 through 5 more than one time through, then add the movement in Step 7 to finish.

Sampler combo #3 — Yoga warm-up or pick-me-up

Jenni Fox and Paul Gould, Santa Cruz, California-based Yoga teachers and owners of Yoga-Nia Adventures, offered this combo of seven Yoga-based movements for a pre-exercise warm-up. (Add some NIA after Step 7 if you want a complete mind-body routine.) Note the specific directions on timing and other tips.

You can finish with the movement in Steps 8 and 9 to make a complete mini-routine. Or, if you just want a pick-me-up, do just Steps 6, 8, and 9 first thing in the morning or in the evening.

1. **Vocalized Breath in Mountain Posture** (Yoga): **Inhale, then say "Aaaah!" with the exhalation to release tension particularly in the throat and face.**

2. **Centering Breath in Mountain Posture** (Yoga): **Join hands together in Namaste. Observe your breath for 1 minute.**

3. **Mountain Posture** (Yoga): **For extension with uplifted arms overhead — 1 minute.**

4. **Tree** (Yoga): **For balance — 30 seconds each side.**

5. **Warrior** (Yoga): **For building heat and strength — 1 minute each side.**

6. **Downward Facing Dog** (Yoga): **For destressing and warming — 30 seconds.**

7. **Seated Forward Bend** (Yoga): **For tuning in — 1 minute.**

   The next two steps are your closing if this entire set is your routine. If you decide to add some other movements, save Steps 8 and 9 for your closing.

8. **Going Horizontal with Legs Up On Wall** (Inversion): **For rejuvenating the entire body — 1 to 5 minutes, but only at the end of a session.**

   Remember to consult with your physician before attempting any exercise that involves inversion.

9. **Corpse** (Yoga): **For relaxing body and mind — 5 to 10 minutes, but as a relaxing ending only.**

Sampler combo #4 — awareness classics

Taking a look at the Modern Classics in Chapter 16, this next set is just to help you build body awareness, either on its own or as a preliminary to another routine.

Repeat all the movements in the following list as you'd like or need.

1. **Sit to Stand I** (Alexander)

2. **Sit to Stand II** (Alexander)

3. **Stand and Be Aware** (Feldenkrais)

4. **Sit, Turn, and Look** (Feldenkrais)

5. **Preparatory Exercise for Creeping to Standing** (Laban)

6. **Creeping to Standing Level for Locomotion** (Laban)

Sampler combo #5 — New Kids combo

Okay, the New Kids contemporary methods need their own set, too! Don't neglect these ideas for a great little workout, with an emphasis here on stretching and feeling the energy flow. Of course, you have so many more movements in the full instructional sets. See the Appendix for the resources to research more about these methods.

1. **Butterfly** (Chi Ball)

2. **Cross-Back Sink Step** (NIA)

3. **Pivot and Sink Stance** (NIA)

4. **Basic Hamstring Rolling** (Body Rolling)

5. **Up Each Side of the Spine** (Body Rolling)

6. **Spinal Roll** (Chi Ball)

Sampler combo #6 — Pilates and Qigong

Qigong, dating back centuries with its gentle centering flow, and Pilates, dating back to a German immigrant in the twentieth century with its emphasis on core and spinal alignment and control, may seem a bit contradictory when used in one routine. But you can work the contrasts to your advantage.

Start and end with two to three Qigong movements so that you find your energy flow, then get it back again after the short Pilates segment.

1. **Standing Like a Tree** (Qigong)

2. **Whole Body Breathing** (Qigong)

3. **Qigong Walking** (Qigong)

4. **Dead Bug Roll, working into Rolling Like a Ball** (both Pilates)

5. **Hundreds, starting with Ab Preps if desired** (both Pilates)

6. **Spine Stretch** (Pilates)

7. **Saw** (Pilates)

8. **Arrow** (Pilates)

9. **Row the Boat** (Qigong)

10. **Standing Like a Tree** (Qigong)

Want more? Do more Pilates and even add some Tai Chi after the first Qigong section if you want!

Your combinations are limited only by your imagination!

Design your own combos

No rules really exist for designing your own exercise combinations. Just make sure you try to create a flow moving from standing to floor or moving from floor to standing, and don't bounce back and forth. Make sure you don't jump into higher intensity, drop down to low-intensity standing and meditating, then push your exercise to very intense again. Of course, you can always do something completely creative and all your own. And you can combine any of these mind-body methods with some traditional workouts, too. For example, your routine can have several variations of intensity to create a sort of graph-like picture. Have you used any exercise equipment where you see a visual of your aerobic intensity measured in dots on a screen? I want you to try to visualize something like that, and I hope the following list helps.

- ✔ **A straight line:** One intensity from start to finish, or really no intensity from start to finish.

- ✔ **A staircase going up then going back down:** Start with low intensity, increase it, then decrease the intensity back down again.

- ✔ **A gentle rolling hill:** Start very light, increase only a bit, then decrease again.

- ✔ **A series of gently rolling hills:** Repeat the above for an undulating workout.

- ✔ **One big mountain peak:** Climb directly from a light beginning into some very intense activity, then climb back down quickly.

- ✔ **A range of tall mountains:** Go very intensely, then let your heart rate drop. (This class is for people doing interval-like work, such as athletes.) For example, you could run a hard interval, then recover with some meditative walking between each one.

Mix and match to your heart's content to devise a mind-body method fit for you!

Part VIII
The Part of Tens

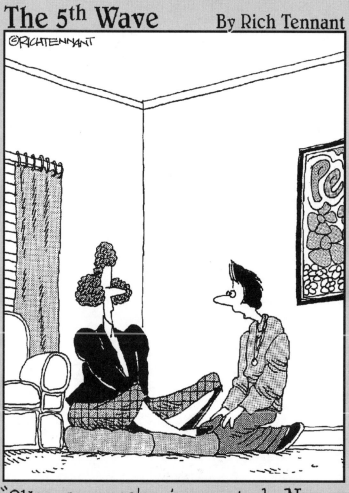

The 5th Wave   By Rich Tennant

@RICHTENNANT

"Okay, your posture's very good. Now relax, concentrate, and slowly let go of your cell phone."

In this part . . .

You like quick hits, quick reads, quick checklists, and a quick way to cut to the quick, quickly: Why do I want to do this? Is it for me? What will I get from it? In this part, I give you the definitive Part of Tens, where you can find lists of the top ten greatest things about mind-body fitness. Okay, okay, definitive based on Therese's two cents. You can always find more and different approaches. Nevertheless, you can take a gander and use these lists to help you sort out your thoughts and make a decision, either before you read the book, during the read, or after.

But take a deep meditative breath first and do it sloooooooowwleeeeeeeee in the proper mind-body way.

Chapter 20

Ten Reasons to Try Mind-Body Workouts

. . . .

In This Chapter

▶ Moving gently

▶ Flowing instead of fighting

▶ Taking it easy

▶ Setting your own goals

▶ Finding inner peace

▶ Enhancing your breathing

▶ Discovering your inner focus

▶ Improving strength, flexibility, and your aerobic condition

. . . .

*M*aybe you aren't quite convinced about this mind-body stuff, either because you can't imagine being so low-key since you're a dedicated endorphin junkie (you run 10 or 20 miles for fun on the weekends) or because you (ssssh!) don't really exercise enough now and don't think a meditative moment will fill the bill.

If you're a workout fanatic, your exercise routine may be one-dimensional. A walk on the less-wild, less-rigid side, could help you discover something new about yourself inside and out. I've been there, and I still have to work to balance the mix of high-power with inner calm, continually fighting the urge to go, go, harder, harder. So listen up, I know what you're feeling. And, yes, I've discovered something inside that not only feels good, but also helps me do better at the high-intensity stuff. The two really do tango. Remember: Mind-body workouts aren't just about meditating!

Maybe you're more prone to being prone mainly because you fear that exercise equals pain. For so long, exercise was supposed to hurt, or else the session wasn't good enough. I remember doing three-hour aerobic classes where the instructor's goal was to make the class so hard that everybody limped away. Well, folks, that's old hat now. Exercise doesn't have to hurt to do you good. Enter mind-body workouts. Less pain, you gain. (See Chapter 21 in The Part of Tens for brief medical and physical benefits if you need more convincing.)

The reasons in this part are more mental, more intuitive, a little more right-brained, a little less academic, and a little more about focus and contemplation. But they still count for a lot. The last three mentioned are the tenets to basic fitness that, in the mind-body context, take on a softer tone than the traditional interpretation. So take a look at some of the best reasons to step up to mind-body.

Experiencing a Softer Movement

Huh? Soft? Exercise? Let me explain: In mind-body workouts, you don't jump, you don't pound, you don't slam yourself against walls, kick or jab invisible competitors, or carry heavy equipment. You just do. You often do it barefoot, with mellow music, and in softly lit rooms. You finish smiling, not gritting your teeth.

Trying Fitness That Flows

Maybe something that's soft is also always flowing — they go together. But maybe they don't go together all the time. I mean, jazz dance flows, but is it soft? Not when you throw in blaring music and a few bumps and grinds. *Flowing* means the movement patterns all have round edges, not hard ones. There are no stop signs, just yield signs. There is no hot and cold, just warm and cozy. One movement just flows into the next. So it feels like a dance. Even if you aren't dancing or you aren't a dancer, you can feel as if you're doing both: a fine feeling.

Relaxing with No Demands for Perfection

Most mind-body methods have a bit of a "whatever" attitude: Whatever you do is perfect. Compare that to something rigid like, say, ballet where every toenail has to be positioned just right. Other than some forms, like Pilates or some styles of Hatha Yoga, that tend to be pretty structured in their positioning with only a flirt with leniency, most mind-body forms encourage you to do whatever feels right for you on any given day. Feeling less flexible? Don't put your leg out so far. You don't have to copy the guy next to you or the instructor on the video tape. Just do what's best for you, and that's utterly divine.

Finding Your Own Limits without an Instructor Yelling In Your Face

Heard about classes called "boot camp" or "sergeant's pride" or any number of names indicating that they're overwhelmingly difficult? Classes where, no matter what you do, the instructor yells that you're a slimy weakling? I just cringe. Why do I want somebody screaming at me nose-to-nose to go faster, harder, or do more?

Well, when you do Yoga, Body Rolling, Chi Ball, or any other mind-body exercise, no one will ever call you a sissy because you can't do enough or do it hard enough.

Enjoying Inner Peace and Calm

Instead of finishing an exercise session feeling hyped up, you finish a mind-body session feeling centered and calm, yet still energetic and ready to face whatever is next on your schedule. You won't have that buzzed and scattered feeling that regular exercise sometimes gives you, or even a major sense of fatigue and the need for a nap. After a mind-body session, you'll feel the relief you would as if you had an ocean's stormy waves swirling high against your insides, slamming around for a way out, and they suddenly give way to the still, deep, blue calm of the peaceful waters you find off the Greek islands so famous in tourist pictures. Sound serene? You bet.

Breathing Better

Yes, just breathing. As simple as it sounds, breathing is something everyone often forgets to do, especially in moments of tension or anxiety. Holding your breath tightens down your insides. All mind-body forms emphasize thorough and continued deep breaths. Breathing alone, and some more esoteric mind-body forms that I don't have room to cover, focus exclusively on breathing and can wash away the cares gnawing at your insides and cleanse your soul.

Finding an Inner Focus

Mind-body methods aren't only about what happens to your muscles, joints, and bones — although lots can happen to your physical body if you do certain methods in the right way. Mindful exercise is more about what happens within you while your muscles, joints and bones are in motion. Put your priority and focus on the inside, and the effects will move outward.

Gaining Strength without Weights

No need to pump dumbbells, press barbells, or pull on elastic cords for a specified number of repetitions. Doing mind-body exercises develops your leg, torso, and upper-body strength, as well as your balance more than you ever imagined — as long as you do the right combination of movements.

Mind-body routines aren't for wimps. I've seen buffed-up macho guys nearly break down in tears during Yoga exercises that can make anyone's muscles quiver.

You will develop lower-extremity, upper-body and torso strength, and balance that you never imagined if you execute the appropriate combination of movements and sequences.

Acquiring Flexibility without Pain

The point of a mind-body workout is to do a particular exercise or movement only as long as it still feels good, so you can avoid pain. Many of us try so hard to stretch overly tight muscles. We've been told all our lives to stretch, usually without being told how, why, or how much! So we stretch, frustrated by our lack of ability and driven into a competition with ourselves to stretch more and harder to attain that flexibility goal. I've been there, tightening my jaw and growling at myself to go farther. You don't do that in mind-body. Yet flexibility still happens.

Getting Aerobic Fitness without Impact

You help your heart and lungs get stronger and healthier by doing mind-body exercises — a little or a lot depending on what you do and how you do it. But you won't, or at least you shouldn't, hurt. No grinding knees, complaining backs, pulled hamstrings, or any of those other miseries often brought on by high-impact exercise. And, here's that nice plus again: Being more fit can mean more calorie-burn, too, since toned and fit muscles demand more calories than fat does.

Chapter 21

Ten Physical Benefits of No-Pain, You-Gain Mind-Body Fitness

· ·

In This Chapter

▶ Lowering your stress level and blood pressure

▶ Finding better balance and posture

▶ Strengthening your muscles (including your heart) and bones

▶ Relieving low back pain

▶ Finding more flexibility

· ·

Some traditionally oriented scientific researchers and physicians may tell you that the benefits of mind-body fitness are all in your mind. And you could answer jokingly, "Why, yes, my mind is why I do mind-body." But slapping your knee gleefully may not sit well in this scenario. All jokes aside, many of the physical gains you can experience through mind-body exercise haven't been proved by academic and scientific research. But that's okay. You know how much better you feel, and that counts for a lot.

This chapter tells you the top 10 benefits to your physical body of mind-body fitness practice according to both the scientific and anecdotal evidence. (For more detailed information about the proven and accepted benefits — or just the mostly accepted ones — by scientists, take a look at Chapter 6. To read more about some of the mindful reasons for trying mind-body fitness, see Chapter 20.)

Reduce Stress and Anxiety

This is probably one of the top benefits you experience even after one class or session of a mind-body practice. After several weeks, months, or even years of practicing one or more of these mind-body exercises, your stress — or should I say, your reaction to a stressful moment — may likely drop dramatically.

Achieve Better Balance

Staying up on two feet, not to mention one foot, is not an inbred skill. Unfortunately, it is common for people who become unsteady in their older years to break their hips and pelvic girdles when they lose their balance and fall. Have you noticed that some elderly people have a shuffling gait? They have lost their sense of balance and may feel insecure even about lifting one foot off the ground when merely walking. Then, of course, there are simple athletic and fitness pursuits that require balance, such as hiking on rocky trails, or just jogging (where you are "balancing" on one foot with every step). Tai Chi Chuan, in particular, is known for its balance-training advantages.

Improve Your Posture

If balance isn't good enough for you, then a fine, upright posture may be. Forget the dowager's hump turning you into a slumped-over older person or even younger person. Keep strong and tall with mind-body fitness that emphasize good posture and spinal alignment.

Develop Strong, Toned Abs

You can get away with letting it all hang out in many regular fitness routines, but not in most mind-body methods. Tightening and strengthening your abdominals is what allows you to move correctly and allows you to accomplish much of what certain methods prescribe. Some methods, of course, put a stronger emphasis on core tightening than others. If that sudden use of the word "core" (Wait, where's the apple?) sounds like Greek to you, take a look at Chapter 4.

Decrease Low Back Pain

Because 8 out of 10 of us will experience low back pain at some point, this benefit is a biggie. Discovering how to use your abdominal muscles, to stand straight, and to keep the right muscles flexible or strong all can lead to less ouch in your low back.

Acquire More Flexible Muscles

Many common aerobic exercises tighten you up, especially in muscles specifically required for that movement, because the workouts often involve repetition of some kind. You use the same muscles the same way every time. Ever notice a step-aerobics instructor's thighs and low back? Many of them end up with over-developed and tight thighs and hip flexors, and therefore have a slight sway and a tight low back because of all of the up-up, down-down movements. Both of those inflexible areas can lead to back pain, too. Of course, not every, or even most, step instructors have this problem, but many can be at risk for it. Mind-body methods, on the other hand, emphasize overall flexibility, not to the point of making you become a pretzel the likes of gymnast Mary Lou Retton, but enough for good health, injury prevention, and comfort. Plus, mind-body fitness has more well balanced and less repetitive programs than some traditional exercise programs.

Increase Your Strength

You may not be able to bench-press 350 pounds, but you'll probably notice muscle tone and strength from ankles to eyelashes with a regular practice of most methods. This is particularly true with more physical forms such as Hatha Yoga or Pilates.

Strengthen Your Bones

Any weight-bearing activity can help your bones stay strong, and that includes the softer movements of many mind-body forms of fitness. You don't have to pound, pound, pound your body, body, body to keep brittle bones at bay.

Acquire a Heartier Heart and Lungs

You can get your heart pumping with many of these mind-body forms, and that helps decrease your risk of heart disease, just as does everyday aerobic exercise, such as running or step aerobics — without the jarring or jostling. Regular participation in mind-body exercise, even at a low-intensity, can reduce your risk of cardiovascular disease by improving your blood pressure, by improving your level of "good" cholesterol (HDL) and lowering your level of "bad" cholesterol (LDL), and by helping you take time out from tense moments in life. When you get a heartier heart and lungs, you may find yourself running for a bus or climbing a flight of stairs comfortably and even perhaps enjoying it more. You may even discover that mind-body fitness has cross-training benefits for something like your next marathon! (Marathon?)

Lower Your Blood Pressure

Any regular and steady aerobic exercise can help drop your blood pressure — and that goes for most mind-body workouts, too. Of course, you want to consult with your doctor first to make sure the mind-body exercise you are leaning toward is right for you, and you certainly don't want to stop any regular medical treatments. But the combination of the traditional medical and the non-traditional mind-body exercise may be the best way to do battle with hypertension.

Chapter 22

Ten Times to Take a Mind-Body Moment

*Y*ou can find a mind-body moment any old time during the day, not just during the specific exercise slot you doodle onto your calendar.

Mind-body exercise feels good, and helps you become healthier. Plus, you can draw on the benefits in some small yet glorious fashion many times during the day. Okay, okay, you won't get sculpted biceps or lose 10 pounds from these smaller fitness tidbits. But you can gain a little more peace of mind, lose a little stress, or simply prepare yourself better for your sweaty workouts later. Darn solid reasons to meddle in mind-body moments.

First of all, I suppose I should clarify: What the heck is a mind-body moment? For me, it means a snippet of seconds any of those umpteen times during a day when you can start to feel your blood pressure inch upward like the mercury in a thermometer on a hot day. For example, when your boss is calling and you already have two calls on hold and a report to finish five minutes ago. Or when you're late for an appointment and traffic has come to a standstill. Or when your spouse suddenly wants to watch Sports Center when you were hoping for a nice chat. Or when . . . I don't need to go on, do I?

In other words, a *mind-body moment* is any time you need a personal time-out, when you can check in with your body, recenter yourself, and take on what's been thrown at you in a calmer manner.

That reminds me of a time not too long ago when I was trying to get to a weekend of speaking engagements on the Gulf Coast in Texas. I flew into Dallas in the early afternoon, scheduled to head out to Corpus Christi an hour later. Little did I know that the heavens had other plans. My flight was the last one that dipped into Dallas and landed just ahead of thunderstorms. The airport then completely shut down, and after waiting around for about 5 hours, I discovered that no flights — yes, that means none at all — were going to go out that night to the Coast. I could have ramped myself into full gear and stormed around the airport like a maniac, demanding the airline agents do something (which of course they couldn't), but what good would that have done except to raise my blood pressure? Instead, I stood in line — the first of many that evening I dare say — and practiced Qigong centering, Yogic breathing and Pilates-style spinal alignment. I rocked back and forth on my feet a little to sense my weight placement. I lifted one foot off the ground and tested my balance. Above all, I breathed. Deeply. (Oh, and I also took every opportunity I had to walk very fast between gates as a little dose of regular exercise, too.)

Take a look at these suggestions for times to practice your own mind-body moment. You can, of course, apply any of the techniques in the book for alignment, centering, breathing, abdominal tightening, balance, or slow knee bends a la Tai Chi that suit your fancy.

Before Going to Sleep

What better time to breathe and center yourself than when you're trying to relax after your day and go to sleep? If you have a family and you find it difficult to take five minutes for yourself without interruption, you can always retreat to the bathroom, lock the door, and say, "I'll be out in a minute!" Then try to tap into your Microcosmic Orbit from Qigong. (Refer to Chapter 11 for more information on this exercise.)

While Waiting in Line

In line, on a line, in a queue . . . whatever you call that art of waiting patiently that has become a rather unavoidable part of everyday modern life. You have a couple of choices: Go wherever you're going when there's no line (that's a pretty good choice, but not always possible), stand there and get aggravated while mumbling nasty things about someone's brain capacity (not really productive), or (here it comes) practice your mind-body moment. It's a perfect time to take a Feldenkrais-ian awareness check (Chapter 16), or get into a modified Yoga Tree posture for balance (Chapter 8).

During Your Shower

Maybe this sounds odd, but isn't the shower sometimes the only place you can get some peace and quiet? So who's going to be the wiser that you're actually working on your Yoga Mountain Pose (Chapter 8), or Tai Chi Bow Stance (Chapter 10) as you splash water around behind the curtain or door?

After a Fight

Admit it, sometimes you have disagreements in your life with your spouse, roommate, parents, siblings, colleagues, or teachers that leave you storming and fuming. This is the perfect time to breathe deeply and find your mind-body connection with some standing Qigong meditation (Chapter 10). What you wanna bet that the reason for the disagreement will become a lot less important than you thought it was?

When You Get Up in the Morning

Maybe morning isn't necessarily your preferred time of day for exercise. But think about it: A mind-body moment can help you pull yourself together before you thunder out to meet the day and its demands. That morning moment could be a couple of Yoga spinal twists (Chapter 8), Feldenkrais awareness moves (Chapter 16), Pilates Ab Preps (Chapter 14), or mind-body pelvic placement drills (Chapter 4) while you're still on your back in bed. Or it could be a little standing work while you're brushing your teeth or while you're waiting for water to boil.

When Warming Up Before Exercise

I use the word "warm-up" loosely here because warming up your mind doesn't really mean sweating and stuff. But you still need to bring your mind to the moment and focus, even if your workout for the day is high-intensity aerobics or a long run or walk. I still take a few moments before I'm about to undertake some higher-intensity activity, like running track intervals, and simply ground myself so I can feel the earth empowering me. That may involve simply closing my eyes and using my feet (and their energy-receiving acupoints . . . refer to Chapter 11 for more information in the Qigong chapter about these) to fill my body with positive energy.

When Cooling Down After Exercise

Well, heck, why not? If it can be enmeshed into your warm-up, it can be a part of the finish, too. Slow down, use your muscles in a different way. You may feel more whole from it. Qigong walking (see Chapter 11) or a slow Tai Chi Chuan form (Chapter 10) may be the perfect, grounding finish.

Before Picking a Fight

You're mad and you ain't gonna take it anymore. You feel like bulleting into the office/room/home (choose one or add your own) of your boss/kids/spouse/parents (choose one or add your own) and giving him/her/them (choose one) a piece of your mind. Or do you? Maybe a short moment to gather yourself can put it all into perspective, change your outlook, and so change your presentation style. Try standing tall and breathing fully and consciously (Refer to Chapter 4 for information about basic concepts like this.)

When You're on Deadline

Isn't this just the time when you feel as if you have no time — not to eat, not to sleep, not to exercise, not to . . . hold on. You gotta have a couple of minutes for you. And if you spend a few minutes (maybe two to five) you'll feel better, be mentally and physically refreshed, and be raring to go. You'll probably be more productive, too. If you're in an office, that may mean just pushing back your chair, folding your arms in your lap and trying a few body awareness lessons from Feldenkrais or Alexander methods (Chapter 16). If you work at home, you could get yourself down on the floor for a Yoga breathing session (Chapters 7 and 8).

While Walking Through a Store

Who says a walk has to be a nonmindful affair? Next time, as you make your way to the banana bin or the home appliance aisle, do it mindfully. Stop holding your breath as you hurry past people, and stop tapping your toes when someone blocks the entire escalator and you can't dash by. Even try a few Tai Chi moves in the elevator (Chapter 10) or slow down your hurry for a little Meditation Walking (Chapter 16).

Use the moments you have many times throughout your day mindfully, and your mental and physical being can benefit even more from your entire exercise regimen.

Chapter 23

Ten Tips for Finding the Best Teacher, Class, or Video

*I*n this chapter I give you some hints about types of instruction to seek for your mind-body journey, but everybody's tastes and personalities are different. One person's preference may be another person's nightmare.

You may not click with one teacher or practitioner — no matter how good that teacher is — and if so, it's all over. If you don't feel good when you step into a studio or club — no matter how popular it is — you may never want to go back. If you don't get the long-distance warm fuzzies from a video you just popped in, it ends up gathering dust on your shelf. So you may as well not force it, but realize that if something doesn't feel right, it won't benefit you to stick with it. Keep searching for what's right for you.

Sure, I talk about training, experience, certificates and blah-de-blah-de-blah; but the first order of business is to find out whether you feel good in a certain place and safe with a certain person. Because I'm talking fitness of mind, body, and spirit here, make sure all parts have an equal say-so.

Checking into a Club, Studio, or Private Training

To help you decide which type of health club, training, or instruction meets your needs, I evaluate the alternatives in the following list.

- ✔ **Health club:** A health club may be a great bet for you if you want to have a class in a facility that motivates you to do other fitness activities, if you want weights and other machinery handy for other workouts or to supplement your class, and if you don't mind walking through weight machines and lots of people to get to a studio.

- ✔ **Mind-body studio:** Perhaps you want a little more calm, with a real focus on the specific method you choose or on mind-body activities in general. Then a method-specific studio or a mind-body studio may be ideal for you. With the popularity of these methods now, studios are popping up everywhere that offer, for example, just Yoga, just Pilates, or just ethnic dance, and others offer many of the mind-body methods from Yoga to NIA all in a one-stop shop. Some may even have special Feldenkrais and Alexander classes. Ask when you call.

- ✔ **Personal training:** Private-training studios are small operations where you meet with an instructor for a one-on-one lesson or a small-group lesson with two to three students. Certainly, you pay more than at other locations, but you get personalized attention — and that can mean more growth for you and gaining experience more quickly.

- ✔ **Private practitioner or analyst:** Feldenkrais, Alexander, and Laban instructors spend many hundreds of hours training, apprenticing, and getting certified. So they often work out of private offices with clients, just as other health care professionals do. You can sometimes find them on college campuses or through special workshops at fitness studios.

Zeroing In on the Right Location

As with any fitness endeavor aimed at personal improvement, if the place or teacher you pick isn't convenient, you'll probably find every excuse in the world not to go there. When considering a club, studio, or instructor for your mind-body practice, decide on the time of day that's right for you to practice, then make sure the location isn't hard to get to due to the traffic at the time of day you plan to do your session. The place of your choice may be:

- ✔ On your way to work
- ✔ On the way home from dropping the kids at school
- ✔ Near work so you can stop in for a class and not sit in commute traffic
- ✔ Near home so you can get there on weekends

You may find a teacher you think makes the world go 'round at a studio 35 minutes away, but the teacher's instruction won't do you any good unless you actually get there.

Deciding On the Method, Style, or Philosophy You're Interested In

After you use this book, try out some material, and perhaps do some other research, you may then have an idea which methods you want to do more of. Make sure when you start calling facilities or dropping in at clubs or studios that they describe to you their method, style, or even philosophy. You may even want to watch a class or talk to other students.

Perhaps you want the more traditional Pilates exercises; in that case, you won't be happy with a method that mixes modern forms with the classic exercises. Perhaps you want an emphasis on relaxation; make sure you find out if the class you would attend is in a fitness club where the music and mania would drive you nuts. Maybe you want meditative martial art; make sure you don't get confused, ask about Chinese martial arts, and end up in a Kung Fu studio instead of a Tai Chi Chuan school!

Inquiring about the Frequency of the Classes

Maybe you want choice in the number of classes offered and the times they're offered, so you know you can drop in just about any day when it fits your schedule. Maybe you want to get your chosen style or class two to three times a week. Make sure you are satisfied with the offerings and the frequency — and that all the teachers at the times of day you may attend also meet your expectations.

Finding Out about the Club's Longevity

Certainly studios are springing up at every corner mall these days — maybe including one around the corner from you — and that may initially seem to offer great convenience. But can you count on the studio to be there next month or next year? Maybe so, if it develops a small and dedicated clientele. But maybe not, if the overhead proves too much and the studio can't compete with the chain health club down the street. Don't overlook a new place, but ask all the right questions about an owner's dedication or any mandated contracts — and don't buy an annual membership in advance.

Avoid paying for more than a month at a time. That way, if the facility shuts its doors all of a sudden, you won't be out much money.

Interviewing Instructors about Their Credentials

This is a tough one. When you choose a doctor, you can look at his or her degree and other fellowships. Even when you choose a group-exercise instructor, you can often ask about the training or certificates he or she may have. This mind-body stuff is a whole different package, partly because some of it is so old and some of it is so, well, new, and for the most part certifications and training protocols aren't standardized.

Figuring out what a certification means

First of all, most of the methods — especially the Early Classics and the Chinese arts — don't truly have certifications. Teachers spout names like "trained under Master ABC or Swami XYZ," which can carry a lot of clout — if you know who the master is. In the old days, someone studied a very long time with a particular guru, and after years or even decades, became good enough to begin to take on students him- or herself.

But, even as certifications begin to develop in areas like Yoga, no standards exist covering:

✔ **What someone must learn or be able to do to say they are "certified":** The instructor may have sat in a workshop for a day, taken a multiple-choice test, and was handed a piece of paper saying they're certified.

✔ **How long an instructor must study or apprentice to earn a certificate:** The instructor may have studied a weekend, weeks, or months. They may have had to prove their teaching ability . . . or just had to show up. These mind-body methods can take years to fully grasp and to be able to pass on fully and safely to others.

Some of the Modern Classic methods — like Feldenkrais, Alexander, and Laban — mandate hours, months, and years of study before you can put out your shingle and call yourself a teacher, practitioner, or movement analyst. They have well-developed schools and apprentice programs. Even NIA, a New Kid contemporary method, requires many hours of schooling and various levels with strict standards to meet before you can call yourself a NIA instructor.

So how do you search for the instructor who is right for you?

✔ If you're looking at a Modern Classic method, make sure the instructor has his or her appropriate certificate and the formal training behind it. You can check with the professional and overseeing organizations and schools for each, listed in the Appendix. This would include Alexander, Feldenkrais, and Laban. NIA also keeps a good oversight on trained teachers, with information available on its web site.

✔ If you're leaning toward any other method, ask about the teacher's experience — number of years they studied, with whom, how long they've been teaching, and his or her background with people who have your particular needs, if any. Usually, at least a year or two helps them learn the specialized teaching skills of these methods. But certainly, the longer they've been doing it, the better. For Yoga, you can check with the Yoga Alliance, a non-profit group that is trying to set standards and register teachers who meet them (see the Appendix for contact information). However, if a teacher isn't listed, that doesn't mean he or she won't still be a fine teacher.

Is the instructor mind-body certified?

Of course, you may hear someone say they are "certified," but currently, since many mind-body methods don't have recognized standards, you should probably just weigh that along with the entire package of experience. If nothing else, that means the instructor has cared enough to take some workshops and further his or her education.

Does the instructor have fitness-leader certification or a related degree?

The legitimate groups that certify fitness instructors — American Council on Exercise (ACE), American College of Sports Medicine (ACSM), National Strength and Conditioning Association (NSCA), for example — require a broad range of knowledge of basic anatomy and physiology, as well as some teaching expertise. So having one of those certifications may be helpful, but certainly not necessary for teaching some of the mind-body methods. Some instructors may actually have college degrees in a health- or fitness-related field, or even advanced degrees, which can be just as good or even better than a certification.

Some of the New Kids methods, such as the above-mentioned NIA programs as well as methods such as Gyrokinesis and Tai Chi Chih, actually run their own training programs. Inquire what type of training program is required to become a teacher.

Is the instructor a health professional?

You may actually find, for example, a nurse, chiropractor, or physical therapist teaching some of these classes. That certainly means the person has had more in-depth instruction in the way the body moves and reacts, at least physically, and could be a plus for safety, especially if you have any special needs, such as an injury, chronic disease, or other disability.

Does the instructor meet certain standards?

Although many mind-body programs don't have recognized standards, there are certain qualities of a competent teacher and the way he or she instructs a class that you can keep an eye out for. These include:

- ✔ Performs adequate assessment of a student's physical abilities and experience before teaching new movements or allowing a student into a class.
- ✔ Avoids movements that may be harmful to muscles, joints, bones, or the heart and lungs, and takes an individual student's needs into consideration about what may be harmful.
- ✔ Individualizes program recommendations and suggests modifications to suit each student.
- ✔ Demonstrates respect for an individual's needs, abilities, and background.
- ✔ Maintains professional competency by taking on-going classes, workshops, conferences, and attending other teachers' programs.

Making Sure the Price Is Right

Remember the adage, "You get what you pay for"? That holds true with fitness-type activities where your fee is also paying for an instructor's fee, and for a club's or studio's upkeep. You probably don't want to choose a place — especially on the phone — based just on having the lowest price. That's not to say that a low price can't offer the best for you. Just weigh all the options and be ready to choose some place or someone who may cost a bit more, but have the credentials or longevity to go with it.

Take a look at the section on credentials, "Interviewing Teachers About Their Credentials." You get what you pay for. . . .

Finding Out Whether You Can Sit In on a Class

Watching a class can be helpful in trying to decide if the method or teacher is right for you. If a facility won't let you at least watch a class before joining — some even let you take your first class for free — then you probably want to reconsider. What do they have to hide?

If the facility is membership-only, ask about a guest pass for your first lesson or two so that you can get a good feeling for what the place has to offer. Talk to students before and after sessions, or even just eavesdrop on conversations about the facility. Finding out how long a student has been around can tell you a little bit about the teacher or facility.

Do have some respect when you sit in or watch a class. A certain feeling of safety is necessary for students taking classes like these. A studio may believe that having someone just sitting and watching may make students feel uncomfortable. You may only be able to watch the first part or peek through a back door, depending on the setup, because some small studios don't have space for an audience.

Using Instructional Videos

Look for almost the same things as you do for teachers and classes. Credentials and experience are still number 1. Make sure a package bio mentions the instructor's background. For a video, having some teaching experience — and not just performing experience — can make or break a good class on the small screen. It isn't easy to get across the message in the video medium. If you can borrow or rent the video before buying it, all the better. Or make sure the retailer has a satisfaction-guaranteed warranty of some sort that allows returns or at least exchanges. Refer to the Appendix for a few places to find videos and audios.

Knowing When It Feels Right

What goes around, comes around. I started out this chapter talking about listening to your feelings, so I now end it with asking you to check back in with your feelings. Throughout the chapter I talk about frequency, location, credentials, fees, and all of those non-mind-body sort of things. Now, go back inside yourself for your final decision. If it doesn't feel right in your gut, don't do it. Listen to the words, then feel the atmosphere. Hear the words, then hear between the words. Ask questions, then eavesdrop on the tone of other conversations. Then go back inside yourself and trust what you hear there.

It must feel right to be the best for you.

Appendix

Your Resource for More Mind-Body Fitness Ideas

• •

*I*n this appendix I list a variety of associations, teachers, studios, catalogs, and other sources with all the information you need to contact them, including the Web site addresses for many of them. Each mind-body category in the Appendix features sources for one or more of the following areas: instruction and networking, publications, Web sites to search, and equipment you may need for that type of fitness program. Remember that Web sites come and go daily. If an address I list doesn't exist, do a search in your favorite search engine for the organization's name to see if it moved its pages.

The four headings and areas of information in this appendix are:

- ✔ **Finding instruction and networking:** In this section you can find resources for classes, instructors, studios, videos/audiotapes, and other instruction, as well as contacts for organizations and associations through which you may find teachers or other information about instruction. Don't miss the Web sites for each group; they often have links to many other resources.

- ✔ **Hitting the library:** If you want to do more reading, here's where you can find information about selected books, journals, and magazines.

- ✔ **Searching the Web:** This is a section listing Web sites that are not associated with a particular group or other resource. They are just helpful Web sites. Many are full of resources, education, and links.

- ✔ **Getting equipped:** Look for contacts here to catalogs, equipment, clothing, and other accessories you may want for your exercise and practice.

This appendix is organized alphabetically by technique.

General Mind-Body and Fitness Sources

Finding instruction and networking

IHRSA, the association of quality health clubs and fitness facilities. Club locators and directories. 263 Summer St., Boston, MA 02210; Phone: 800-228-4772; Internet: www.ihrsa.org.

National Center for Complementary and Alternative Medicine, a division of the government's National Institutes of Health. Conducts and supports research and provides information to the public. Phone: 888-644-6226; Internet: www.nccam.nih.gov.

Hitting the library

ACE Fitness Matters, fitness newsletter and other publications for consumers by the non-profit American Council on Exercise. 5820 Oberlin Drive, Suite 102, San Diego, CA 92121-3787; Phone: 800-825-3636; Internet: www.acefitness.org.

IDEA Source, journal of IDEA, the association for fitness professionals. Covers fitness, trends, information and products for instructors, trainers, and enthusiasts. Other publications and instructional tapes, such as *Introduction to the Art and Science of Mind-Body Fitness* (teacher continuing education credits). 6190 Cornerstone Ct. East, Suite 204, San Diego, CA 92121-3773; Phone: 800-999-4332; Internet: www.ideafit.com.

Meditation For Dummies, by Stephan Bodian. Indianapolis, IN; IDG Books Worldwide, Inc., 1998.

Nutrition For Dummies, **2nd Edition,** by Carol Ann Rinzler. Indianapolis, IN; IDG Books Worldwide, Inc., 1999.

Power Eating, by Susan Kleiner. Human Kinetics Publishers, 1998.

The Psychobiology of Mind-Body Healing: New Concepts of Therapeutic Hypnosis (revised edition), by E. Rossi. W. W. Norton & Company, 1993.

Somatics: Reawakening the Mind's Control of Movement, Flexibility, and Health, by Thomas Hanna. Reading, MA; Addison-Wesley, 1988.

The Relaxation Response, by Herbert Benson. New York, NY; Avon Books, 1976.

Wherever You Go, There You Are, by Jon Kabat-Zinn. New York: Hyperion, 1995.

Tao of Pooh, by Benjamin Hoff. New York, NY; Penguin Books, 1982.

Zen and The Brain, by James Austin. MIT Press, 1998.

Surfing the Web

Total Fitness Network, Web site of general fitness and training advice from Therese Iknoian, author of *Mind-Body Fitness For Dummies.* Internet: www.totalfitnessnetwork.com.

Getting equipped

Hugger Mugger, Yoga props and products, including mats, bolsters, blocks, straps, and Yoga clothing. 3937 S. 500 W., Salt Lake City, UT 84123; Phone: 800-473-4888; Internet: www.huggermugger.com.

Living Arts, Yoga and mind-body props, clothing, accessories, and instructional video tapes, including tapes by David-Dorian Ross, Patricia Walden, John Friend, and Rodney Lee. Phone: 877-989-6321; Internet: www.livingarts.com or www.gaiam.com.

Collage Video, catalog of fitness-oriented music, audio, and videotapes. 5390 Main St. NE, Minneapolis, MN 55421-1128; Phone: 800-433-6769; Internet: www.collagevideo.com.

Dynamix Music, producer and distributor of workout music and instructional audio and videotapes. 9411 Philadelphia Rd., Baltimore, MD 21237; Phone: 800-843-6499; Internet: www.dynamixmusic.com.

Fitness First, catalog of fitness products, including a large assortment of mats. P.O. Box 251, Shawnee Mission, KS 66201; Phone: 800-421-1791; Internet: www.fitness1st.com.

Planet Earth Music, producer and distributor of music appropriate for mind-body arts. Phone: 800-825-8656; Internet: www.planet-earth-music.com.

YogaMats, mats, bolsters, cushions, room screens, lamps, bamboo flooring, and other accessories. P.O. Box 885044, San Francisco, CA 94188; Phone: 800-720-YOGA; Internet: info@yogamats.com.

Alexander

Finding instruction and networking

Alexander Technique International, professional organization, workshops, articles, books, Web site links and resources. 1692 Massachusetts Ave., 3rd floor, Cambridge, MA 02138; Phone: 888-668-8996; Internet: www.ATI-net.com.

Robert Rickover, author and instructor. His Web site is rich with links and articles. 2434 Ryons St., Lincoln, NB 68502; Phone: 402-475-4433; Internet: www.alexandertechnique.com; E-mail: robert@alexandertechnique.com.

Hitting the library

The Alexander Technique, by J. Leibowitz and B. Connington. New York, NY: Harper & Row, 1990.

Fitness Without Stress: A Guide to the Alexander Technique, by Robert Rickover. Metamorphous Press, 1988.

How to Learn the Alexander Technique: A Manual for Students, by Barbara Conable. Andover Press, 1995.

Surfing the Web

Nicholas Brockbank, author and instructor. Articles and reviews on his Web site give good insights and sample instruction. Internet: www.dodman.freeserve.co.uk/alex.htm.

Body Rolling

Finding instruction and networking

Body Logic studio, founded by Body Rolling creator Yamuna Zake. The source for Body Rolling videotapes, books, and audiotapes, plus schedules of classes and workshops. 295 W. 11th St., Suite 1F, New York, NY 10014; Phone: 888-226-9616. Internet: www.bodylogic.com.

Hitting the library

Body Rolling, by Yamuna Zake and Stephanie Golden. Rochester, VT; Healing Arts Press, 1997.

An Experiential Approach to Complete Muscle Release, by Yamuna Zake and Stephanie Golden. Inner Traditions International, Limited; October 1997.

Chi Ball Method

Finding instruction and networking

International Fitness Promotions Pty Ltd., headquarters of founder Monica Linford and source for books, videos, and instructional or training information. P.O. Box 542, Mitcham, South Australia 5062, or 15 Ashenden Road, Aldgate, South Australia 5154; Phone: 618 8272 8453; Internet: www.chiball.com; E-mail: Monica@chiball.com.

Hitting the library

Awaken Your Body, Balance Your Mind, by Monica Linford with Jennai Cox. Hammersmith, London UK; Thorsons, 2000.

Feldenkrais

Finding instruction and networking

Feldenkrais Guild of North America, an international organization of certified practitioners, training program, practitioner directory, and sample movement lessons online. 3611 SW Hood, Suite 100, Portland, OR 97201; Phone: 503-221-6612 or 800-775-2118; Internet: www.feldenkrais.com.

Michael Purcell and Alison Rapp, Guild-certified practitioners and worldwide teacher trainers. 444 S. Auburn St., Grass Valley, CA 95945; Phone: 530-274-9977.

Feldenkrais Resources, workshops, classes, books, training programs, sample lessons online. 830 Bancroft Way, Suite 112, Berkeley, CA 94710; Phone: 800-765-1907; Internet: www.feldenkrais-resources.com.

Somatic Options, Feldenkrais classes, books, tapes, online lessons. P.O. Box 194, Pacific Palisades, CA 90272; Phone: 310-454-8322; Internet: www.somatic.com.

Reese Movement Institute, training programs. 2187 Newcastle Ave., Suite 102, Cardiff, CA 92007; Phone: 760-436-9087; Internet: www.feldenkraisglobal.com.

Hitting the library

Awareness Through Movement, by Moshe Feldenkrais. New York, NY; HarperCollins, 1990.

Relaxercise, by D. Zemach-Bersin, K.Z. Bersin, and M. Reese. (based on the work of Moshe Feldenkrais); San Francisco, CA; Harper & Row; 1990.

Inversion Therapy

Equipping yourself

Body Slant, gravity inversion tools invented by Larry Jacobs, founder and director of Age in Reverse, Inc. P.O. Box 1667, Newport Beach, CA 92663; Phone: 800-443-3917; Internet: www.ageeasy.com.

Hang Ups International, inversion chairs, tables, and boots. 10004 162nd Street, Ct. East, Puyallup, WA 98375; Phone: 800-847-0143; Internet: www.inversiontherapy.com.

Laban

Finding instruction and networking

Laban/Bartenieff Institute of Movement Studies, center for training and certifying instructors and finding information. 234 Fifth Ave., Room 203, New York, NY 10001; Phone: 212-477-4299; Internet: www.limsonline.org; E-mail: limsinfo@erols.com.

Janet Hamburg, author, professor of dance, researcher and trained Laban Movement Analyst, The University of Kansas, Department of Music and Dance, 452 Murphy Hall, Lawrence, KS 66045-2279; Phone: 785-864-5168; E-mail: jhamburg@ukans.edu.

Hitting the library

Body Code: The meaning in movement, by W. Lamb and E. Watson. Princeton, NJ; Princeton Book Company, 1987.

Laban for Actors and Dancers: Putting Laban's Movement into Practice: A Step-By-Step Guide, by Jean Newlove. Theatre Arts Books, 1993.

Body Movement: Coping with the Environment, by Irmgard Bartenieff with Dori Lewis. New York, NY: Gordon and Breach Science Publishers, 1980.

Discovering Your Expressive Body, by Peggy Hackney. An instructional video. Princeton Books.

NIA

Finding instruction and networking

The NIA Technique, headquarters of founders Debbie and Carlos Rosas and source of videos, books, workshops and other instruction. Web site lists other certified classes and teachers around the world, plus gives history and background. 6244 SW Burlingame Ave., Portland, OR 97201; Phone: 800-762-5762; Internet: www.nia-nia.com.

Yoga Nia Adventures, classes, teacher training, book. Jennifer Fox and Paul Gould, 1710 Ocean St., Santa Cruz, CA 95060; Phone: 831-427-2370; Internet: www.Yogania.com.

Pilates

Finding instruction and networking

PhysicalMind Institute, classes, teacher training, videotapes, and books. Joan Breibert, president. 1807 2nd St. #15/16, Santa Fe, NM 87505; Phone: 505-988-1990; Internet: www.the-method.com.

Polestar Education, education for health professionals and fitness instructors, plus videos and accessories. Elizabeth Larkam, co-founder. 500 Monza Avenue, Suite 350, Coral Gables, FL 33146; Phone: 800-387-3651 or 305-666-0037; Internet: www.polestareducation.com; E-mail: info@polestareducation.com.

Stott Conditioning, classes, teacher training, videotapes for all levels, and equipment. Moira Stott, co-founder and program director. 2200 Yonge Street, Suite 1402, Toronto Ontario, Canada; Phone: 800-910-0001 or 416-482-4050; Internet: www.stottconditioning.com; E-mail: stott@stottconditioning.com.

Synergy Systems Fitness Studio, classes, teacher training, videotapes for all levels. Cathleen Murakami, founder and director. 555 2nd St., Encinitas, CA 92024; Phone: 760-632-677; Internet: www.synergypilates.com.

The Pilates Studio, Pilates, Inc. On-line, class and teacher training and information. Phone: 800-474-5283; Internet: www.pilates-studio.com.

Hitting the library

Pilates' Return to Life Through Contrology, by Joseph H. Pilates and Judd Robbins (editor). One of Pilates' original books re-released. Presentation Dynamics Inc., 1998.

The Pilates Body, by Brooke Siler. New York, NY; Broadway Books, 2000.

Your Health: A Corrective System of Exercising That Revolutionizes the Entire Field of Physical Education, by Joseph H. Pilates and Judd Robbins (editor). A re-release of an original Pilates book. Presentation Dynamics Inc., 1998.

Surfing the Web

Pilates-Cancel, a Web site established about the Pilates lawsuits and class action suits as well as background information about the disagreements. This site may disappear once the suits are resolved. Internet: www.pilates-cancel.com.

Equipping yourself

Stamina Products, makers of Pilates equipment for the home. P.O. Box 1071, Springfield, MO 65801-1071; Phone: 800-375-7520; Internet: www. staminaproducts.com/pilates.html.

Balanced Body, maker of Pilates equipment for the home and club. 7500 14th Ave., Suite 23, Sacramento, CA 95820-3539; Phone: 800-745-2837; Internet: www.balancedbody.com.

Tai Chi Chuan and Qigong

Finding instruction and networking

Bingkun Hu, master Qigong instructor. Holds regular weekend classes. Instructional videotape, *12 Qigong Treasures for Beginners* (1999). 2114 Sacramento St., Berkeley, CA 94702; Phone: 510-841-6810.

David-Dorian Ross, creator of videos including Tai Chi Basics, A.M. Chi for Beginners, Energy Chi, and others. Zenergy — Enlightened Fitness, a studio teaching mind-body arts in La Jolla, CA. 7712 Fay Ave., La Jolla, CA 92037; Phone: 858-729-0494; Internet: www.thebodymind.com E-mail: drtaichi@aol.com.

Manny Fuentes, a master instructor offering classes, lectures, and work-shops for health professionals and the public. P.O. Box 53464, Lafayete, LA 70505; Phone: 337-261-1278; E-mail: Mannyfuentes@hotmail.com.

The Qigong Institute, a non-profit educational and research institute and resource for teachers. Good place to find other information and links or refer-rals. Kenneth Sancier, founder. 561 Berkeley Ave., Menlo Park, CA 94025; Phone: 415-323-1221; Internet: www.qigonginstitute.com.

Hitting the library

The Way of Qigong: The Art and Science of Chinese Energy Healing, by Kenneth S. Cohen. New York, NY; Ballantine Books, 1997.

Tai Chi Chuan & Qigong: Techniques & Training, by Wolfgang Metzger and Peifang Zhou with Manfred Grosser. New York, NY; Sterling Publishing, 1996.

The Complete Book of Tai Chi Chuan, by Wong Kiew Kit. Boston, MA; Element Books, 1996. Also includes a section on Qigong.

The Healer Within: The Four Essential Self-Care Techniques for Optimal Health, by Roger O.M.D. Jahnke. San Francisco, CA; Harper, 1999.

Surfing the Web

New Age Directory, an online resource for finding associations, instruction, and links to other groups. Internet: www.newagedirectory.com/qigong.htm or www.newagedirectory.com/tai_chi.htm.

Yoga

Finding instruction and networking

Astanga Yoga, offers Power Yoga, an athletic and precise approach to Hatha Yoga. 325 East 41st Street, Suite 203, New York, NY 10017; Phone: 212-661-2895.

International Association of Yoga Therapists, publishes an annual journal. P.O. Box 1386, Lower Lake, CA 95457; Phone: 707-928-9898; Fax: 707-928-4738; E-mail: mail@Yogaresearchcenter.org.

Wild Mountain Yoga Center, a studio in the heart of California's Gold Country in the Sierras, offers classes and special workshops in Yoga and other mind-body arts. 574 Searls Ave., Nevada City CA 95959; Phone: 530-265-4072; Internet: www.wildmountainyogacenter.com.

Yoga Alliance is a voluntary non-profit alliance of Yoga organizations and teachers that has established voluntary national standards for Yoga teachers. Teacher registry, 234 South 3rd Avenue, West Reading, PA 19611; Phone: 877-964-2255 or 610-376-4421.

Yoga Biomedical Trust, publishes a quarterly newsletter and research reports. Offers Yoga and therapy classes, teacher training courses, and Yoga therapy diploma courses. 60 Great Ormand Street, London WCIN, Great Britain; Phone: 0171-419-7195; Fax: 0171-419-7196.

Yoga Research Center, dedicated to research and education on all branches and aspects of Hindu, Buddhist, and Jaina Yoga. Publishes a quarterly newsletter and other publications. Source for Georg Feuerstein's audiotape, *Introducing Yoga: Its Purposes and Approaches.* P.O. Box 1386, Lower Lake, CA 95457; Phone: 707-929-9898; Fax: 707-928-4738; Internet: www.yrec.org; E-mail: mail@Yogaresearchcenter.org.

YogaFit International, trains fitness and health professionals and fitness enthusiasts on how to structure a user-friendly fitness-oriented Yoga class. Also offers books, music CDs, videos, and Yoga clothing and props. 332 Hermosa Avenue, Hermosa Beach, CA 90254; Phone: 310-376-1036; E-mail: info@Yogafit.com.

Yoga Nia Adventures, offers classes, teacher training, and a book. Jennifer Fox and Paul Gould, 1710 Ocean St., Santa Cruz, CA 95060; Phone: 831-427-2370; Internet: www.Yogania.com.

Hitting the library

Explorations in Stillness, by Richard Miller, co-founder of the International Association of Yoga Therapists. P.O. Box 1673, Sebastopol, CA 95473; Phone: 415-456-3909; Internet: www.nondual.com.

Hatha Yoga: The Hidden Language, by Swami Sivananda Radha. Porthill, ID; Timeless Books, 1987.

Living Your Yoga, by J. Lasater. Berkeley, CA; Rodmell Press; 2000.

Office Yoga: Simple Stretches for Busy People, by Darrin Zeer. Chronicle Books, 2000.

Power Yoga: The Total Strength and Flexibility Workout, by Beryl Bender Birch. New York, NY; Fireside Books, 1995.

YogaFit, a training program in book format by Beth Shaw. Champaign, IL; Human Kinetics, 2000.

Yoga For Dummies, by Georg Feuerstein and Larry Payne. Indianapolis, IN; IDG Books Worldwide, 1999.

Yoga Journal, The most widely distributed magazine on Yoga in the world. 2054 University Avenue, Berkeley, CA 94704.

Yoga Journal's Yoga Basics: The Essential Beginner's Guide to Yoga for a Lifetime of Health and Fitness, by Mara Carrico. Henry Holt, 1997.

The Yoga Tradition: Its History, Literature, Philosophy and Practice, by Georg Feuerstein. Prescott, AZ; Hohm Press, 1998.

Surfing the Web

Samata Yoga Center, Web site of Larry Payne's User Friendly Yoga Program. Includes color photos of annual retreats, and offers a series of "user friendly" Yoga videos, audiotapes, and books. Internet: www.samata.com.

Yoga Teacher Directory, a list of names and addresses of participating Yoga teachers in the United States. Internet: www.Yogasite.com/teachers.html.

Other Methods

Brain Gym, find out about the method and where classes are held. Phone: 800-356-2109; Internet: www.braingym.org.

E-motion, a modern combination of mind-body methods geared to the mainstream and fitness world. Phone: 415-990-6402; Internet: www.bodymindfitness.net.

The 5 Rhythms, rhythm and dance by Gabrielle Roth. Phone: 212-760-1381; Internet: www.ravenrecording.com.

Gyrotonic XS and Gyrokinesis, founder Juliu Horvath's Web site explains the two techniques and has pictures. 560 W 43rd. St., Suite 40E, New York, NY 10036; Phone: 212-594-5025; Internet: www.gyrotonic.com.

Rosen Method, several education and certifying centers around the world. Information from The Berkeley Center, Berkeley, CA; Phone: 510-845-6606; Internet: www.rosenmethod.org.

Tai Chi Chih, a contemporary method with some relationship to classical Tai Chi Chuan. Book from Good Karma Publishing (1996) called *Tai Chi Chih: Joy Thru Movement*). Also video and audiotapes. P.O. Box 6460, San Rafael, CA 94903-0460; Internet: www.taichichih.com.

Watsu Water Therapy, Phone: 707-987-3834; Internet: www.waba.edu.

Yogarobics, one place to find information about a contemporary and aerobic form of Yoga. Internet: www.Yogarobics.com.

Index

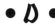

• Z •

Notes